Quick Reference Dictionary

for Massage Therapy and Bodywork

Quick Reference Dictionary for Massage Therapy and Bodywork

Ed Denning, MEd, LMT
Formerly of Stark State College of Technology
North Canton, Ohio

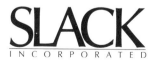

An innovative information, education, and management company
6900 Grove Road • Thorofare, NJ 08086

10/2005

Library of Congress Cataloging-in-Publication Data

Denning, Ed.
  Quick reference dictionary for massage therapy and bodywork / Ed Denning.
    p. ; cm.
  Includes bibliographical references.
  ISBN-13: 978-1-55642-646-9 (alk. paper)
  ISBN-10: 1-55642-646-1 (alk. paper)
  1. Massage therapy--Dictionaries.
    [DNLM: 1. Massage--Dictionary--English. 2. Massage--Terminology--English. 3. Musculoskeletal Diseases--therapy--Dictionary--English. 4. Musculoskeletal Diseases--therapy--Terminology--English. 5. Musculoskeletal System--Dictionary--English. 6. Musculoskeletal System--Terminology--English. WB 15 P411q 2005] I. Title.
    RM721.D386 2005
    615.8'22'03--dc22
                                        2004026597

Printed in the United States of America.

Published by: SLACK Incorporated
                     6900 Grove Road
                     Thorofare, NJ 08086 USA
                     Telephone: 856-848-1000
                     Fax: 856-853-5991
                     www.slackbooks.com

Last digit is print number: 10 9 8 7 6 5 4 3 2 1

DEDICATION

This work is dedicated to all those massage therapists who work their miracles on their patients each day. It is the culmination of all that I've learned from my teachers, mentors, colleagues, students, friends, and relatives.

CONTENTS

Dedication . . . .*v*
Acknowledgments . . . .*ix*
About the Author . . . .*xi*
Preface . . . .*xiii*

Dictionary of Terms .1
Bibliography 188
List of Appendices .190

Appendix 1:   AMTA Code of Ethics 191
Appendix 2:   ABMP Professional
               Code of Ethics 196
Appendix 3:   IMA Group Code of Ethics. . 200
Appendix 4:   The Benefits of Massage 202
Appendix 5:   Safety and Hygiene. 204
Appendix 6:   Suggested Reading 209
Appendix 7:   General Acronyms and
               Abbreviations 215
Appendix 8:   Organization Acronyms 242
Appendix 9:   Selected National and
               International Massage
               Associations. 254
Appendix 10:   Medical Roots: Etymology . . 257
Appendix 11:   Massage Techniques and
               Modalities Contact
               Information 284
Appendix 12:   Range of Motion 330
Appendix 13:   Bones of the Body 332
Appendix 14:   Muscles of the Body 333
Appendix 15:   Metric System 363
Appendix 16:   Weight and Measure
               Conversions. 365

Appendix 17: Peripheral Nerve Innervations:
              Upper Extremity 369
Appendix 18: Peripheral Nerve Innervations:
              Lower Extremity 372
Appendix 19: Diseases, Pathologies, and
              Syndromes Defined. 378
Appendix 20: Licensure by State 451
Appendix 21: Canada Licensure by
              Province 463
Appendix 22: Medical Codes for Massage
              Therapy 466

Acknowledgments

My thanks to a higher power whose influence in my life must be acknowledged. Otherwise, I cannot explain the many crystal clear lessons of life that I have been privileged to learn through my lifetime. It is easy to reflect back and see how many of those lessons have placed me in the position of doing this project.

Carrie Kotlar, Acquisitions Editor at SLACK Incorporated, asked me to work on the *Quick Reference Dictionary for Massage Therapy*. After many e-mails back and forth, we agreed to change the name to The *Quick Reference Dictionary of Massage Therapy and Bodywork*. Carrie has been instrumental in the decisions regarding focus, placement of materials and information, and of great help in moving the project forward.

Additional appreciation is extended to John Bond, Publisher; Amy McShane, Editorial Director; Lauren Biddle Plummer, Managing Editor; Michelle Gatt, Marketing Manager; and Jessica Sycz, Assistant Project Editor; for their support and encouragement.

Special thanks go out to my professional friends and colleagues who have been supportive of my efforts. The influences of my relationships with American Massage Therapy Association, Associated Bodywork and Massage Professionals, and International Massage Association have been instrumental in many of the choices I have made.

Special thanks to my good friend and part-time secretary, Judi Martin, whose gracious acceptance of my idiosyncrasies is greatly appreciated, along with the hours of typing and office work she has done for me over the years and for this book. I knew without asking that I could count on her encouragement and support.

Special thanks to my friend and colleague, Cheryl Davis O'Neill, LMT, who did lots of reading and research into the benefits of massage and the contraindications for massage. Her cheerful countenance did not allow for negativity or discouragement. Cheryl also has provided many skillful massage sessions to support my efforts.

Special thanks to my partner and best friend, Brenda K. Maurer, for her patience during this project. Brenda spent hours researching, printing, and verifying information regarding modalities of massage and bodywork. Her love and support were instrumental in the creation of this work.

There are many others who have influenced my professional and personal life who deserve mention: my friends and colleagues at Stark State College of Technology; my friends and colleagues in The Massage Focus Group; my son, Gary, for his love and support and our regular Tuesday morning breakfast, which helps keep me grounded; Tom Benge, LMT; Dennis Gibbons, LMT; Carol Carlton, LMT; Phil Klem, LMT; and the many other massage therapists I know whose touch and friendship is treasured.

ABOUT THE AUTHOR

Ed Denning, MEd, LMT, taught for 26 years and has a Master's Degree in Elementary Education. As a teacher, he held additional certifications as a library/media specialist and a computer instructor. Ed has been a practicing licensed massage therapist in Ohio since 1993 and is involved with massage and bodywork education. He was president of the Ohio State Massotherapy Association in 1995 and was a founding member of the Ohio Massage Schools Council in 1999. Ed was selected to be on the Massage Therapy Advisory Committee for the State Medical Board of Ohio from 1999 to 2003, and the Committee for Insurance Issues for the American Massage Therapy Association from 2000 to 2003. He was the coordinator of the massage therapy program at Stark State College of Technology from 1998 to 2003, after which he was an instructor in the Massage Therapy Program at Stark State College of Technology. He has conducted workshops in coding every year since 1997.

Ed has written and published works in the massage therapy field, including writing and publishing the first edition of *The Medical Code Manual For Massage Practitioners* in 1995 and several articles in national massage magazines. He created and maintains www.massagecpt.com, a Web site devoted to massage therapy medical coding issues.

Ed is a member of American Massage Therapy Association, Associated Bodywork and Massage Professionals, Ohio State Massotherapy Association, and Massage Focus Group. He is a life member of The American Association of Retired Persons, Akron Bicycle club, and the League of American Wheelmen.

In Ed's spare time he enjoys traveling, walking, power boating, and bicycling. Ed has been a life-long resident of the Akron-Canton, Ohio area.

Preface

In the pursuit of <u>Excellence</u>, One must
<u>Care</u> beyond what others think is wise,
<u>Envision</u> more than most feel is practical,
<u>Chance</u> beyond what others see as safe,
And <u>anticipate</u> more than others think is possible.

An adaptive verse by MR Mittelstadt

Whenever we decide to do something we've not done before, we face the attitudes within us that may determine our success or failure. If we grow up afraid to take a chance, we may never be able to express in our lives the gifts and talents awaiting our self-discovery.

Let the purpose of this book be to provide basic information about massage and bodywork. To introduce information about the massage and bodywork professions to minds ready to stretch beyond current boundaries might lead them into a journey of self-discovery regarding their own bodies and the bodies of others. In such a journey may be found a lifelong passion.

It is hoped that for the professional massage therapist and bodyworker, the contents of this book will provide basic information, sources of information, and a ready reference. May it serve as a handy reference to the thousands of massage therapists and bodyworkers who have dedicated their lives to the health and wellness of their family, friends, and patients.

Ed Denning, MEd, LMT

A

abduction (ABD): Movement of a body part (usually the limbs) away from the midline of the body.

abnormal: Not normal. Not average. Not typical or usual. An irregularity.

abortion: Any loss of pregnancy before the 28th week, either accidentally or intentionally.

absorption: Process by which a substance is made available to the body fluids for distribution.

abstract thinking: Ability to derive meaning from an event or experience beyond the tangible aspects of the event itself.

acceleration: Increase in the speed or velocity of an object or reaction.

accessibility: Degree to which an exterior or interior environment is available for use, in relation to an individual's physical and/or psychological abilities.

accessory movers: Muscles capable of performing a motion; assist prime movers.

accommodation: Process of adapting or adjusting a thing or set of things to another.

accreditation: Process used to evaluate educational programs against a set of standards that represent the knowledge, skills, and attitudes needed for competent practice.

acromion process: Outer projection of the spine of the scapula; considered to be the highest part of the shoulder, it connects laterally to the clavicle.

acrosage: A combination of massage, yoga, and acrobatics developed by Benjamin Marantz. The client is placed in an inverted pose atop the acrosager's feet, allowing the client's head to hang freely. With no pressure on the neck or spine, the client's difficult points can be easily massaged.

active assistive range of motion (AAROM): Amount of motion at a given joint achieved by the person using his or her own muscle strength with assistance.

active joint movements: Movements initiated by an individual and controlled through an individual's nervous system. Also known as voluntary movements.

active listening: Skills that allow a person to hear, understand, and indicate that the message has been communicated.

active range of motion (AROM): Amount of motion at a given joint achieved by the person using his or her own muscle strength.

active stretch: Stretch produced by internal muscular force.

activity: The nature and extent of functioning at the level of the person. Productive action required for the development; maturation; and use of sensory, motor, social, psychological, and cognitive functions.

acuity: Ability of the sensory organ to receive information. Keenness of thought or vision.

acupressure: Use of touch at specific points along the meridians of the body to release the tensions that cause various physical symptoms. Based on the principles of acupuncture. An ancient healing art developed in Asia over 5 000 years ago that uses the fingers to press key points on the surface of the skin to stimulate the body's natural self-curative abilities.

acupuncture: Chinese practice of inserting needles into specific points along the meridians of the body to relieve pain and induce anesthesia. It is used for preventive and therapeutic purposes.

acute: A very serious, critical period of short duration in illness.

acu-yoga: A system of exercises integrating the knowledge of 2 holistic methods of health maintenance—acupressure and yoga.

adamantine particles: Pure particles that form all the elements of the universe. They are energized by only 1 energy form—love.

adamantine system: An advanced complementary energy therapy based on adamantine particles.

adaptation: Satisfactory adjustment of individuals within their environment over time. Successful adaptation equates with quality of life.

adduction (ADD): Movement toward the midline of the body.

adhesion: Fibrous band holding parts together that are normally separated.

adhesive capsulitis: Inflammation of the joint capsule, which causes limitations of mobility or immobility of the joint.

administrative controls: Decisions made by management intended to reduce the duration, frequency, and severity of exposure to existing workplace hazards. It leaves the hazards at the workplace, but attempts to diminish the effects on the worker (eg, job rotation or job enlargement).

adrenal gland: A pair of endocrine organs lying immediately above the kidney, consisting of an inner medulla, which produces epinephrine and norepinephrine, and an outer cortex, which produces a variety of steroid hormones.

adverse effects: Undesired consequences of chemical agents resulting from toxic doses or allergies.

advocacy: Actively supporting a cause, an idea, or a policy (eg, speaking in favor); recommending accommodations under the Americans with Disabilities Act.

aerobic activity/exercise/conditioning: Any physical exercise or activity that requires additional effort by the heart and lungs to meet the increased demand by the skeletal muscles for oxygen. The performance of therapeutic exercise and activities to increase endurance.

aerobic capacity: A measure of the ability to perform work or participate in activity over time using the body's oxygen uptake and delivery and energy release mechanisms.

aerobic metabolism: Energy production utilizing oxygen.

aerobic training/exercise: Exercise of sufficient intensity, duration, and frequency to improve the efficiency of oxygen consumption during activity or work. Endurance-type exercise that relies on oxidative metabolism as the major source of energy production.

affect: Emotion or feelings conveyed in a person's face or body; the subjective experiencing of a feeling or emotion. To influence or produce a change in.

afferent: Conducting toward a structure.

afferent neuron: A nerve cell that sends nerve impulses from sensory receptors to the central nervous system.

age-appropriate activities: Activities and materials that are consistent with those used by nondisabled age mates in the same culture.

agglutination: Act of blood cells clumping together.

aging: Passage of years in a person's life; the process of growing older.

aging in place: Where older adults remain in their own homes, retirement housing, or other familiar surroundings as they grow old.

agonist: Muscle that is capable of providing the power so a bone can move.

agoraphobia: An abnormal fear of being in an open space.

alchemia: A form of channeling involving the activation of Universal Fifth Dimension Energy.

alcoholism: A chronic disease characterized by an uncontrollable urge to consume alcoholic beverages excessively to the point that it interferes with normal life activities.

aldosterone: A steroid hormone produced by the adrenal cortex glands and the chief regulator of sodium, potassium, and chloride metabolism, thus controlling the body's water and electrolyte balances.

Alexander technique: Movement education in which the student is taught to sit, stand, and move in ways that reduce physical stress on the body.

allied health: Broad field of study encompassing diverse health professionals with special training in such fields as physical therapy, occupational therapy, respiratory therapy, speech pathology, and health information services, as well as laboratory, radiology, and dietetic services. It does not include physicians, nurses, dentists, or podiatrists.

alopecia: Absence or loss of hair; baldness.

alternative therapies: Interventions to provide holistic approaches to the management of diseases and illnesses such as acupuncture, massage, or nutrition.

altruism: Unselfish concern for the welfare of others.

alveolar: A general term used in anatomical nomenclature to designate a small sac-like dilatation, such as the sockets in the mandible and maxilla in which the roots of the teeth are held, or the small outpocketings of the alveolar sacs in the lungs, through whose walls the gaseous exchange takes place.

ambience: One's surroundings. Also, the atmosphere created by those surroundings.

ambulate: To walk from place to place.

ambulatory care: Care delivered on an outpatient basis.

American Journal of Physical Therapy: The official journal of the American Physical Therapy Association. It provides literature on physical therapy research, education, and practice.

American National Standards Institute (ANSI): Clearinghouse and coordinating body for voluntary standards activity on the national level.

American Society of Hand Therapists (ASHT): Established in 1978, the ASHT is concerned with hand rehabilitation education and research among practitioners in this area. The *Journal of Hand Therapy* is a publication resulting from the work of the ASHT.

amma/amna: Amma (sometimes spelled amna) is the traditional word for massage in the Japanese language and is more than 5 000 years old. The amma techniques encompass myriad pressing, stroking, stretching, and percussive manipulations with the thumbs, fingers, arms, elbows, knees, and feet on acupressure points along the body's 14 major meridians.

amnesia: Dissociative disorder characterized by memory loss during a certain time period or of personal identity.

amniocentesis: A low-risk prenatal diagnostic procedure of collecting amniotic fluid and fetal cells for examination through the use of a needle inserted into the abdominal wall and uterus to determine the fetal age and genetic characteristics after 4 months of gestation.

amputation: Partial or complete removal of a limb; may be congenital or acquired.

anaerobic exercise/activity: Exercise or activity without oxygen; oxygen intake cannot keep up with level of exercise/activity, so oxygen debt occurs.

analgesic: Drug for reducing pain. Some mild analgesics are nonsteroidal anti-inflammatory drugs (eg, Motrin [McNeil-PPC, Inc, Ft. Washington, Pa]), and some analgesics are narcotics (eg, morphine).

analog: Continuous information system (eg, a clock with dials that move continuously on a continuum, as opposed to a digital clock).

analysis: An examination of the nature of something for the purpose of prediction or comparison.

analysis of covariance (ANCOVA): Controlling the effects of any variable(s) known to correlate with the dependent variable.

analysis of variance (F ratio or ANOVA): Establishing whether or not a significant difference exists among the means of samples.

anaphylactic shock: Condition in which the flow of blood throughout the body becomes suddenly inadequate due to dilation of the blood vessels as a result of allergic reaction.

anatomical position: Standing erect, arms at the sides, with palms facing forward.

anatomy: Area of study concerned with the internal and external structures of the body and how these structures interrelate.

anatripsis: Use of friction as a treatment modality for a medical condition.

androgens: Substances that produce or stimulate the development of male characteristics.

anemia: A condition in which there is a reduction of the number or volume of red blood corpuscles or the total amount of hemoglobin in the bloodstream, resulting in paleness and generalized weakness.

anesthetic: Drug that reduces or eliminates sensation. It can either affect the whole body (eg, nitrous oxide, a general anesthetic) or a particular part of the body (eg, xylocaine, a local anesthetic).

aneurysm: A sac formed by local enlargement of a weakened wall of an artery, a vein, or the heart, caused by disease, anatomical anomaly, or injury. Massage therapy is contraindicated due to the potential for excessive bleeding. Refer to a physician.

angina pectoris: Chest pain due to insufficient flow of blood to the heart muscle.

angiography: Injection of a radioactive material so that the blood vessels can be visualized.

animal massage: Massage specifically designed for pets or performance animals.

ankylosis: Condition of the joints in which they become stiffened and nonfunctional. Abnormal immobility and consolidation of a joint.

anointing: Rubbing olive oil or oil essences on the body.

anomaly: Pronounced departure from the norm.

ANOVA (analysis of variance): Abbreviation for statistical method used in research to compare sample populations.

anoxemia: Absence or deficiency of oxygen in the blood.

anoxia/anoxic: Absence or deficiency of oxygen in the tissues.

antagonist: Muscle that resists the action of a prime mover (agonist).

anterior: Toward the front of the body.

anterior fontanel: Region of the head that is found as a membrane-covered portion on the top of the head, generally closing by the time a child reaches 18 months. *Synonym*: the soft spot.

anterior horn cell: Motor neuron located anteriorly which is similar in shape to a pointed projection such as the paired processes on the head of various animals.

anthropometric: Human body measurements such as height, weight, girth, and body fat composition.

antibiotic: Chemical substance that has the ability to inhibit or kill foreign organisms in the body.

antibody: A protein belonging to a class of proteins called immunoglobins. A molecule produced by the immune system of the body in response to an antigen and which has the particular property of combining specifically with the antigen that induced its formation. Antibodies are produced by plasma cells to counteract specific antigens (infectious agents like viruses, bacteria, etc). The antibodies combine with the antigen they are created to fight, often causing the death of that infectious agent.

antigen: A substance foreign to the body. An antigen stimulates the formation of antibodies to combat its presence.

anti-inflammatory: Counteracting or suppressing inflammation.

antimicrobial: Designed to destroy or inhibit the growth of bacterial, fungal, or viral organisms.

antioxidant: A substance that slows down the oxidation of hydrocarbon, oils, fats, etc, and helps to check deterioration of tissues.

antisocial personality disorder: Personality disorder resulting in a chronic pattern of disregard for socially acceptable behavior, impulsiveness, irresponsibility, and lack of remorseful feelings. *Synonyms*: sociopathy, psychopathy, antisocial reaction.

anxiety: Characterized by an overwhelming sense of apprehension; the expectation that something bad is happening or will happen; class of mental disorders characterized by chronic and debilitating anxiety (eg, generalized anxiety disorder, panic disorder, phobias, and post-traumatic stress disorder).

aortic aneurysm: Aneurysm of the aorta.

aortic heart disease: A disease affecting the main artery of the body, carrying blood from the left ventricle of the heart to the main arteries of the body.

apnea: Temporary cessation of breathing.

aponeurosis: Fibrous or membranous tissue that connects a muscle to the part that the muscle moves.

appendicular skeleton: Bones forming the limbs, pectoral girdle, and pelvic girdle of the body.

applied kinsiology: A healing system that evaluates and treats an individual's structural, chemical, and mental aspects through the use of nutrition, manipulation, diet, acupuncture, exercise, and education. Muscle testing is used to determine the individual's structural, chemical, and mental health. Treatment may include nutritional counseling, manipulation, acupressure, and exercise.

applied physiology: A muscle monitoring technique that allows the body to express what is out of balance and provide information to restore that balance.

apprenticeship: Learning process in which novices advance their skills and understanding through active participation with a more skilled person.

aquatherapy: The use of water as a therapeutic measure (eg, hydrotherapy, whirlpools, pools for exercise).

arm sling: Orthosis used to provide support to the proximal upper extremity.

aromatherapy: The skilled and controlled use of essential oils for physical and emotional health and well being.

arousal: Internal state of the individual characterized by increased responsiveness to environmental stimuli.

arrhythmia: Variation from the normal rhythm, especially of the heartbeat.

arterial embolism/thrombosis: The obstruction of an arterial blood vessel by an embolus too large to pass through it or a thrombosis caused by the coagulation and fibrosis of blood at a particular site.

arteriosclerosis: Thickening and hardening of the arteries.

arteriovenous: Designating arteries or veins or arterioles and venules.

arteritis: Inflammation of an artery.

arthritis: Inflammation of the joints, which may be chronic or acute.

arthrography: Injection of dye or air into a joint cavity to image the contours of the joint.

arthrokinesiology: The study of the structure and function of skeletal joints.

arthropathy: Disease of a joint.

arthroplasty: Surgical replacement, formation, reformation, or reconstruction of a joint.

arthroscopy: Procedure in which visual equipment can be inserted into a joint so that its internal parts can be viewed.

articular cartilage: The tough, elastic tissue that separates the bones in a joint.

articulation: The joining or juncture between 2 or more bones.

ASCII (American Standard Code for Information Interchange): Standardized coding scheme that uses numeric values to represent letters, numbers, symbols, etc. ASCII is widely used in coding information for computers (eg, the letter "A" is "65" in ASCII).

Ashatsu Oriental Bar therapy: A combination of the elements of traditional Thai massage, barefoot shiatsu, and Keralite foot massage (Chavutti Thirummal) for the treatment of low back pain.

asphyxia: Condition of insufficient oxygen.

aspirate: To inhale vomitus, mucus, or food into the respiratory tract.

aspiration: Inhaling fluids or solid substances into the lungs.

assertiveness: Behavior aimed at claiming rights without denying the rights of others.

assessment: Process by which data are gathered, hypotheses formulated, and decisions made for further action; a subsection of the problem-oriented medical record. The measurement or quantification of a variable or the placement of a value on something (not to be confused with examination or evaluation).

assignment: Process through which a provider agrees to accept the amount the insurer pays as payment in full. The only amounts the patients/clients may be billed for are copayments and deductibles.

assimilation: Expansion of data within a given category or subcategory of a schema by incorporation of new information within the existing representational structure without requiring any reorganization or modification of prior knowledge.

assisted-living facility: Medium- to large-sized facilities that offer housing, meals, and personal care, plus extras such as housekeeping, transportation, and recreation. Small-sized facilities are known as board and care homes.

assistive devices: A variety of implements or equipment used to aid patients/clients in performing tasks or movements. Assistive devices include crutches, canes, walkers, wheelchairs, power devices, long-handled reachers, and static and dynamic splints.

assistive-living settings: A type of living situation in which persons live in community housing with attendant care provided for those parts of the day or those activities where assistance is required.

assistive technology: Any item, piece of equipment, or product system, whether acquired commercially off the shelf, modified, or customized, that is used to increase, maintain, or improve functional capabilities of individuals with disabilities.

assistive technology services: Any service that assists an individual with a disability in the selection, acquisition, or use of an assistive technology device.

association learning: Form of learning in which particular items or ideas are connected.

assumption: Proposition or supposition; a statement that links or relates 2 or more concepts to one another.

asthenia: Chronic lack of energy and strength.

asthma: Respiratory disease in which the muscles of the bronchial tubes tighten and give off excessive secretions. This combination causes obstruction of the airway and results in wheezing; characterized by recurring episodes. Massage therapy may not be applied during episodes. Application of massage to muscles already in spasm may cause the symptomology to increase in severity.

Aston-patterning: An educational process, developed by Judith Aston in 1977, combining movement coaching, bodywork, ergonomics, and fitness training.

asymmetric body balance: A combination of Paul St. John's neuromuscular therapy and traditional Hatha yoga.

asymmetrical: Lack of symmetry.

asymptomatic: Showing or causing no symptoms.

ataxia: Poor balance and awkward movement.

atherosclerosis: Deposits of fatty substance in arteries, veins, and the lymphatic system.

athetosis: Type of cerebral palsy that involves involuntary purposeless movements which fall into 1 of 2 classes: nontension involves contorted movements and tension involves blocked movements and flailing.

atonic: Absence of muscle tone.

atopic dermatitis: A clinical hypersensitivity of the skin.

atrioventricular block: Disruption in the flow of electrical impulse through the atrium wall of the heart leading to arrhythmias, bradycardiac, or complete cardiac arrest.

atrophy: Due to lack of use or deficient nutrition, the decrease in size of a normally developed organ or tissue.

atropine: Drug that inhibits actions of the autonomic nervous system, relaxes smooth muscle, is used to treat biliary and renal colic, and reduces secretions of the bronchial tubes, salivary glands, stomach, and intestines.

attachment: Deep affective bond between individuals or a feeling that binds one to a thing, cause, ideal, etc.

attendant care: Services that provide individuals with nonmedical, personal health and hygiene care, such as preparing meals, bathing, going to the bathroom, getting in and out of bed, and walking.

attention: Ability to focus on a specific stimulus without distraction.

attention span: Length of time an individual is able to focus or concentrate on a task or thought.

attitude: The position or posture assumed by the body in connection with an action, feeling, or mood. One's disposition, opinion, or mental set.

attunement: A noninvansive therapy incorporating nontouch and occasional light touch that balances the physiologic and energetic functions of the body. Attunement opens the sacred space for health, healing, and well being.

auditory: Pertaining to the sense or organs of hearing.

auditory defensiveness: Oversensitivity to certain sounds (eg, vacuum cleaners, fire alarms).

aura: Subjective sensation preceding a paroxysmal attack; a subtly pervasive quality or atmosphere seen as coming from a person, place, or thing.

autoimmunity: Condition in which the body has developed a sensitivity to some of its own tissues.

automatic processes: Processes that occur without much attentional effort.

automatization: When a learned motor skill is performed with little conscious thought.

autonomic nervous system: Part of the nervous system concerned with the control of involuntary bodily functions.

autonomy: State of independence and self-control.

avocational: Leisure pursuits.

avoidance: Psychological coping strategy whereby the source of stress is ignored or avoided.

avoidance learning: Form of learning through stimuli avoidance and cause and effect (eg, negative reinforcement).

axial skeleton: Bones forming the longitudinal axis of the body; consists of skull, vertebral column, thorax, and sternum.

axilla: Area located dorsal to the humerus and gleno-humeral joint. It is the site where the cords of the brachial plexus pass through in order to innervate the muscles of the arm, superficial back, and superficial thoracic region.

axis: A line, real or imaginary, running through the center of the body; the line about which a part revolves.

axon: Long part of a nerve cell that sends information away from the cell, across a synapse, to the dendrites of another cell.

axonotmesis: Interruption of the axon with subsequent wallerian degeneration; connective tissues of the nerve, including the schwann cell basement membrane, remains intact.

Ayurvedic massage: One part of the traditional detoxification and rejuvination program of India called Pancha Karma, in which the entire body is vigorously massaged with large amounts of warm oil and herbs to remove toxins from the system.

B

baby boom generation: People born between the years of 1946 and 1964.

back disorder/injury: Injury to or diseases of the lower lumbar, lumbosacral, or sacroiliac region of the back.

back labor: Pain arising from pressure on the lumbar and sacral nerve roots, experienced in some women as the baby's head descends in the birth canal.

back school: A structured educational program about low back problems, usually offered to a group of patients/clients.

bacterial diseases: Diseases resulting from infection by bacteria.

bacterial pneumonia: Inflammation caused by a bacterial infection in the lungs.

bactericidal: Able to kill bacteria.

balance: Ability to maintain a functional posture through motor actions that distribute weight evenly around the body's center of gravity, both statically (eg, while standing) and dynamically (eg, while walking).

Balinese massage: A combination of stretching, long strokes, skin rolling, and palm and thumb pressure techniques.

ballistic stretching: A method of stretching which uses bouncing to increase the amount of stretch. No longer recommended due to potential injury to the soft tissue.

barbiturate: Sedative that can cause both physiological and psychological dependence. *Trade/Generic names*: Seconal/secobarbital (Ranbaxy Pharmaceuticals, Princeton, NJ), Nembutal/pentobarbital (Ovation Pharmaceuticals, Deefield, Ill).

barriers: The physical impediments that keep patients/clients from functioning optimally in their surroundings, including safety hazards (eg, throw rugs, slippery surfaces), access problems (eg, narrow doors, high steps), and home/office design difficulties (eg, excessive distance to negotiate, multi-story environment).

basal ganglia: A collection of nuclei at the base of the cortex including the caudate nucleus, putamen, globus pallidus, and functionally include the substantia nigra and subthalamic nucleus.

baseline: Known value or quantity representing the normal background level against which a response to intervention can be measured.

base of support: The body surfaces, such as the plantar surface of the feet, around which the center of gravity is maintained via postural responses.

basic activities of daily living: Tasks that pertain to self-care, mobility, and communication.

battery: Assessment approach or instrument with several parts.

B cell: A type of lymphocyte capable of producing antibody. The B cell is a white cell which is able to detect the presence of foreign agents and, once exposed to an antigen on the agent, differentiates into plasma cells to produce antibodies.

beating: A type of tapotement. The body is struck by the palmer surface of a half closed fist, the terminal phalanges of the fingers and the heel of the hand.

behavioral modification: Process of reinforcing desirable responses; food, praise, and tokens may be used.

behavioral setting: Milieu in which the specific environment dictates the kinds of behaviors that occur there, independent of the particular individuals who inhabit the setting at the moment.

behavioral theory: Developmental theory that suggests that learning is a relationship between certain stimuli and their subsequent responses. This learning theory sees the individual as a result of present and past environments. Behaviorists believe that learning occurs through the processes of classical or operant conditioning.

behaviorism: Theory of behavior and intervention that holds that behavior is learned, that behaviors that are reinforced tend to recur, and those that are not reinforced tend to disappear.

belly: Midsection of a muscle (usually produces a bulge) between its 2 ends.

benchmark: Standard against which something else is judged.

beneficence: The quality of being kind or doing good; a charitable act or generous gift. Doing good resulting in benefit to others.

benefit: Sum of money that an insurance policy pays for covered services, under the terms of the policy.

benefit period: Time during which an insurance policy provides payments for covered benefits.

bereavement: Normal grief or depression commonly associated with the death of a loved one.

bilateral integration: Ability to perform purposeful movement that requires interaction between both sides of the body in a smooth and refined manner.

bilingual: Used to describe a person who speaks 2 languages fluently.

bindegewebsmassage: German for connective tissue massage or reflexive therapy of the connective tissue. The therapist strokes the subcutaneous fascia by pulling or dragging the tissues. Primarily used in Europe as a form of medical massage.

binocular: Pertaining to both eyes.

bio sync: A system of hands-on movement education. Also known as the Lamm technique.

bioethics: Application of ethics to health care.

biofeedback: A training technique that enables an individual to gain some element of voluntary control over muscular or autonomic nervous system functions using a device that produces auditory or visual stimuli.

biological age: Definition of age that focuses on the functional age of biological and physiological processes rather than on calendar time.

biomechanics: Study of anatomy, physiology, and physics as applied to the human body.

biorhythm: Biological or cyclical occurrence or phenomenon (eg, sleep cycle, menstrual cycle, or respiratory cycle).

bipolar disorder: Disorder characterized by an unstable self-image, abrupt mood swings, and poor impulse control.

birth asphyxia: Stopping of the pulse and loss of consciousness as a result of too little oxygen and too much carbon dioxide in the blood leading to suffocation during the birthing process.

birth trauma: Injury during delivery of an infant.

blastema: Immature substance from which cells and tissues are created.

blister: Epidermal loss considered second degree due to a burn.

blood-borne pathogen: Infectious disease spread by contact with blood (eg, AIDS, hepatitis B).

blood pressure (BP): Pressure of the blood against the walls of the blood vessels. Normal in young adults is 120 mmHg during systole and 70 mmHg during diastole.

blood thinner: Drugs used to thin the blood increase the risk of subdermal bleeding. Thus, massage therapy may be applied only under the supervision of a physician.

Blue Cross/Blue Shield Association (BC/BS): Nationwide federation of local, nonprofit insurance organizations that contract with hospitals and other health care providers to make payments for health care services to their subscribers.

boarding homes or board and care homes: Smaller sized housing for older adults offering supervised housing, meals, and personal care, plus housekeeping, transportation, and recreational activities.

body alignment technique: Energy blockages are released through balancing vibrational energy points associated with organs, glands, and systems of the body.

body image: Subjective picture people have of their physical appearance.

body logic: A self-care technique utilizing a 6 to 10 inch ball to stretch muscles, release restrictions, increase blood flow, and promote healing.

body mechanics: The interrelationships of the muscles and joints as they maintain or adjust posture in response to environmental forces.

body-mind centering: Developed by Bonnie Bainbridge Cohen. Body-mind centering is an integrated approach to transformative experience through movement re-education and hands-on patterning.

body-oriented psychology: A holistic therapy that incorporates traditional therapy with techniques that free energy blocks.

body righting reflex: Neuromuscular response aimed at restoring the body to its normal upright position when it is displaced.

body rolling: A 10 inch ball is used to stretch muscles for the purpose of releasing restrictions, increasing blood flow, and promoting healing.

BodyTalk: A combination of advanced yoga, advaitic philosophy, the insights of modern physics and mathematics, acupuncture, applied kinesiology, and Western medical expertise.

bolster: A specialized supportive device in varying forms and sizes. Used to support body parts during massage procedures.

bone grafts: Transplantation of bone.

bone marrow: Tissue filling the porous medullary cavity of the diaphysis of bones.

bone scan: Radiographic scan that evaluates skeletal involvement related to connective tissue disease.

Bonnie Prudden Myotherapy: A hands-on, drugless, noninvasive method of relieving muscle-related pain, which emphasizes a speedy, cost-effective recovery and active patient participation for long-term relief.

borderline personality: Disorder characterized by abrupt shifts in mood, lack of coherent sense of self, and unpredictable, impulsive behavior.

botulism: Fatal toxemia caused by ingestion of botulinum neurotoxin, which causes muscle weakness and paralysis.

Bowen technique: A hands-on, light touch body therapy consisting of gentle rolling movements over muscle bellies and tendons to stimulate the body's own healing mechanisms.

brachial plexus: Network of nerves that originates as roots C5, C6, C7, C8, and T1 and terminates as nerves that innervate the upper extremity.

bradycardia: Slowness of heartbeat (eg, less than 60 beats/minute).

bradykinesia: Slowness of body movement and speech.

Braille: Standardized system for communicating in writing with persons who are blind. Grade II Braille is standard literary Braille.

brain death: Irreversible destruction of the cortex and brainstem. Ways to determine are: lack of responsiveness, apnea, absence of reflexes, dilation of pupils, flatline electroencephalogram, and absence of cerebral blood flow for a given period of time.

brain gym: A program of physical activities that enhance learning ability by developing the brain's neural pathways through movement.

brain scan: Nuclear medicine diagnostic procedure used to detect tumors, cerebrovascular accidents, or other lesions in the brain.

brain tumors: Abnormal growth of cells within the cranium that may cause headaches, altered consciousness, seizures, vomiting, visual problems, cranial nerve abnormalities, personality changes, dementia, and sensory and motor deficits.

Braxton Hicks contractions: Intermittent contractions of the uterus during pregnancy.

breast massage: Specific kneading, rubbing, and/or squeezing strokes applied to the soft tissue of the breast to increase lymph and blood flow. The application of massage therapy principles to massage of the female breast tissues. Specific training is needed to avoid damage to sensitive tissues and to respect possible boundary issues.

breath therapy: Circular and conscious breathing techniques and exercises are used to bring physical and emotional stress to the surface for release and integration.

Breema bodywork: Nurturing touch, tension-relieving stretches, and rhythmic movements are used to create physical, emotional, and mental balance.

bruise: An injury with an escape of fluid into subcutaneous tissue; skin is discolored but not broken. Massage of bruised area is contraindicated to prevent increasing the amount of fluid moving into the bruised area. Nearby tissues may be massaged.

bruxism: Grinding of teeth.

Budzek medical massage therapy: A combination of 12 different bodywork techniques applied in specific sequences.

bunion: A swelling of the bursa mucosa of the first metatarsal head with callousing of the overlying skin and lateral migration of the great toe.

burn: A lesion caused by the contact of heat.

burnout: State of mental fatigue that results in the inability to generate energy from one's occupational performance areas.

bursa: Sac that contains synovial fluid. Bursae are located in superficial fascia, in areas where movement takes place and aid in decreasing friction.

bursectomy: Excision of bursae.

bursitis: Inflammation of a bursa resulting from injury, infection, or rheumatoid synovitis. It produces pain and tenderness and may restrict movement at a nearby joint.

byte: Unit of information in computer programming equal to 1 character.

C

cachectic: Marked state of poor health and malnutrition secondary to disease, treatment, or poor nutrient intake.

calcification: The deposition of calcium salts in body tissues. A calcified substance or structure.

calibration: Determination of what the output of a measuring instrument means, then compared with known values.

callousities: Hardened, thickened places on the skin.

cancer: A malignant tumor of potentially unlimited growth that expands locally by invasion and systemically by metastasis; massage therapy is contraindicated for cancers which might metastasize. Apply massage only if you have the approval of a physician.

candidiasis: Infection by fungi of the genus candida, most commonly involving the skin, oral mucosa, respiratory tract, and vagina.

cane: Stick or short staff used to assist one during walking; can have a narrow or broad base depending on the amount of support needed.

capacitance: Elastic capacity of vessels and organs of the body.

capacity: One's best, includes present abilities as well as potential to develop new abilities.

capitation: Method of payment for health services in which a provider receives a fixed, prepaid, per capita amount for each person enrolled in the health plan for whom the provider has responsibility for all necessary health care services.

capsular restriction: Limitation of mobility and range due to tightness or rigidity of the joint capsule.

carbuncle: A painful bacterial infection deep beneath the skin having a network of pus-filled boils.

carcinogen: Any substance or agent that produces or increases incidence of cancer..

carcinoma: Any of the several kinds of cancerous growths deriving from epithelial cells.

cardiac arrest: Cessation of effective heart action.

cardiac arrhythmias: Irregularity in the rhythm of the heartbeat.

cardiac contusion: Bruising of the heart due to direct trauma or injury to the myocardium.

cardiac output: Volume of blood pumped from the heart per unit of time. Cardiac output is the product of heart rate and stroke volume.

cardiomyopathy: A subacute or chronic disorder of heart muscle of unknown or obscure etiology, often with associated endocardial, and sometimes with pericardial involvement, but not atherosclerotic in origin.

cardiopulmonary: Pertaining to the heart and lungs.

cardiotonic: Drug that promotes the force and efficiency of the heart.

cardiovascular (CV): Pertaining to the heart and blood vessels.

cardiovascular insufficiency: Inability of the cardiovascular system to perform at a level necessary for basic homeostasis of the body.

cardiovascular pump: Structures responsible for maintaining cardiac output, including the cardiac muscle, valves, arterial smooth muscle, and venous smooth muscle.

cardiovascular pump dysfunction: Abnormalities of the cardiac muscles, valves, conduction, or circulation that interrupt or interfere with cardiac output or circulation.

cardioversion: The use of electrical current to convert irregular rhythms or no rhythms to an active, regular, rhythmical heartbeat.

caregiver: One who provides care and support to a person.

carpals: Bones of the wrist; there are 8 carpal bones in each wrist.

carrier (eg, Medicare): Private contractor to Health Care Financing Administration that administers claims processing and payment for Medicare B services.

cascade effect: Ability of the blood to clot via multiple factors.

case management: Uses a legally mandated case manager to oversee the coordination of services for a patient/client. This manager, whose roles may include helper, teacher, planner, and advocate, assists in facilitating the needs of a patient/client and his or her family.

case manager: Individual who assumes responsibility for coordination and follow-up on a given patient/client case.

cataplexy: Sudden episodes of loss of muscle function.

cataract: Abnormal progressive condition of the lens of the eye characterized by loss of transparency.

catastrophic health insurance: A type of health insurance that provides protection against the high cost of treating severe or lengthy illnesses or disabilities.

catatonia: Motor abnormality usually characterized by immobility or rigidity, in which no organic base has been identified.

categorization: Ability to classify; to describe by naming or labeling.

cathartic: Drug that relieves constipation and promotes defecation for diagnostic and operative procedures.

cauda equina: Spinal nerves descending in the spinal column below the level of L2.

caudal: Away from the head or toward the lower part of a structure.

causalgia: A condition of severe burning pain usually caused by a peripheral nerve injury.

cause and effect: When something occurs as a result of a motion or activity.

cellulitis: An inflammation of connective tissue, especially subcutaneous tissue.

centering: A meditative activity that is used to focus one's energy so that it can be channeled more effectively into whatever activity is desired.

center of gravity: Point at which the downward force created by mass and gravity is equivalent or balanced on either side of a fulcrum.

central nervous system (CNS): Consists of all the neurons of the brain, brainstem, and spinal cord.

central tendency: The typical, middle, or central scores in a distribution.

centrifugal control: Brain's ability to regulate its own input.

centrifuge: Separates components of blood for further testing through high speed, rotational movement.

centripetal: From the center, movements made from the heart or in the direction of arterial flow.

cephalad: Toward the head or upper portion of a part or structure. *Synonym*: superior.

cerclage: A purse string ring suture placed around an incompetent cervix at the level of the os at 12 to 14 weeks of gestation to prevent premature delivery from an incompetent cervix.

cerebral angioplasty: Injection of dye into the cerebrovascular system to observe its function.

cerebral atrophy: Deterioration of the cerebral tissue.

cerebral contusion: Bruising of brain tissue.

cerebral degeneration: Deterioration or loss of function or structure in the cerebral region of the brain.

cerebral embolism: The obstruction of a blood vessel by an embolus in the brain.

certification: Process developed to ensure that each practitioner has the knowledge, skills, and attitudes required for competent professional service in an area of specialization (eg, geriatrics, pediatrics, massage therapy, orthopedics, neurology).

cervicalgia: Any disorder causing pain in the cervical region.

cervical spondylosis: Dissolution of the cervical vertebrae.

cervical vertebrae: Seven small neck bones between the skull and thoracic vertebrae; they support the head and allow movement.

cervix: The neck of the uterus, which leads into the vagina and thins out and dilates during labor.

Cesarean section: Delivery of a child by abdominal surgery.

chair massage: A brief bodywork session done in a special chair in which the client sits facing the cushion, exposing the scalp, shoulders, neck arms, back, and hips. Also known as on-site massage.

champissage: A 1 000 year old form of head massage practiced in India.

CHAMPUS (Civilian Health and Medical Program of the Uniformed Services): Program paid for by the Department of Defense; pays for care that civilian health providers deliver to retired members and dependents of active and retired military personnel. This program does not charge premiums but has cost-sharing provisions.

characteristic behavior: Behavior typical of one's performance under everyday conditions.

checklist: Type of assessment approach whereby a list of abilities, tasks, or interests is presented and those items meeting a designated criterion are checked. An interest checklist, for example, might list a number of activities in varied categories and ask the respondent to check those that are viewed as most interesting.

chemotherapy: The use of drugs or pharmacologic agents that have a specific and toxic effect on a disease-causing pathogen.

chest pain: Angina resulting from ischemia of the heart tissue.

chickenpox: An acute communicable disease caused by a virus and marked by slight fever and an eruption of macular vesicles which appear as a rash.

chilblains: A localized itching and painful erythema on the skin which is a disease of the small blood vessels of the skin and may result in ulceration and necrosis.

chi gong: The process of exercising mental intent to direct one's internal energy through the body. *Alternate spellings*: qi gong, chi kung.

chi kung: *See* chi gong.

chi nei tsang: A wholistic approach of Taoist origin that integrates the physical, mental, emotional and spiritual aspects of the self.

child abuse: Intentional physical or psychological injury inflicted upon children by caretaker(s).

child neglect: Inadequate social, emotional, or physical nurturing of children.

chi square (2): A statistical test used to establish whether or not frequency differences have occurred on the basis of chance.

cholecystectomy: Removal of the gallbladder.

chondrocyte: Cartilage cell embedded in lacunae within the matrix of cartilage connective tissue.

chondromalacia: Softening of the articular cartilages.

chorea: Abrupt irregular movements of short duration involving the fingers, hands, arms, face, tongue, or head.

chromosome: Thread-like structure made up of genes; there are 46 chromosomes in the nucleus of each cell of a human.

chronic bronchitis: Chronic inflammation of the bronchial tubes. A long-continued form, often with a more or less marked tendency to recurrence after stages of quiescence. Diagnosis is made when a chronic cough for up to 3 months in 2 consecutive years is present.

chronic disorders: Characterized by slow onset and long duration; rarely develop in early adulthood, increase in middle adulthood, and become common in late adulthood.

chronic fatigue: Long continued fatigue not relieved by rest, may be indicative of disease. Only light massage therapy due to an already overburdened excretory system.

chronic respiratory disease: Lung diseases resulting from constrictive or obstructive conditions of the airways.

chronological: Individual's age; definition of age that relies on the amount of calendar time that has passed since birth.

circulation: Movement in a regular or circutious course, as the movement of blood through the heart and blood vessels.

circumduction: Movement in which the distal end of a bone moves in a circle while the proximal end remains stable, acting like a pivot.

claim: Request to an insurer for payment of benefits under an insurance policy.

claim adjudication: Determination of payment on a claim based on type of contract, type of coverage, and present use.

class: Group containing members who share certain attributes such as economic status, social identifications, or cultural identity.

class I lever system: Lever system in which the fulcrum is between the force and the resistance (eg, seesaw). The mechanical advantage can be less than, more than, or equal to 1.

class II lever system: Lever system in which the resistance is between the fulcrum and the force. The mechanical advantage is always greater than 1.

class III lever system: Lever system in which the force is between the fulcrum and the resistance. The mechanical advantage is always less than 1.

classical conditioning: Method of eliciting specific responses through the use of stimuli that occur within a period of time that permits an association to be made between them. Also called Pavlovian conditioning, after the Russian scientist who made the technique famous.

classification: Arrangement according to some systematic division into classes or groups.

claudication: Lameness, limping; usually caused by poor circulation of blood to the leg muscles. *Intermittent* claudication is a complex of symptoms characterized by absence of pain or discomfort in a limb at rest or the commencement of pain, tension, and weakness with walking that intensifies with continued walking and is relieved by rest. Usually seen in occlusive arterial diseases of the limbs.

clavicle: Bone that acts as a brace to hold the upper arm free from the thorax to allow free movement and serves as a place for muscle attachment. *Synonym*: collarbone.

clients: Individuals who are not necessarily sick or injured but who can benefit from a therapist's consultation, professional advice, or services. Clients are also businesses, school systems, and others to whom therapists offer services.

clinical guidelines: Systematically developed statements to assist practitioner and patient decisions about appropriate health care for specific clinical circumstances.

clinical reasoning: Thinking that directs and guides clinical decision making; reflective thinking.

clinical trial: Studies with human subjects.

clinical utility: Factors such as clarity of instruction, cost, and facileness in using the assessment determine the amount of the assessment's utility.

clonus: Spasmodic alternation of contraction and relaxation of muscles.

closed-chain movements: The distal end of a kinematic chain is fixed or stabilized, and the proximal end (origin) moves (eg, push-ups). Also called closed kinetic chain, usually involving multiple joints.

closed question: Question that asks for a specific response (eg, one that may be answered with a "yes" or "no").

close supervision: Contact that is daily, direct, and given on the work premises.

clubbing: A proliferative change in the soft tissues about the terminal phalanges of the fingers or toes with no osseous changes.

clubfoot: Birth defect in which the soles of the feet face medially and the toes point inferiorly; occurs in about 1 out of 1 000 births and may be caused genetically or by the folding of the foot up against the chest during fetal development. *Synonym*: talipes.

clubhand: Medical condition seen in children in which the hand is radically displaced; the radius bone may be partially formed or may be absent.

cluster trait sample: Assesses a number of traits inherent in a job or various jobs, such as dexterity, strength, endurance, range of motion, and speed.

coagulation: The process of blood clot formation.

coccyodynia: Painful coccyx usually resulting from an injury, making sitting difficult.

cocontraction: Simultaneous contraction of agonistic and antagonistic muscle groups, which act to stabilize joints.

codeine: Narcotic derived from the opium family that is highly addictive.

code of ethics: Statement that a certain group follows; sets the guidelines so that a high standard of behavior is maintained.

codependence: Condition in which substance dependence is subtly supported by the codependent who meets some need through the continued dependence of the individual.

cognition: Mental processes that include thinking, perceiving, feeling, recognizing, remembering, problem solving, knowing, sensing, learning, judging, and metacognition. The act or process of knowing, including both awareness and judgment.

cognitive development: Process of thinking and knowing in the broadest sense, including perception, memory, and judgment.

cognitive disability: Physiologic or biochemical impairment in information-processing capacities that produce observable and measurable limitations in routine task behavior.

cognitive learning: Form of learning that encompasses the forming of mental plans of events and objects.

cohesiveness: Growth of interpersonal harmony and intimacy within a group.

coinsurance: Component of a health insurance plan that requires the insurer and patient/client each to pay a percentage of covered costs.

Colles' wrist fracture: Transverse fracture of the distal end of the radius (just above the wrist).

colloid osmotic pressure: The pressure exerted by substances capable of influencing osmosis of water across membranes.

coma: Abnormally deep unconsciousness with the absence of voluntary response to stimuli.

commitment: Degree of importance attached to an event by an individual, based on his or her beliefs and values. The degree of commitment is an important element in motivation.

communication: The act of transmitting thoughts or ideas. Giving or exchanging of information, signals, or messages by talk, gestures, or writing. A system of sending or receiving messages.

community forum: A needs assessment technique that invites residents/members of the target population to discuss their concerns at open "town hall" type meetings.

community rehabilitation programs: Structured daily social alternatives, including daily, evening, and weekend programs, as well as prevocational and vocational skills development. They provide supported employment, work adjustment, and job placement, and also include leisure programs.

community/work integration or reintegration: The process of assuming or resuming roles in the community or at work.

comorbidity: Characterized by the presence of symptoms of more than 1 ailment (eg, depression and anxiety).

competence: Achievement of skill equal to the demands of the environment; also a legal term referring to the soundness of one's mind.

competition: Rivalry for objects, resources, facilities, or position in an organization.

compliance: Subservient behavior that implies following orders or directions without self-direction or choice. Also related to respiratory mechanics with change in respiratory volume over pressure gradient. Refers to the elasticity and expandability of the lungs.

components: Fundamental units; in relation to activities refers to processes, tools, materials, and purposefulness.

comprehensive battery: Battery of tests that measure different components of cognitive functioning and perceptual and motor functioning.

compression: Squeezed together; being pressed together.

compression therapy: Treatment using devices or techniques that decrease the density of a part of the body through the application of pressure.

compulsion: A repetitive, distressing act that is performed to relive obsession-related fear.

computer-assisted tomography (CAT): Scanning procedure that combines x-rays with computer technology to show cross-sectional views of internal body structures.

computerized assessment: Assessment that includes the administration, scoring, and interpretation of test results done by a sophisticated computer program.

concentration: Ability to maintain attention for longer periods of time in order to keep thoughts directed toward completing a given task.

concentric contraction: Muscular contraction during which the muscle fibers shorten in an attempt to overcome resistance.

concept: Mental image, abstract idea, or general notion.

concussion: Resulting from impact with an object (usually to the brain).

conditioning: Learning process that alters behavior through reinforcements or associating a reflex with a particular stimulus to trigger a desired response. Also a cardiovascular effect related to exercise and the overall improvement of functional endurance.

conduction: Conveying energy (eg, heat, sound, or electricity).

conference committee: Committee of legislators with the purpose of working out compromises between different versions of a bill.

confidentiality: Maintenance of secrecy regarding information confided by a patient/client.

conflict of interest: Situation in which a person may have hidden or other interests that conflict or are inconsistent with providing services to a patient/client or agency.

congenital: Present or existing at birth.

congenital amputation: Child is born without part or all of a limb or limbs.

congenital anomalies/disorders: Structural abnormalities resulting from birth defects or genetic disorders.

congenital defects: Abnormalities or deformations of the skull or vertebrae where there is a failure to enclose the neural structures or a complete absence of different parts of the brain itself.

congested: The presence of an abnormal amount of blood or fluid.

congregate housing: Housing for unrelated individuals, often older persons, usually sponsored by government or nonprofit organizations.

conjunctivitis: Inflammation of the conjunctiva of the eye.

connective tissue: Structural material of the body that connects tissues and links anatomical structures together.

connective tissue massage: A type of massage of the superficial and middle layers of fascia that creates effects within the central nervous system.

consensus: A common center or agreement.

consent: Agree to participate.

conservation: Cognitive skill that requires the realization that a quantity of a substance remains constant regardless of changes in form.

constipation: Difficult defecation; characterized by dry, hard fecal matter.

construct: Conceptual structure used in science for thinking about the factors underlying observed phenomena.

construct validity: In research, the extent to which a test measures the construct (mental representation) variables that it was designed to identify.

consultation: Process of assisting a patient/client, an agency, or other provider by identifying and analyzing issues, providing information and advice, and developing strategies for current and future actions.

consumer price index (CPI): Published by the U. S. Department of Labor, a measure of increases in the price of a market basket of goods and services by region of the country.

contact dermatitis: Inflammatory response of the skin due to contact with a toxic or caustic agent (eg, chemical, poison ivy).

contagious disease: An infectious disease readily transmitted from one person to another. Massage is contraindicated due to potential to spread the condition from one person to another.

context: Refers to the social, physical, and psychological milieu of a situation.

continuing education: Educational programming that provides opportunities for certification or training to improve an individual's knowledge and practices.

contract: Agreement, usually written, between practitioner and agency that specifies the services to be provided and the responsibilities of each party.

contractile protein: A substance produced to remove waste at an intra- and extra-cellular level.

contractions: Shortening and tightening of the uterine muscle fibers during and after labor.

contracture: Static shortening of muscle and connective tissue that limits range of motion at a joint.

contraindication: Condition that deems a particular type of treatment undesirable or improper.

contralateral: Pertaining to, situated on, or affecting the opposite side.

contrast bath: The immersion of an extremity in alternating hot and cold water.

contributory insurance: Type of group insurance in which the employee pays for all or part of the premium and the employer or union pays the remainder.

control group: Comparison group in research.

contusion: A bruise.

convergence: Ability of the brain to respond only after receiving input from multiple sources.

convulsion: Paroxysms of involuntary muscular contractions and relaxation; spasm.

coordinated care: Term Health Care Financing Administration often uses, more or less generically, for managed care plans, particularly if they are gatekeepers.

coordination: Property of movement characterized by the smooth and harmonious action of groups of muscles working together to produce a desired motion.

copayment: Specified amount of money per visit or unit of time that the patient/client pays, while the insurer pays the rest of the claim.

coping: Process through which individuals adjust to the stressful demands of their daily environment.

copious: Large amounts.

core energetics: A form of psychotherapy developed by John C. Pierakos. Core energetics focuses on unifying and connecting the body, emotions, mind, will/intent, and spiritual self into a unified whole expressing the complete reality of the person.

correlation coefficient: The relationship among 2 or more variables.

corticorubrospinal pathway: Descending pathway that serves limb control; from the motor cortex through the red nucleus in the brain stem and onto the spinal cord.

corticospinal pathway: Oversees the finely tuned movements of the body by controlling finely tuned movements of the hands; this pathway travels from the motor cortex to the spinal neurons that serve the hand muscles.

cortisone: Hormone produced in the cortex of the adrenal gland that aids in the regulation of the metabolism of fats, carbohydrates, sodium, potassium, and proteins.

cost-benefit analysis: Process used to evaluate the economic efficiency of new policies and programs by comparing an outcome and the costs required to achieve it.

cost containment: Approach to health care that emphasizes reduced costs.

cost effectiveness: Extent to which funds spent to improve health and well being reduce overall cost of care.

cost sharing: Requirement in health insurance plans for the patient/client to pay part of the cost of care.

counterculture: Subculture that rejects important values of the dominant society.

countertransference: Developing an inappropriate emotional relationship with a client; the therapist may lose objectivity.

cranial nerve: Nerve extending from the brain.

craniosacral therapy: A holistic therapy that involves the manipulation of the cranial bones and the sacrum. A gentle hands-on method of evaluating and enhancing the function of a physiological body system called the craniosacral system—comprised of the membranes and cerebrospinal fluid that surround and protect the brain and spinal cord.

credentialing: Process that gives title or approval to a person or program such as certification, registration, or accreditation.

crepitation: Dry, crackling sound or sensation, such as made by the ends of 2 bones grating together.

crepitus: The noise of gas discharged from the intestines.

cretinism: Condition in which an individual is small, unusual looking, and has severe mental retardation as a result of the lack of thyroid hormone.

criterion: Particular standard or level of performance or expected outcome.

criterion-referenced tests: Goal of these tests is to evaluate specific skills or knowledge where the criterion is full mastery of them.

criterion validity: Test that measures and predicts the specific behaviors required to function in, meet the standards of, and be successful in daily life.

critical inquiry: Important investigation or examination.

cross-linking: Theory that aging is caused by a random interaction among proteins that produce molecules that make the body stiffer.

cross-sectional research: Nonexperimental research sometimes used to gather data on possible growth trends in a population.

cryotherapy: Therapeutic application of cold (eg, ice). Cold water immersions or ice packs are used to alleviate blood flow, swelling, and inflammation, by contraction of blood vessels.

crystal arthropathies: Diseases of the joints that result in crystalization such as gout and pseudogout.

crystaldyne therapy: A self-activiting crystal stimulator is used to electrically stimulate the acupressure, acupuncture, and reflexology points.

cue: Subjective and objective input that serves as a signal to do something. A secondary stimulus that guides behavior.

cueing: Hints or suggestions that facilitate the appropriate response.

culture: Patterns of behavior learned through the socialization process, including anything acquired by humans as members of society (eg, knowledge, values, beliefs, laws, morals, customs, speech patterns, economic production patterns). The system of meanings and customs shared by some identifiable group or subgroup and transmitted from one generation of that group to the next.

curvature of the spine: Structural deformity of the spine resulting in scoliosis, kyphoscoliosis, lordosis, or kyhposis.

custom: Habitual practice that is adhered to by members of the same group or geographical region.

cyanosis: Blue discoloration of the skin and mucous membranes due to excessive concentration of reduced hemoglobin in the blood.

cyst: Closed sac or pouch with a definite wall that contains fluid, semifluid, or solid material.

D

database: Collection of data organized in information fields in electronic format.

daytime splint: Splint used during the daytime that must be designed in such a way that it may be removed several times a day so that the patient/client can prevent joint stiffening by moving the joint(s) to the full range of motion.

death rates: Number of deaths occurring within a specific population during a particular time period, usually in terms of 1 000 persons per year.

debility: Weakness or feebleness of the body.

debridement: Excision of contused and necrotic tissue from the surface of a wound. *Autolytic*: Self-debridement, that is, removal of contused or necrotic tissue through the action of enzymes in the tissues. *Sharp*: Debridement using a sharp instrument.

decision making: The process of making decisions (eg, the choice of certain preferred courses of action over others).

declarative memory: The registration, retention, and recall of past experiences, sensations, ideas and thoughts, knowledge through the hippocampal nuclear structures or the amygdala which result in long-term memory.

decubitus ulcer: Open sore due to lowered circulation in a body part. Usually secondary to prolonged pressure at a bony prominence.

deductible: Amount of loss or expense that an insured or covered individual must incur before an insurer assumes any liability for all or part of the remaining cost of covered services.

deductive reasoning: A serial strategy where conclusions are drawn on the basis of premises that are assumed to be true.

deep tissue massage: Techniques that utilize deep tissue/deep muscle massage and are administered to affect the sub-layer of musculature and fascia. These techniques require more advanced training and a more thorough understanding of anatomy and physiology.

deep vein thrombosis: A blood clot in a deep vein.

defense mechanisms: Unconscious processes that keep anxiety producing information out of conscious awareness (eg, compensation, denial, rationalization, sublimation, and projection).

defibrillation: The stoppage of fibrillation of the heart. The separation of the fibers of a tissue by blunt dissection.

defibrillator: An apparatus used to counteract fibrillation by application of electric impulses to the heart.

defibrination syndrome: A syndrome resulting from a deprival of fibrin.

deficiency disease: A disease caused by a dietary lack of vitamins, minerals, etc, or by an inability to metabolize them.

deficit: Inadequate behavior or task performance. A lack or deficiency. *Developmental*: The difference between expected and actual performance in an aspect of development (eg, motor, communication, social).

degrees: In reference to the measurement of range of motion, the amount of movement from the beginning to the end of the action.

degrees of freedom: The options or directions available for movement from a given point.

degriefing: The mental and physical pain of grief is treated with a combination of somatic and psychotherapeutic tools.

dehydration: Absence of water. Removal of water from the body or a tissue. A condition that results from undue loss of water.

deinstitutionalization: Transfer to a community setting of patients/clients who have been hospitalized for an extended period of time, usually years.

delay of gratification: Postponement of the satisfaction of one's needs.

delirium: Characterized by confused mental state with changes in attention, hallucinations, delusions, and incoherence.

delusion: Inaccurate, illogical beliefs that remain fixed in one's mind despite having no basis in reality.

delusional disorder: Psychosis characterized by the presence of persistent delusions often involving paranoid themes in an individual whose behavior otherwise appears quite normal.

dementia: State of deterioration of personality and intellectual abilities, including memory, problem-solving skills, language use, and thinking that interferes with daily functioning.

demography: Scientific study of human populations particularly in relation to size, distribution, and characteristics of group members.

demyelinating disease: Diseases that destroy or damage the myelin sheath of the nerves.

demyelination: The destruction of myelin, the "white lipid" covering of the nerve cell axons. The loss of myelin decreases conduction velocity of the neural impulse and destroys the "white matter" of the brain and spinal cord.

dendrite: Short processes found on the end of a nerve cell that send or receive information from another neurotransmitter.

dendritic growth: New evidence indicating growth (rather than the common descriptions of decline) in the brains of the elderly.

Department of Health and Human Services (DHHS): Department within the U.S. government that is responsible for administering health and social welfare programs.

dependence: Need to be influenced, nurtured, or controlled; relying on others for support.

dependent: Person who can be claimed on insurance.

depolarization: The process or act of neutralizing polarity, such as in a heart beat.

depression: Characterized by an overwhelming sense of sadness that may be brought on by an event or series of events, but lasts far longer than a reasonable time.

depth perception: Ability to determine the relative distance between self and objects and figures observed.

dermatome: Area on the surface of the skin that is served by one spinal segment.

dermatomyositis: Systemic connective tissue disease characterized by inflammatory and degenerative changes in the skin. Leads to symmetric weakness and some atrophy.

developmental: Pertaining to gradual growth or expansion, especially from a lower to a higher stage of complexity. Pertaining to development.

developmental assessment: Evaluation of a child with disorders that should be repeated every 2 months until the child reaches age 2.

developmental delay: The failure to reach expected age-specific performance in one or more areas of development (eg, motor, sensory-perceptual). Wide range of childhood disorders and environmental situations where a child is unable to accomplish the developmental tasks typical of his or her chronological age.

developmental disabilities: A physical or mental handicap or combination of the two that becomes evident before age 22 and is likely to continue indefinitely, resulting in significant functional limitation in major areas of life.

developmental skills: Skills that are developed in childhood, such as language or motor skills.

deviance: Behavior that is in contrast to acceptable standards within a community or culture.

dexterity: Skill in using the hands or body, usually requiring both fine and gross motor coordination. *Synonym*: agility.

diabetes mellitus: A disorder of carbohydrate metabolism resulting from inadequate production or utilization of insulin. Massage therapy may be applied under the supervision of a physician.

diabetic retinopathy: Complication of diabetes in which small aneurysms form on renal capillaries.

diagnosis (Dx): Technical identification of a disease or condition by scientific evaluation of history, physical signs symptoms, laboratory tests, and procedures.

diagnostic interview: Interview used by a professional to classify the nature of dysfunction in a person under care.

dialysis: The process of separating crystalloids and colloids in solution by the difference in their rates of diffusion through a semipermeable membrane; crystalloids pass through readily, colloids very slowly or not at all.

diaphoresis: Perspiration, especially profuse perspiration.

diaphragmatic breathing: The use of the diaphragm to draw air into the bases of the lungs.

diaphragmatic hernia: A hernia in the diaphragm.

diarrhea: The passage of unformed watery bowel movements; massage is contraindicated as it may over stimulate the digestive system.

diastole: Period of time between contractions of the atria or the ventricles during which blood enters the relaxed chambers from the systemic circulation and lungs; significant in blood pressure readings.

diffuse: Spread out or dispersed. Not concentrated.

diffusion: The process of becoming diffused, or widely spread. Dialysis through a membrane.

digital: Discrete form of information (eg, a clock that displays only digits at given moment, as opposed to analog).

dignity: Importance of valuing the inherent worth and uniqueness of each person.

dilation (dilatation): The stretching and enlarging of the cervical opening to 10 cm to allow birth of the infant.

dilation and curettage (D&C): Widening of the cervical canal with a dilator and the scraping of the uterine endometrium with a curette.

diminutive: Suffix added to a medical term to indicate a smaller size, number, or quantity of that term.

diplegia: Involvement of 2 extremities.

direct service: Treatment or other services provided directly to one or more patients/clients by a practitioner.

disability: The inability to engage in age-specific, gender-related, and sex-specific roles in a particular social context and physical environment. Any restriction or lack (resulting from an injury) of ability to perform an activity in a manner or within the range considered normal for a human being.

disablement: Used as an umbrella term to cover all the negative dimensions of disability together or separately.

discharge: The process of discontinuing interventions included in a single episode of care, occurring when the anticipated goals and desired outcomes have been met. Other indicators for discharge: the patient/client declines to continue care, the patient/client is unable to continue to progress toward goals because of medical or psychosocial complications, or the therapist determines that the patient/client will no longer benefit from therapy.

discharge planning: To enhance continuity of care, plans are made to prepare the patient/client for moving from one setting to another, usually a multidisciplinary process.

disclosure: In dealing with informed consent, the patient/client has to be informed of what he/she is going to do for a study in which he/she participates.

disc prolapse: Displacement of intervertebral disc tissue from its normal position between vertebral bodies; also referred to as slipped, herniated, or protruded disc.

discrimination: Act of making distinctions based on differences in areas such as culture, race, gender, or religion.

disease (DZ): Deviation from the norm of measurable biological variables as defined by the biomedical system; refers to abnormalities of structure and function in body organs and systems.

disinhibition: Inability to suppress a lower brain center or motor behavior, such as a reflex, indicative of damage to higher structures of the brain.

dislocation: Displacement of bone from a joint with tearing of ligaments, tendons, and articular capsules. Symptoms include loss of joint motion, pain, swelling, temporary paralysis, and occasional shock. To avoid increased aggravation of the condition, massage is contraindicated without medical supervision.

disorder: Disruption or interference with normal functions or established systems.

disorientation: Inability to make accurate judgments about people, places, and things.

disruption: To disrupt or interrupt the orderly course of events.

distal: From anatomical position, located further from the trunk.

distractibility: Level at which competing sensory input are able to draw attention away from tasks at hand.

distraction: Linear separation of joint surfaces without rupture of the binding ligaments and without displacement.

distress: The state of being in pain, uncomfortable, or suffering. Any affliction that is distressing.

distribution: Refers to manner through which a drug is transported by the circulating body fluids to the sites of action.

disuse atrophy: The wasting degeneration of muscle tissue that occurs as a result of inactivity or immobility.

diuresis: Increased secretion of urine.

divergence: Brain's ability to send information from one source to many parts of the central nervous system simultaneously.

diversity: Quality of being different or having variety.

do-in: A therapy that combines some of the principles of shiatsu and acupressure with stretches, exercises, breathing, and meditation techniques.

Doctor Vodder Manual Lymphatic Drainage: Stimulates the lymphatic system to remove congestion and stagnation from within the body thus returning it to a healthy condition.

documentation: Process of recording and reporting the information gathered and intervention performed on a patient/client. It ensures that the patient/client receives adequate services and that the provider is reimbursed for them.

domain: Specific performance area of work (including education), self-care and self-maintenance, and play and leisure.

dormant: Time period when a disease remains inactive.

dorsal: From anatomical position, located toward the back.

dorsal column tracts: Afferent ipsilateral ascending tracts for fine discriminative touch, vibratory sense, and kinesthesia.

dorsal splint: Splint applied to the dorsal aspect of the hand to prevent full extension of the wrist or any of the finger joints.

double-blind study: Strategy used in research that attempts to reduce one form of experimental error.

draping: An organized system of cover used to provide modesty cover for a client while providing access to the body for therapeutic and/or Swedish massage.

drug half-life: The time required for half the drug remaining in the body to be eliminated.

dual diagnosis: Presence of more than one diagnosis at the same time, most often a combination of a substance use disorder and some other condition, but may include any situation in which comorbidity exists.

durable power of attorney: Legal instrument authorizing one to act as another's agent for specific purposes and/or length of time.

dyad: Relationship between 2 individuals in which interaction is significant.

dyadic activity: Activity involving another person.

dynamic equilibrium: The ability to make adjustments to the center of gravity with a changing base-of-support.

dynamic flexibility: Amount of resistance of a joint(s) to motion.

dynamics: Study of objects in motion.

dynamic splint: Orthosis that allows controlled movement at various joints; tension is applied to encourage particular movements.

dynamic strength: Force of a muscular contraction in which joint angle changes.

dynamic systems theory: Theory concerning movement organization that was derived from the study of chaotic systems. It theorizes that the order and the pattern of movement performed to accomplish a goal comes from the interaction of multiple, nonhierarchical subsystems.

dynamometer: Device used to measure force produced from muscular contraction.

dynamometry: Measurement of the degree of muscle power.

dysethesias: Sensation of "pins and needles" such as that experienced when one's extremity "goes to sleep."

dysfunction: Complete or partial impairment of function.

dysfunctional hierarchy: Levels of dysfunction including impairment, disability, and handicap.

dyskinesia: Impairment of voluntary motion.

dyslexia: Impairment of the brain's ability to translate images received from the eyes into understandable language.

dysmenorrhea: Pain experienced during menstrual periods.

dyspepsia: Poor digestion.

dysreflexia: A life-threatening uninhibited sympathetic response of the nervous system to a noxious stimulus that is experienced by an individual with a spinal cord injury at T-7 or above.

dysrhythmia: Disturbance in rhythm in speech, brain waves, or cardiac irregularity.

dystonia/dystonic: Distorted positioning of the limbs, neck, or trunk that is held for a few seconds and then released.

E

early childhood education: School or other educational program for children ages 3 to 5 years.

early intervention: Multidisciplinary, comprehensive, coordinated, community-based system for young children with developmental vulnerability or delay from birth to age 3 years and their families. Services are designed to enhance child development, minimize potential delays, remediate existing problems, prevent further deterioration, and promote adaptive family functioning.

eccentric contraction: Muscular contraction during which the muscle generates tension while lengthening. Eccentric exercise occurs mainly in stabilizing the body against gravity.

ectoderm: Layer of cells which develop from the inner cell mass of the blastocyst. Eventually this layer develops into the outer surface of the skin, nails, part of teeth, lens of the eye, the inner ear, and central nervous system.

ectopia: Displacement or malposition.

eczema: An inflammatory skin disease characterized by lesions varying greatly in character, with vesiculation, infiltration, watery discharge, and the development of scales and crusts.

edema: Accumulation of large amounts of fluid in the tissues of the body.

education: The process of training and developing knowledge, skill, mind, and character. Formal schooling at an educational institution.

educational approaches: Interventions that make use of factual learning/teaching to change behaviors.

effectiveness: Degree to which the desired result is produced.

efferent: Conducting away from a structure, such as a nerve or a blood vessel.

efferent neuron: Includes motor neurons.

efficacy: Having the desired influence or outcome.

effleurage: Deep or gentle stroking; from a French term meaning to touch lightly.

effusion: Escape of fluid into a joint or cavity.

ego: In psychoanalytic theory, 1 of 3 personality structures. It controls and directs one's actions after evaluating reality, monitoring one's impulses, and taking into consideration one's values and moral and ethical code. The executive structure of the personality.

elastic stiffness: The amount of tissue force produced when a tissue is deformed and held at a given length.

elder: Term used to refer to individuals in the later years of the life span, arbitrarily set between the age 65 to 70 and beyond.

elder abuse: Intentional physical or psychological injury inflicted upon older adults by caretakers.

electrical potential: The amount of electrical energy residing in specific tissues.

electrical stimulation: Intervention through the application of electricity.

electroencephalography: Study of the electrical activity of the brain.

electrolytes: Mineral salts which conduct electricity in the body when in solution.

electromyography (EMG): The examining and recording of the electrical activity of a muscle.

electrotherapy: The use of electrical stimulation modalities in treatment.

embolism: Sudden blocking of artery by clot of foreign material (embolus) brought to site of lodging via blood stream.

EMF balancing technique: The electromagnetic field technique utilizes intent and precise adjustments to the EMF to balance, strengthen and increase the connectivity to the Universal Calibration Lattice (UCL).

empathy: While maintaining one's sense of self, the ability to recognize and share the emotions and state of mind of another person.

emphysema: An abnormal swelling of the lung tissue due to the permanent loss of elasticity or the destruction of the aveoli, which seriously impairs respiration.

empirical base: Knowledge based upon the observations and experience of master clinicians.

empowerment: To enable.

encephalitis: Disease characterized by inflammation of the parenchyma of the brain and its surrounding meninges usually caused by a virus.

encephalopathy: Any disease that affects the tissues of the brain and its surrounding meninges.

encoding (cognitive): Processes or strategies used to initially store information in memory.

end feel: Sensation imparted to the hands of the clinician at the end point of range of motion.

endocarditis: Inflammation of the endocardium, a disease generally associated with acute febrile or rheumatic diseases, and marked by dyspnea, rapid heart action, and peculiar systolic murmurs.

endocardium: The thin endothelial membrane lining the cavities of the heart.

endocrine: Designating or of any gland producing one or more hormones, such as the thyroid and its hormone thyroxine.

endogenous: Growing from within. Developing or originating within the organism.

endometriosis: Abnormal proliferation of the uterine mucus membrane into the pelvic cavity.

endothelial: Pertaining to the epithelial cells that line the heart cavities, blood vessels, lymph vessels, and serous cavities of the body.

end-systolic volume: The amount of blood remaining in each ventricle after each heartbeat.

endurance: The ability of a muscle to sustain forces or to repeatedly generate forces.

endurance testing: Used to determine the capacity of an individual to sustain the energy output needed to fulfill a task.

energetic integration: *See* Rolfing structrural integration.

engagement: Signifies that the fetus has firm head-down position within the mother's pelvis, and is no longer floating above the bony pelvis.

engineering controls: Changes to the workstation, equipment, or tools to eliminate hazards at the sources.

enteric: Pertaining to the intestines.

entry level: Individual with less than 1 year of work experience.

environment: External social and physical conditions or factors that have the potential to influence an individual.

environmental approaches: Interventions based on changing the environment (eg, changing support systems, modifying job, home).

environmental assessment: Process of identifying, describing, and measuring factors external to the individual that can influence performance or the outcome of treatment. These can include space and associated objects, cultural influences, social relationships, and system available resources.

environmental barrier: Any type of obstacle that interferes with a person's ability to achieve optimal occupational performance.

environmental contingencies: Factors in the environment that influence the patient's/client's performance during an evaluation.

environmental factors: The background of a person's life and living, composed of components of the natural environment (weather or terrain), the human made environment (tools, furnishing, the built-environment), social attitudes, customs, rules, practices, and institutions, and other individuals.

environmental fit: The process of matching the individual's capacity with opportunities for action in the physical, social, and cultural environments.

environmental support: Any environmental element that facilitates an individual's ability to attain his/her optimum occupational performance.

enzyme: A protein functioning as a biochemical catalyst, necessary for most major body functions.

epicardium: The layer of the pericardium that is in contact with the heart.

epidemiology: A study of the relationships of the various factors determining the frequency and distribution of diseases in a human environment. Science concerned with factors, causes, and remediation as related to the distribution of disease, injury, and other health-related events.

epidural: Anesthesia injected into the epidural space of the spine, which can produce loss of sensation from the abdomen to the toes.

epilepsy: Group of disorders caused by temporary sudden changes in the electrical activity of the brain that results in convulsive seizures or changes in the level of consciousness or motor activity.

epinephrine: A hormone secreted by the adrenal medulla in response to splanchnic stimulation, and stored in the chromaffin granules, being released predominantly in response to hypoglycemia. It increases blood pressure, stimulates heart muscle, accelerates the heart rate, and increases cardiac output.

episodic memory: Memory for personal episodes or events that have some temporal reference.

epistemology: Dimension of philosophy that is concerned with the questions of truth by investigating the origin, nature, methods, and limits of human knowledge.

Epstein-Barr virus (EBV): A virus that causes infectious mononucleosis. It is spread by respiratory tract secretions (eg, saliva, mucous).

equality: Requires that all individuals be perceived as having the same fundamental rights and opportunities.

equilibrium reaction: Reaction that occurs when the body adapts and posture is maintained, and when there is a change of the supporting surface; any of several reflexes that enables the body to recover balance.

equine massage: Soft tissue manipulation applied to horses.

equipment: Device that usually cannot be held in the hand and is electrical or mechanical (eg, table, electrical saw, or stove); devices can be specifically designed to assist function or compensate for absent function or they can be labor-saving and convenience gadgets.

ergonomics: Field of study that examines and optimizes the interaction between the human worker and the non-human work environment. The relationship among the worker, the work that is done, the tasks and activities inherent in that work, and the environment in which the work is performed. Ergonomics uses scientific and engineering principles to improve the safety, efficiency, and quality of movement involved in work.

erythemia: First degree reddening of the skin due to a burn or injury.

esalen massage: A combination of Oriental and Swedish massage techniques developed in the 1960s at the Esalen Institute in Big Sur, California

Escherichia coli (E. coli): A species of organisms constituting the greater part of the intestinal flora. In excess, causes urinary tract infections and epidemic diarrheal disease.

esoteric healing: Various balancing techniques are used to bring an individual's energy field to a more flowing, healthy, harmonious state.

essential fat: Stored body fat that is necessary for normal physiologic function and found in bone marrow, the nervous system, and all body organs.

essential hypertension: High blood pressure that is idiopathic, self-existing, having no obvious external cause. Also called intrinsic hypertension.

ethical dilemma: Conflict of moral choices with no satisfactory solution, which is often caused by attempting to balance 2 or more undesirable alternatives with no overriding principle to tell an individual what to do.

ethical relativism: View that each person's values should be considered equally valid.

ethical research practice: Refers to the investigator's obligations to respect the individual's freedom to decline to participate in research or to discontinue participation at any time.

ethics: System of moral principles or standards that govern personal and professional conduct.

ethnic: Member of, or pertaining to, groups of people with a common racial, national, linguistic, religious, or cultural history.

ethnicity: Component of culture that is derived from membership in a racial, religious, national, or linguistic group or subgroup, usually through birth.

ethnocentrism: Process of judging different cultures or ethnic groups only on the basis of one's own culture or experiences.

ethnogerontology: Study of ethnicity in an aging context.

etiology: Dealing with the causes of disease.

etiquette: Particular behaviors that are observed by a certain society as being acceptable.

eucapnic breath retraining: A combination of guided breathing exercises with musculoskeletal therapy to release and normalize the function of the thorax, diaphragm, and other muscles of breathing.

euthanasia: The deliberate ending of life of a person suffering from an incurable disease; has been broadened to include the withholding of extraordinary measures to sustain life, allowing a person to die.

evaluation: A dynamic process in which the physical therapist makes clinical judgments based on data gathered during the examination.

eversion: Turning outward.

evidence-based practice: Practice founded on research that supports its effectiveness.

evisceration: Removal of the contents of a cavity.

exacerbation: Increase in the severity of a disease or any of its symptoms.

examination: The process of obtaining a history, performing relevant systems reviews, and selecting and administering specific tests and measures.

excretion: Process through which metabolites of drugs (and the active drug itself) are eliminated from the body through urine and feces, evaporation from skin, exhalation from lungs, and secretion into saliva.

excursion: A range of movement regularly repeated in performance of a function.

exercise therapy: Manages musculoskeletal disorders by restoring strength to weakened muscles, restoring mobility or increased range of motion, correcting postural faults, preventing joint deformity, and improving joint stability.

exerssage: A kind of facial yoga.

exertional angina: Paroxysmal thoracic pain due most often to anoxia of the myocardium precipitated by physical exertion. *Synonym*: angina.

exhaustion: Depletion of energy with consequent inability to respond to stimuli.

exocrine: Secreting outwardly (the opposite of endocrine).

expectorate: To expel mucus or phlegm from the lungs; to spit.

expertise: The possession of a large body of knowledge and procedural skill that allows the solution of most domain problems effectively and efficiently.

extended care facility (ECF): Facility that is an extension of hospital care; derived from Medicare legislation.

extension (EXT): Straightening a body part.

external applications: Massage or massage topical preparations applied to the outside portions of the body.

external stimulation: Factors in the area where the activity is being performed that may enhance or impede performance.

external validity: The degree to which an experimental finding is predictable to the population at large.

extinction: Behavioral approach to discouraging a particular behavior by ignoring it and reinforcing other more acceptable behaviors.

extrafusal muscle: Striated muscle tissue found outside the muscle spindle.

extremities: The arms and legs.

extrinsic: Coming from or originating outside.

extrinsic motivation: Stimulation to achieve or perform that initiates from the environment.

exudate: Material, such as fluid, cells, or cellular debris, which has escaped from blood vessels and been deposited in tissues or on tissue surfaces, usually as a result of inflammation. An exudate, in contrast to a transudate, is characterized by a high content of protein, cells, or solid materials derived from cells.

F

face validity: Dimension of a test by which it appears to test what it purports to test.

fact: Truth or reality.

factor analysis: Statistical test that examines relationships of many variables and their contribution to the total set of variables.

family therapy: Intervention that focuses on the context of the entire family system.

fascia: A thin layer of connective tissue covering, supporting, or connecting the muscles or inner organs of the body.

fascial mobilization: Restrictions in the fascial layers are addressed in order to produce a balanced symmetrical musculoskeletal system.

fasciculation: A small local contraction of muscles, visible through the skin, representing a spontaneous discharge of a number of fibers innervated by a single motor nerve filament.

fascitis: Inflammation of a fascia.

fatigue: State of exhaustion or loss of strength and endurance; decreased ability to maintain a contraction at a given force.

feedback: Knowledge of the results of an individual's performance to the extent that the individual's behavior is changed or reinforced in a desirable direction.

feedback control: Refers to the postural control mechanism of automatic responses that occurs when there is a displacement of one's center of gravity that is not under voluntary control. Automatic postural responses.

feedforward control: Refers to the postural control mechanism of automatic responses that occurs during an intentional displacement of the center of gravity, as during voluntary movement.

fee-for-service: Payment method by which a health care provider is reimbursed for each encounter or service rendered.

fee schedule: List of accepted charges or established allowances for specified medical or dental procedures.

Feldenkrais: A sophisticated method of communicating with the unconscious through movement.

fever: A rise in body temperature to 100 degrees Fahrenheit (37.8°C) or above. Massage is contraindicated; fevers may be life threatening and should be managed by a physician.

fibrillation: Small, local, involuntary muscle contraction.

fibrin: A whitish, insoluble protein formed from fibrinogen by the action of thrombin, as in the clotting of blood. Fibrin forms the essential portion of a blood clot.

fibroblast: Chief cell of connective tissue responsible for forming the fibrous tissues of the body, such as tendons and ligaments.

fibrosis: Formation of fibrous tissue; fibroid degeneration.

fidelity: Duty to be faithful to the patient/client and his/her best interests; includes the mandate to keep all patient/client information confidential.

figure ground: Person's ability to distinguish shapes and objects from the background in which they exist.

fine motor coordination: Motor behaviors involving manipulative, discreet finger movements, and eye/hand coordination. Dexterity.

fine motor pattern of development: Mastery of smaller muscles (ie, fingers); takes place after gross-motor development.

fiscal management: Method of controlling the economics of problems at hand. It is concerned with discovering, developing, defining, and evaluating the financial goals of a department.

fissure: Any cleft or groove.

five element shiatsu: A hands-on Japanese technique based upon Chinese medicine. The 5 elements found in the earth and within us are wood, earth, fire, metal, and water.

fixator: Muscle that contracts to brace 1 bone, to which a mover attaches.

flaccidity: State of low tone in the muscle that produces weak and floppy limbs.

flagellation: The stroking action in massage therapy.

flexibility: Range of motion at a joint or in a sequence of joints.

flexion (FLEX): Act of bending a body part.

floppy disk: Magnetic storage medium used in a computer for electronic information of high or low density, single- or double-sided, and sizes of 3 1/2 and 5 1/4 inches.

folkways: Social customs to which people generally conform; traditional patterns of life common to a people.

foot-drop splint: Splint used to prevent the development of plantarflexion contractures.

foot zone therapy: A 10 zone therapy that claims that pressure exerted anywhere within a zone affects other areas within the same zone. A theory later developed into reflexology.

force: Product of mass and acceleration; a kinematic measurement that encompasses the amount of matter, velocity, and its rate of change of velocity; also strength, energy, and power.

force couple: Body being acted upon by 2 equal and parallel forces from opposite directions; the points of application of these forces must be on opposite sides of the object and be operating at some distance apart from one another.

four hand massage: A coordinated massage session performed by 2 therapists on 1 client.

fracture (Fx): Pertaining to a broken bone. Avoid massage over affected area so as not to interfere with proper bone healing or cause re-breaking; should seek medical clearance.

frail elderly: The elderly who are physically weak. Massage therapy needs to be applied with sensitivity to the condition of the patient.

frame of reference: Organization of interrelated, theoretical concepts used in practice.

freedom: Allows the individual to exercise choice and to demonstrate independence, initiative, and self-direction.

free radicals: Any molecule that contains 1 or more unpaired electrons. Changes in cells that result from the presence of free radicals are thought to result in aging.

friction: Movement of the hand, in whole or part over the surface of the body.

frontal plane: Runs side to side, dividing the body into front and back portions.

frostbite: To injure the tissues of the body by exposure to intense cold. Massage therapy to damaged tissue is contraindicated as further damage could result. Healthy nearby tissues may be massaged.

fulcrum: The intermediate point of force application of a three- or four-point bending construction; entity on which a lever moves.

function: Those activities identified by an individual as essential to support physical, social, and psychological well being and to create a personal sense of meaningful living. Performance; action.

functional assessment: Observation of motor performance and behavior to determine if a person can adequately perform the required tasks of a particular role or setting.

functional limitation: Restriction of the ability to perform a physical action, activity, or task in an efficient, typically expected, or competent manner.

functional mobility: The ability to perform functional activities and tasks without restriction.

functional muscle testing: Performance-based muscle assessment in particular positions simulating functional tasks and activities and usually under specific test conditions.

G

gag reflex: Involuntary contraction of the pharynx and elevation of the soft palate elicited in most normal individuals by touching the pharyngeal wall or back of the tongue.

gait: The manner in which a person walks, characterized by rhythm, cadence, step, stride, and speed.

galvanic skin response (GSR): Change in the electrical resistance of the skin as a response to different stimuli.

ganglion: A mass of nerve cells serving as a center from which impulses are transmitted. A cystic tumor on a tendon sheath.

gangrene: Decay of tissue in a part of the body when the blood supply is obstructed by disease or injury.

gastric intubation: Forced feeding, usually through a nasogastric tube.

gastric lavage: Washing out the stomach with repeated flushings of water.

gate control theory: The pain modulation theory developed by Melzak and Wall, who proposed that presynaptic inhibition in the dorsal gray matter of the spinal cord results in blocking of pain impulses from the periphery.

gatekeeper: A primary care physician responsible for coordinating all services.

gender identity: Realization of a child that males and females are different due to physical characteristics. *Synonym*: core gender identity.

generalization: Skills and performance in applying specific concepts to a variety of related solutions.

general systems theory: Conceptualizes the individual as an open system that evolves and undergoes different forms of growth, development, and change through an ongoing interaction with the external environment.

genes: Biological unit that contains the hereditary blueprints for the development of an individual from one generation to the next.

genetic: Pertaining to reproduction or to birth of origin; hereditary traits.

genotype: The genetic constitution of an organism or group.

geriatric day care: Ambulatory health care facility for older adults.

geriatric massage: A form of massage designed specifically for the needs of the elderly (65-70 and up). Before applying massage, pay close attention to any physical conditions or medications that could be contraindicated for massage therapy.

geriatrics: Area of study concerned with care of individuals in old age. The branch of medicine that treats all problems unique to old age and aging, including the clinical problems associated with senescence and senility.

gerontological tripartite: Approach to the study of aging which collectively combines 3 phenomena of the aging process: the biological capacity for survival, the psychological capacity for adaptation, and the sociological capacity for the fulfillment of social roles.

gerontology (GER): Area of study concerned with care, health issues, and special problems of growing old.

gestation: Total period of time the baby is carried in the uterus, approximately 40 weeks in humans.

globin: The protein constituent of hemoglobin; also any member of a group of proteins similar to the typical globin.

glomerulus: A tuft or cluster; used in anatomical nomenclature as a general term to designate such a structure, as one composed of blood vessels or nerve fibers.

glottis: The vocal apparatus of the larynx, consisting of the true vocal cords and the opening between them (rima glottisdis).

glucagon: A hyperglycemic-glycogenolytic factor thought to be secreted by the pancreas in response to hypoglycemia or stimulation by the growth hormone of the anterior pituitary gland.

glucocorticoid: Hormone from the adrenal cortex that raises blood sugar and reduces inflammation.

glucose: A thick, syrupy, sweet liquid generally made by incomplete hydrolysis of starch.

glucosuria: Presence of glucose in the urine. Secretion of excess sugar into the urine is often a sign of diabetes mellitus.

glycogenesis: The formation or synthesis of glycogen.

glycogenolysis: The splitting up of glycogen in the body tissue.

glycoprotein: A substance produced metabolically that creates osmotic force.

Golgi tendon organ (GTO): Sensory receptors in the tendons of muscles that monitor tension of muscles.

goniometer: Instrument for measuring movement at a joint.

goniometry: Measurement of the angle of the joint or a series of joints.

gout: Painful metabolic disease that is a form of acute arthritis; characterized by inflammation of the joints, especially of those in the foot or knee.

grand mal: Type of seizure in which there is a sudden loss of consciousness immediately followed by a generalized convulsion.

granulation tissue: The formation of a mass of tiny red granules of newly formed capillaries, as on the surface of a wound that is healing.

granulocyte: Any cell containing granules, especially a granular leukocyte. A heterogeneous class of leukocytes characterized by a multilobed nucleus and intracellular granules. Granulocytes include neutrophils, eosinophils, basophils, and mast cells.

granulocytosis: Increase in circulating granulocyte number.

gratification: Ability to receive pleasure, either immediate (immediately upon engaging in an activity) or delayed (after completion of the activity).

gravity: Constant force that affects almost every motor act characterized by heaviness or weight. The tendency toward the center of the earth.

gray matter: Area of the central nervous system that contains the cell bodies.

Grinberg method: A preventive technique that uses touch, movement, breathing, attention to the body, techniques of description, and different exercises to increase a person's well being.

grip force: Pressure exerted on a held object or in lifting an object.

gross motor coordination: Using large muscle groups for controlled, goal-directed movements. Motor behaviors concerned with posture and locomotion.

gross motor pattern of development: Mastery of larger muscles (proximal musculature); takes place before fine motor development.

group: Three or more individuals who are in contact with one another, take each other into account, and are aware of some common goal.

group dynamics: Forces that influence the interrelationships of members and ultimately affect group outcome.

group process: Interpersonal relationship among participants in a group.

group therapy: Any intervention directed toward groups of individuals rather than an individual alone.

gua sha: An ancient Chinese method of promoting chi (bioelectric vital life energy), blood circulation, and removal of toxic heat, stagnant blood, and lymph fluid from the body.

gustatory: Pertaining to the sense of taste.

habit: Performed on an automatic, preconscious level.

habit spasm: Tic that lasts for a long period of time and develops habitually.

habituate: Process of accommodating a stimulus through repeated diminishing exposure.

hakomi: A body-centered form of psychotherapy. *See also* body-oriented psychology.

half-life: Measure of the amount of time required for 50% of a drug to be eliminated from the body. The time in which the radioactivity originally associated with an isotope will be reduced by one half through radioactive decay.

hallucinate: Sense (eg, see, hear, smell, or touch) of something that does not exist externally.

handicap: Disadvantage, resulting from an impairment or disability, that limits or prevents the fulfillment of a role that is normal (depending on age, sex, and social and cultural factors) for that individual. The social disadvantage of a disability.

handicapping situation: A barrier to the performance of an activity (a non-accessible building, an attitude discrimination, a policy that denies access).

Hanna Somatic education: A system of neuromuscular education that requires the client to recognize, release and reverse chronic pain patterns resulting from injury, stress, repetitive motion, or habituated postures.

hazard: State that could potentially harm a person or do damage to property.

head injury (HI): Caused by direct impact to the head, most commonly from traffic accidents, falls, industrial accidents, wounds, or direct blows.

healing touch: An energy-based therapeutic approach to healing that uses touch to restore harmony and balance in the energy system to help the person to self-heal.

health: Physical and mental well being with freedom from disease, pain, or defect, and normalcy of physical, mental, and psychological functions.

health care policy: A principle, plan, or course of action to manage health care in the United States as pursued by a government organization or individual.

health education: A combination of educational, organizational, economic, and environmental supports for behavior conducive to health.

health maintenance: Screening and intervention for potential health risks to prevent disease and promote health and well being.

health maintenance organization (HMO): Prepaid organized health care delivery system.

health policy: Set of initiatives taken by government to direct resources toward promoting, improving, and maintaining the health of its citizens.

health promotion: Programs put in place to promote the physical, mental, and social well being of the person. Includes a focus on the individual's ability to function optimally in her/his environment and a balance in mind and body across all of an individual's life experiences.

heart disease: Any of the diseases of the heart.

heart failure: The inability of the heart to pump enough blood to maintain an adequate flow to and from the body tissues.

heart-lung machine: Performs functions of the heart and lungs during open heart surgery so these organs may be operated on.

heart problems: The heart is the main circulatory pump for the fluids of the body. Massage therapy is contraindicated for any heart condition without expressed approval of a physician.

heat therapy: Application of heat on a body part used to relieve the symptoms of musculoskeletal disorders.

heavy work: Exerting up to 50 to 100 pounds of force occasionally, or 25 to 50 pounds of force frequently, or 10 to 20 pounds of force constantly to move objects.

Hellerwork: A combination of movement education and deep-tissue bodywork that emphasizes vertical realignment of the body and the release of chronic stress and tension.

helplessness: Psychological state characterized by a sense of powerlessness or the belief that one is not capable of meeting an environmental demand competently.

hemianesthesia: Total loss of sensation to either the left or right side of the body.

hemianopsia: Blindness in one half of the field of vision in 1 or both eyes.

hemiparesis: Weakness of the left or right side of the body.

HEMME approach: HEMME is an acronym for history, evaluation, modalities, manipulation, exercise. HEMME is a home study course in manual therapy.

hemoglobin: The oxygen-carrying pigment of the erythrocytes, formed by the developing erthrocyte in bone marrow.

hemorrhage: The escape of large quantities of blood from a blood vessel; heavy bleeding. Massage therapy is contraindicated for situations where hemorrhaging may occur.

hemothorax: A collection of blood in the pleural cavity.

hepatitis: Inflammation of the liver.

hereditary: The genetic transmission of a particular quality or trait from parent to offspring.

hernia: The protrusion of all or part of an organ through a tear in the wall of the surrounding structure such as the protrusion of part of the intestine through the abdominal muscles. Massage therapy is contraindicated for large hernias. Further displacement of the herniated tissues needs to be avoided.

herniated vertebral disc: Weakness in annulus allowing nucleus pulposus to protrude; sometimes presses against nerve root and spinal cord, causing radicular symptoms.

heroin: Highly addictive narcotic from the opium family.

heuristic: Clinical reasoning strategies, or shortcuts, that simplify complex cognitive tasks.

hierarchy: A ranking system having a series of levels running from lowest to highest.

high blood pressure (hypertension): Systolic pressure consistently above 140 mmHg, diastolic pressure consistently above 100 mmHg. Massage therapy is contraindicated for high blood pressure if the patient is on medications; consult with a physician before applying massage therapy.

high risk pregnancy: A pregnancy where the mother or fetus is in danger of a compromised outcome.

Hilton's law: The trunk of a nerve not only sends branches to a particular muscle, but also sends branches to the joint moved by that muscle and to the skin overlying the insertion of the muscle.

hilus: A depression or pit at that part of an organ where the vessels and nerves enter.

hippocampus: A nuclear complex forming the medial margin of the cortical mantle of the cerebral hemisphere forming part of the limbic system.

hirsutism: Excessive growth of hair in unusual places, especially in women.

histogram: Bar graph.

history (Hx): An account of past and present health status that includes the identification of complaints and provides the initial source of information about the patient/client. The history also suggests the individual's ability to benefit from massage therapy services.

holism: View of the human mind and body as being one entity.

holistic: A concept in which understanding is gained by examination of all parts working as a whole.

home health program: Health or rehabilitation services provided in a patient's/client's home.

homeostasis: Physiological system's ability to maintain internal processes and constancy of the internal metabolic balance despite changes in the environment.

homogeneity of variance: Assumption that the variability within each of the sample groups should be fairly similar.

horizontal plane: Runs transversely across, dividing the body into upper and lower parts. Parallel to the ground.

hormones: Chemical substances, produced in the body, that have a specific effect on the activity of a certain organ; applied to substances secreted by endocrine glands and transported in the blood stream to the target organ on which their effect is produced.

Hoshino therapy: 250 acupuncture points are used to improve Biomechanical functioning. Pressure is applied to the points with the first knuckle of the thumb and with whole hand contact.

hospice programs: Care for terminally ill patients/ clients and emotional support for them and their families.

human development: Ongoing changes in the structure, thought, or behavior of a person that occur as a function of both biologic and environmental influences.

human immunodeficiency virus (HIV): Virus that causes AIDS, which is contracted through exposure to contaminated blood or bodily fluid (eg, semen or vaginal secretions).

human subject: Living individual about whom an investigator conducting research obtains data through intervention or interaction.

humerus: Long bone of the upper arm.

humoral: Pertaining to any fluid or semifluid in the body.

Huna Kane: Hawaiian therapy utilizing massage and a form of counseling.

hydration: Providing adequate water.

hydrocephaly: Condition characterized by abnormal accumulation of cerebrospinal fluid within the ventricles of the brain, which leads to enlargement of the head.

hydrostatic weighing: Underwater weighing to determine body volume; body volume is used to determine body density, from which body composition can be calculated.

hydrotherapy: Intervention using water. The use of water in the treatment of disease. Hydrotherapy is contraindicated where circulatory, kidney, or skin conditions are present due to potential of increased stress on those tissues.

hylaronic acid: Substance that under compressive forces lubricates cells.

hyperglycemia: Abnormally increased content of sugar in the blood.

hypermobility: Condition of excessive motion in joints.

hyperplasia: Increased number of cells.

hypertension: Any abnormally high blood pressure or a disease of which this is the chief sign.

hyperthesias: Abnormally increased sensitivity to stimulation.

hypertonus: Muscular state wherein muscle tension is greater than desired; spasticity. Hypertonus increases resistance to passive stretch.

hypertrophic scarring: Excessive markings left by the healing process in the skin or an internal organ.

hypertrophy: Increased cell size leading to increased tissue size. The morbid enlargement or overgrowth of an organ or part due to an increase in size of its constituent cells (eg, hypertrophic cardiomyopathy).

hyperventilation: Increased expiration and inspiration potentially caused by anxiety.

hypnotic: Drugs or conditions that produce drowsiness or sleep.

hypochondriasis: In the absence of medical evidence, a sustained conviction that one is ill or about to become ill; abnormal concern about one's health.

hypokinetic disease: Complications arising from inactivity. *Synonym*: disuse syndrome.

hypoplasia: Defective or incomplete development (eg, osteogenesis imperfecta).

hypotension: Abnormally low blood pressure.

hypothesis: Conclusion drawn before all the facts are known; working assumption which serves as a basis for further investigation; a plausible explanation or best guess about a situation.

hypotonicity: Decrease in the muscle tone and stretch reflex of a muscle resulting in decreased resistance to passive stretch and hyporesponsiveness to sensory stimulation.

hypotonus: Muscular state wherein muscle tension is lower than desired; flaccidity. Hypotonus decreases resistance to passive stretch.

hypovolemia: Abnormally decreased volume of circulating fluid (plasma) in the body.

hypoxia: Deficiency of oxygen in the blood. *See* anoxia.

hysterectomy: Surgical removal of the uterus.

ICD code: *International Classification of Diseases* code used for billing and reimbursement purposes.

icing: Ice is applied in small, overlapping circles for 5 to 10 minutes until skin flushing and numbness occur.

id: In psychoanalytic theory, the unconscious part of the psyche that is the source of primitive, instinctual drives and strives for self-preservation and pleasure. The primary process element of personality.

ideation: An internal process in which the nervous system gathers information from stimuli in the environment or recruits information from memory stores to formulate an idea about what to do.

identity: Gradually emerging, and continually changing, sense of self; used in Erik Erikson's theory of development.

idiopathic: Designating a disease whose cause is unknown or uncertain.

illness: Experience of devalued changes in being and in social function. It primarily encompasses personal, interpersonal, and cultural reactions to sickness.

imbalance: Lack of balance, as in proportion, force, and functioning.

immediate recall: Ability to recall information within a short time after information has been received.

immersion: To plunge, dip, or drop into a liquid.

immunoglobin (Ig): Glycoprotein found in blood and other body fluids that may exert antibody activity. All antibodies are Ig molecules, but not all Ig exhibit antibody activity.

immunosuppression: Decrease in responsiveness of the immune system with an imbalance of the antigen-antibody relationship.

impairment: A loss or abnormality of psychological, physiological, or anatomical structure or function. Impairments that originate from other, preexisting impairments.

impingement: To trap and compress.

impotence: Weakness, especially the inability of the male to achieve or maintain erection.

impulsive: To act without planning or reflection.

incidence: During a specified time period, the number of new cases of a certain illness or injury in a population. It is demonstrated as the number of new cases divided by the total number of people at risk.

incompetence: Failing to meet requirements; incapable; unskillful. Lacking strength and sufficient flexibility to transmit pressure, thus breaking or flowing under stress.

incontinence: Inability to control excretory functions.

independence: Lack of requirement or reliance on another; adequate resources to accomplish everyday tasks.

independent variable: Antecedent variable.

individual education plan (IEP): Interdisciplinary plan required for special education students in the United States under the provisions of Public Law 94-142. Allows parents or guardians to examine all school records and to participate with professionals in making educational placement decisions and in developing written diagnostic-prescriptive plans for school-aged children.

inductive fallacy: Overgeneralizing on the basis of too few observations.

inductive reasoning: Generation and testing of a hypothesis on the basis of evidence to indicate its validity.

industry: According to Erik Erikson and his theory of development, this is when children in elementary school focus on applying themselves in doing certain activities that are reflective of being successful in the adult world.

infancy: Time of development of a child from a few weeks after birth until the second year of life.

infant massage: Massage applied to a child less than 1 year of age. Massage needs to be both delicate and appropriate; training is advisable.

infection: The state of being infected especially by the presence in the body of bacteria, protozoans, viruses, or other parasites.

infective: To cause infection; infectious.

inference: Possible result or conclusion that could be deduced from evaluation data.

inferential (predictive) statistics: Utilizing the measurements from the sample to anticipate characteristics of the population.

inferior: From anatomical position, located below the head.

inflammation: The condition into which tissues enter as a reaction to injury including signs of pain, heat, redness, and swelling. Tissue reaction to injury. The succession of changes which occurs in living tissue when it is injured. Massage of inflamed area is contraindicated to avoid further injury to affected tissue; nearby healthy tissues may be massaged.

inflammatory: Pertaining to or characterized by inflammation.

informal social network: People who provide support but who are not connected with any formal social service agency.

informant interview: Interview in which a therapist gathers information about the patient/client or environment from significant others.

informational support: A type of social support which informs, thereby reducing anxiety over uncertainty.

informed consent: Requirement that the person must be given adequate information about the benefits and risks of planned treatments or research before he/she agrees to the procedures.

Ingram method: Zone therapy applied to the feet.

inguinal: Pertaining to the groin.

inhibition: Arrest or restraint of a process.

injury: Physical harm or damage to a person.

innate goodness: View presented by Swiss-born French philosopher Jean-Jacques Rousseau, who stressed that children are inherently good.

inpatient: Services delivered to the patient/client during hospitalization.

inquiry: An investigation or examination.

insertion: Distal attachment of a muscle that exhibits most of the movement during muscular contraction.

inservice education: In-house seminars or special training sessions, either inside or outside the facility.

insight: Self-understanding. Understanding of consequences/ramifications of a situation or an action.

insight bodywork: A combination of massage, movement, and meditation.

in situ: Localized site, confined to 1 place (eg, cancer that has not invaded neighboring tissues).

instability: Description of a joint that has lost its structural integrity and is overtly hypermobile.

instinctual drives: Aspect of the psychodynamic theory in which Freud believes that there are 2 primary instinctual impulses that demand gratification: sex and aggression.

institution: Any public or private entity or agency.

institutionalization: Effects of dehumanizing and depersonalizing characteristics of the environment that result in apathy, a significant decrease in motivation and activity, and increased passivity of an individual. *Synonym:* confinement.

insufficiency: Deficiency or inadequacy. The failure or inability of an organ or tissue to perform its normal function.

insurance denial: When a third party has denied payment for a service; organizations may appeal denials if they believe the criteria have not been equitably applied.

intake interview: Interview in which the therapist identifies the patient's/client's needs and his or her suitability for treatment.

integrated Kabbalistic healing: A 2-part healing session based upon Judaic traditions. A session consists of a discussion regarding problems followed by a hands-on healing.

integrative manual therapy: A combination of physical therapy, osteopathic medicine, homeopathy, audiology, massage therapy, etc; used to locate and alleviate health challenges to the individual body systems.

integration: Unifying or bringing together; in children, the developmental ability to link successive actions, instead of viewing each action as a separate, unrelated event; usually acquired by 2 years of age.

integumentary: Pertaining to or composed of skin.

intelligence: Potential or ability to acquire, retain, and use experience and knowledge to reason and problem solve.

intention tremor: Rhythmical, oscillatory movement initiated with an arm or hand.

interdependence: A concept that recognizes the mutual dependencies of individuals within social groups.

interface: Program or device that links the way 2 or more pieces of equipment or person/machine units work together.

interferon (IFN): A class of unrelated cytokine proteins formed when cells are exposed to viruses. It is an antiviral chemical, secreted by an infected cell, which strengthens the defenses of nearby cells not yet infected.

intermediate care facilities (ICF): Designed to give personal care, simple medical care, and intermittent nursing care.

intermittent positive-pressure breathing: Mechanical device that uses air pressure to inflate and deflate the lungs for breathing.

internal: Having to do with the inner nature of a thing.

internal postural control: Ability of the body to support and control its own movement without reliance on supporting structures in the environment.

internal validity: The cause and effect relationship can be identified by the results of an experiment.

***International Classification of Diseases* (ICD):** Disease classification system developed by the World Health Organization.

interneuron: Nerve cell that links motor and sensory nerves.

internodal: The space between 2 nodes; the segment of a nerve fiber connecting 2 nodes (often called internodal bundles or pathways).

interoceptive: Receptors activated by stimuli from within visceral tissues and blood tissues.

interpolar: Situated between 2 poles.

interval data: Measurements that are assigned values so the order and intervals between numbers are recognized.

intervertebral disks: Pads of fibrous elastic cartilage found between the vertebrae. They cushion the vertebrae and absorb shock.

intoxication: The overindulgence of alcoholic beverages or poisoning by a toxic substance. Massage therapy is contraindicated due to the possible over taxing of the liver by toxins within the system.

intracranial: Occurring within the cranium.

intrafusal muscle: Striated muscle tissue found within the muscle spindle.

intravascular: Directly into a vessel.

intubation: The insertion of a tube; especially the introduction of a tube into the larynx through the glottis, performed for the use of an external source of oxygen.

inventory: Assessment comprised of a list of items to which the person gives responses.

inversion: Turning inward or inside out.

involuntary movement: Movement that is not done of one's own free will; not done by choice. Unintentional, accidental, not consciously controlled movement.

iodine: Element important for the development and functioning of the thyroid gland.

iontophoresis: Introduction of ions into tissues by means of electric current.

ipsilateral: Situated on or affecting the same side.

ischemia: Reduced oxygen supply to a body organ or part. Deficiency of blood in a part, due to functional constriction or actual obstruction of a blood vessel.

ischemic heart disease: Lack of blood supply to the heart.

Islets of Langerhans: Irregular structures in the pancreas composed of cells smaller than the ordinary secreting cells. These masses (islands) of cells produce an internal secretion, insulin, which is connected with the metabolism of carbohydrates, and their degeneration is one of the causes of diabetes.

isokinetic strength: Force generated by a muscle contracting through a range of motion at a constant speed.

isometric contraction: Static muscle contraction in which the muscle generates tension but does not change length.

isometric strength: Force generated by a contraction in which there is no joint movement and minimal change in muscle length.

isotonic contraction: Contraction of a muscle during which the force of resistance remains constant throughout the range of motion.

isotonic strength: Force of contraction in which a muscle moves a constant load through a range of motion.

isthmus: Narrow structure connecting 2 larger parts.

itinerant: Traveling from place to place.

J

Jamu massage: A combination of Hindu, Chinese, and European influences with herbal oils and lotions added.

Japanese restoration therapy: An ancient Japanese therapy whose 2 goals are to balance the energy in the body and to break down soft tissue areas that have been injured. Most therapy is done with the therapist's elbow.

jaundice: A condition in which the eyeballs, the skin, and the urine become abnormally yellowish as a result of increased amounts of bile pigments in the blood. Usually secondary to conditions such as hepatitis or liver failure. Massage therapy is contraindicated.

Jin Shin Do: A combination of the use of gentle yet deep finger pressure on acu-points with simple body focusing techniques to release physical and emotional tension.

Jin Shin Jyutsu: A healing method using 26 safety energy locks which when held gently free up energy blocks in the body.

job description: Provides a written statement of a particular position in order to identify, define, and describe its parameters.

joint capsule: Any sac or membrane enclosing the junction of the bones.

joint mobility: Functional joint play and flexibility allowing for freedom of joint movement.

joint mobilization: A manual therapy employing mobilization techniques that include graded passive oscillations at the joint to improve joint mobility.

joint protection: Application of procedures to minimize joint stress.

joint range of motion (JROM): Freedom of motion in joints. A goniometer is used to measure joint mobility on a 180 degree scale.

joint receptor: Anatomically localized in joint capsules and ligaments, they include the Golgi-type endings, Golgi-Mazzoni corpuscles, Ruffini's corpuscle, and free nerve endings. In general, they detect joint movement in the gravitational field causing the discharge of receptors in the somatic, visual, and vestibular afferent systems to maintain posture and balance.

joints: Junctures in the body where bones articulate. The classifications are synarthrosis (nonmoving joints), amphiarthrosis (slightly moving joints), and diarthrosis (freely moving joints).

judgment: The ability to use data or information to make a decision.

jump sign: A test that screens for binocular vision, which is when both eyes cannot focus on a single point or target. The patient/client focuses on an object, the therapist then covers one eye; if the uncovered eye "jumps" to refocus on the object, this is a positive jump sign. An involuntary shortening of a fibrous band of muscle, also known as a twitch response.

justice: Notion that all cases should be treated alike and fairly in accord with general standards of right and wrong.

juvenile: Pertaining to youth or childhood diseases, such as juvenile diabetes or juvenile arthritis.

K

Kentro body balance: Gentle centering and balancing movements that stretch, exercise, relax, limber, and strengthen every area of the body.

keratin: A scleroprotein that is the principle constituent of epidermis, hair, nails, and the organic matrix of the enamel of the teeth.

keratosis: Any horny growth such as a wart or callousity.

ketone: Any compound containing a carbonyl group, CO.

ketosis: A condition characterized by an abnormally elevated concentration of ketone (acetone) bodies in the body tissues and fluids causing an acidosis. Also referred to as ketoacidosis.

kidney disease: Pathological changes in the functioning of the kidneys resulting in clinical signs and symptoms and laboratory findings, which identify the condition as abnormal functioning of the kidneys. Massage therapy is contraindicated for kidney disease due to the potential for increasing the level of stress on the functioning of the kidneys.

kinematics: Area of kinesiology that is not concerned with cause, but rather with measuring, describing, and recording motions.

kinesics: The study of body movements, gestures, and postures as a means of communication. *Synonym*: body language.

kinesiology: The study of the mechanics and anatomy related to human body movement.

kinesthesia: Person's sense of position, weight, and movement in space. The receptors for kinesthesia are located in the muscles, tendons, and joints.

kinesthetic: Sense derived from end organs located in muscles, tendons, and joints and stimulated by movement. *Synonym*: proprioception.

kinetic awareness: A type of movement therapy for improving alignment; preventing injuries; and enjoying strength, flexibility, and coordination.

kinetics: Area of kinesiology that is concerned with cause, as well as the forces that produce, modify, or stop a motion.

kneading: A technique used to relax muscles; the therapist wraps his or her hands around a body part and using firm pressure moves his or her hands in opposite directions.

knee/ankle/foot orthosis (KAFO): Devices applied externally to control knee, ankle, and foot motion and position.

Korean martial therapy: An ancient Korean healing art combining massage, energy work, pressure points, and body mechanics.

Kreb's cycle: Tricarboxylic acid cycle which results in the energy production of ATP.

Kripalu bodywork: An integrative approach to stress and tension release blending Swedish massage, pressure point, energy balancing, and breathing techniques.

Kriya massage: A blending of the intuitive ability of the therapist with the art of massage to provide for the needs of the individual client.

Kundalini energization: A process of cleaning the chakras and energy bodies followed by light physical touch and manipulation of the chakras and energy bodies.

kyphosis: Abnormal anteroposterior curving of the spine; hunchback or roundback.

L

labor: Refers to the uterine contractions that produce dilation and effacement of the cervix, assisting in descent of the fetus and delivery through the vaginal opening.

labyrinthine righting reflexes: Begins at birth and continues through life. The head orients to a vertical position with the mouth horizontal when the body is tipped or tilted. Tested with the eyes closed.

laissez faire style: Low involvement.

laminectomy: Surgical excision of the posterior arch of the vertebra.

lastone therapy: Dense stones heated to 140 degrees or cooled as low as 32 degrees are applied to the body.

latent period: Time during which a disease is in existence but does not manifest itself.

latent phase: Early phase of the first stage of labor which ends when the cervix is fully effaced and 3 to 4 cm dilated.

latent stage (latency): Fourth of Freud's stages of psychosexual development, characterized by the development of the superego (conscience) and by loss of interest in sexual gratification; typically occurs from the age of 6 to 11 years in Western cultural groups. Also, latency in the duration of effectiveness following cessation of a treatment or intervention.

lateral: From anatomical position, located away from the midline of the body.

laterality: Tendency toward one side or the other (eg, right-handedness, left-handedness). Dominant side.

lateralization: The tendency for certain processes to be more highly developed on one side of the brain than the other. In most people, the right hemisphere develops the processes of spatial and musical thoughts, and the left hemisphere develops the areas for verbal and logical processes.

lateral trunk flexion: Ability to move the trunk from side to side without moving the legs, which is essential for maintaining balance.

learned helplessness: Process in which the person attributes his or her lack of performance to external factors rather than lack of effort.

learned nonuse: A process that occurs after an injury such as a cerebrovascular accident. Immediately following the injury, motor function is extremely impaired due to diaschisis (cortical shock). Attempts to use the affected limb at this time fail, and the patient/client learns that the limb is useless. Compensation with the unaffected limb begins and produces successful results (a reward behavior), and further attempts at using the involved limb continue to be unsuccessful (a punished behavior). This pattern of reinforcement results in a strong learned response of not trying to use the affected limb. Thus, the patient/client does not realize that a return of function of the affected limb may have gradually occurred.

learning: Enduring ability of an individual to comprehend and/or competently respond to changes in information from the environment and/or from within the self. As one learns about the environment, alterations occur in the definition of the self and possible behaviors.

learning disability: Learning problem that is not due to environmental causes, mental retardation, or emotional disturbances, often associated with problems in listening, thinking, reading, writing, spelling, and mathematics.

learning environment: All the conditions (internal and external), circumstances, and influences surrounding and affecting the learning of the patient/client.

learning stations: Activities or special equipment placed around the room for an individual to use and be evaluated on for therapeutic feedback or educational achievement.

learning theory: Theoretical base behind the behavioral frame of reference in which behavior is best learned when environmental influences are introduced.

least restrictive environment: Most normal learning environment where a person with a disability can have his/her educational needs met.

legislative review: Review of a bill by the legislature when they perceive that an agency has misinterpreted the intent or has excessively revised existing regulations.

leg length discrepancy: Asymmetrical length of the lower extremities when one is compared to the other.

leisure: Category of activities for which freedom of choice and enjoyment are the primary motives.

Lenair technique: A physical treatment. It involves changes in the bioelectrical and electromagnetic properties within the client's body.

length of stay (LOS): The duration of hospitalization, usually expressed in days.

lesion: Injury to the central or peripheral nervous system that may prevent the expression of some functions and/or allow the inappropriate, uncoordinated, or uncontrolled expression of other functions.

leukocyte: White cell; colorless blood corpuscles that function to protect the body against micro-organisms causing disease.

leukocytosis: Increase in circulating lymphocyte number.

leukopenia: Decreased white blood cell count.

levator ani syndrome: Spasm of the muscles surrounding the anus causing severe rectal pain.

level: Even. No slope.

level of arousal: An individual's responsiveness and alertness to stimuli in the environment.

levels of processing: Durability of the memory trace is a function of the level to which the information was encoded.

lever system: System consisting of a rigid bar (lever), an axis (fulcrum), a force, and a resistance to that force. The distance between the axis and the point of application of force is known as the force arm; the distance between the axis and the point of application of resistance is known as the resistance arm.

licensure: Process established by a governmental agency to determine professional qualification.

life cycle: From conception to death of an organism.

life expectancy: Number of years in the lifespan of an individual in a particular cultural group.

life review: Process in which one looks back at one's life experiences, evaluating, interpreting, and reinterpreting them.

life roles: Daily life experiences that occupy one's time, including roles of student, homemaker, worker (active or retired), sibling, parent, mate, child, and peer.

lifespan perspective: Makes 7 basic contentions about development: it is lifelong, multidimensional, multidirectional, plastic, historically embedded, multidisciplinary, and contextual.

lifestream massage technique: A method of bodywork with the benefits of deep tissue massage without the discomfort. Lifestream trains the therapist to work efficiently to prevent injury and burnout.

lifestyle: Pattern of daily activities over time that are stable and predictable, through which an individual expresses their self-identity.

ligament: Inelastic, fibrous thickening of an articular capsule that joins one bone to its articular mate, allowing movement at the joint. Massage therapy is contraindicated for torn ligaments. Torn ligaments are a serious condition requiring surgery.

ligation: Application of a ligature (a ligature being any material used for tying a vessel or to constrict a part).

light work: Exerting up to 20 pounds of force occasionally, or up to 10 pounds of force frequently, or a negligible amount of force constantly to move objects.

limbic system: Primitive central nervous system associated with emotional and visceral functions in the body. A group of brain structures that include amygdala, hippocampus, denate gyrus, cingulate gyrus, and their interconnections with hypothalamus, septal areas, and brainstem.

limitation: Act of being restrained or confined.

limits-of-stability: The boundary or range that is the farthest distance in any direction a person can lean away from vertical (midline) without changing the original base of support (eg, stepping, reaching, etc) or falling.

linear processing: Learning or solving a problem using a step-by-step process in which each step is dependent on what goes on before.

line of pull: Attachments of a muscle, direction of its fibers, and the location of its tendons at each joint at which the muscle crosses.

local twitch response: *See* jump sign.

localized inflammation: Swelling, redness, and increased temperature that is isolated to the injured or infected part of the body.

locomotion: The ability to move from place to place.

locus of control: Psychological term referring to one's orientation to the world of events. Persons with an internal locus of control believe they can influence the outcome of events. Those with an external locus of control, conversely, believe that the outcome of events is largely a matter of fate or chance (ie, that they cannot have influence over the outcome of events).

lomi lomi: A system of massage that utilizes very large, broad movements. Two-handed, forearm, and elbow application of strokes that cover a broad area is characteristic of lomi lomi.

Lonsdale method of lymphatic massage: A unique integration of osteopathic visceral manipulation, stroking, and both superficial and deep lymphatic drainage.

longevity: Long life or life expectancy.

longitudinal research: Studies in which subjects are measured over the course of time to gather data of potential trends.

long-term care (LTC): Array of services needed by individuals who have lost some capacity for independence because of a chronic illness or condition.

long-term memory: Permanent memory storage for long-term information.

long-term support system: Ensuring that individuals have access to the services that are needed to support independent living.

loose associations: Thoughts shift with little or no apparent logic.

Looyen work: A painless approach to deep-tissue therapy, working with the connective tissue and facial components. It is a combination of several restructuring systems, including Rolfing, postural integration, and Aston-patterning.

lordosis: Abnormal forward curvature of the lumbar spine; swayback.

lower motor neuron (LMN): Sensory neuron found in the anterior horn cell, nerve root, or peripheral nervous system.

low technology: Electronic or non-electronic products or systems that have assumed a more commonplace role and accessibility in society.

lubricant: An oil used to allow the therapist's hands to move smoothly over the client's skin.

lumbar rotation: Rotating the patient's/client's pelvis away from the painful side; technique to treat spinal pain.

lumbar stabilization: Exercises whose objective is to strengthen the deep spine muscles as a foundation for good trunk stability.

lumpectomy: Excision of a small primary breast tumor leaving the rest of the breast intact.

lung: The organ of respiration.

lutenizing hormone (LH): A gonadotropic hormone of the anterior pituitary that acts with the follicle-stimulating hormone to cause ovulation of mature follicles and secretion of estrogen by thecal and granulosa cells. It is also concerned with corpus luteum formation and, in the male, stimulates the development and functional activity of interstitial cells.

lymph drainage therapy: Techniques used to manually attune the specific rhythm, pressure, quality, and direction of the lymph flow by using a combination of precise anatomical science and distinct manual techniques.

lymphatic system: The system containing or conveying lymph.

lymphedema: Swelling of an extremity caused by obstruction of the lymphatic vessels.

lymphoblast: T-lymphocytes that have been altered during a viral attack to release a variety of chemicals, which encourage greater defensive activity by the immune system.

lymphocyte: A particular type of white blood cell which is involved in the immune response and produced by lymphoid tissue.

lymphoma: Any of the various forms of cancers of the lymphoid tissue.

lypossage: A combination of manual deep tissue massage, lymphatic drainage, and the principles of structural integration. It is used to combat cellulite.

M technique: A series of stroking movements performed in a set sequence. Each movement is repeated 3 times.

macrobiotic shiatsu: A combination of healthy food preparation (macrobiotics) with the healing physical modality of shiatsu meridians.

macrophage: A phagocyte cell residing in tissues and derived from the monocyte.

macular degeneration: Common eye condition in which the macula is affected by edema, pigment is dispersed, and the macular area of the retina degenerates. It is the leading cause of visual impairment in persons older than 50.

magnet therapy: The use of magnets to treat a variety of physical and emotional disorders.

magnetic resonance imaging (MRI): A scanning technique using magnetic fields and radio frequencies to produce a precise image of the body tissue; used for diagnosis and monitoring of disease.

main effects: The action of 2 or more independent variables each working separately.

maintenance massage: A massage session designed to maintain the client's level of fitness.

major depressive disorder: Mood disorder characterized by features such as downcast mood, loss of interest in activities, insomnia, and feelings of fatigue and worthlessness that cause impairment in daily functioning.

major medical insurance: Type of insurance designed to offset the heavy medical expenses resulting from a prolonged illness or injury.

make test: Form of muscle testing in which the therapist provides resistance against a muscle while it is moving through its range.

malaise: A vague feeling of bodily discomfort or uneasiness, as early in an illness.

malposition: Faulty or abnormal position.

managed care: Integrated delivery systems. Cost containment approach that enables the payer to influence the delivery of health services prospectively (ie, before services are provided).

management: The act, art, or manner of managing, or handling, controlling, or directing.

management by objectives: Managerial system that improves the productivity of an organization by setting goals of progress that can be periodically measured, and using time tables and time limits to adhere to productivity goals.

management strategies: A strategic plan for managing, handling, controlling, or directing businesses or services.

management styles: The beliefs and value system of the manager; the personality of the manager.

mandated reporter: Person who, in the practice of his/her profession, comes in contact with children, and must make a report or see that a report is made when he/she has reason to believe that a child has been abused.

mania: Excessive activity, flight of thought, and grandiosity.

manipulate: The use of the hands in the treatment of soft tissue problems.

manipulation: A passive therapeutic movement, usually of small amplitude and high velocity at the end of the available range.

manipulative therapy: Passive movement technique that can be classified into either joint manipulation or mobilization. Manipulation is a sudden small thrust that is not under the patient's/client's control, while mobilization is a passive movement technique where the patient/client can control the movement.

manual lymphatic drainage: *See* Doctor Vodder Manual Lymphatic Drainage.

manual therapy: A broad group of skilled hand movements used to mobilize soft tissues and joints for the purpose of modulating pain, increasing range of motion, reducing or eliminating soft tissue inflammation, inducing relaxation, improving contractile and noncontractile tissue extensibility, and improving pulmonary function.

MariEL: A transformational healing energy that works at the cellular level to help clients discover and release emotional and physical traumas.

marked crossing: Crosswalk or other identified path intended for pedestrian use in crossing a vehicular way.

marketing: Managerial process by which individuals and groups obtain what they want by creating and exchanging products, services, or ideas with others.

mass: Amount of space an object takes up without regard to gravity; a kinematic measurement.

massage: Manipulation of the soft tissues of the body for the purpose of affecting the nervous, muscular, respiratory, and circulatory systems.

masseur: French term for a man who practices massage.

masseuse: French term for a woman who practices massage.

master care plan: Treatment plan that includes the list of patient/client problems and identifies the treatment team's intervention strategies and responsibilities.

mastery: Achievement of skill to a criterion level of success.

mastication: Chewing; tearing and grinding food with the teeth while it becomes mixed with saliva.

material culture: Artifacts, industry, architecture, and other material aspects of a particular society.

maturation: Sequential unfolding of behavioral and physiological characteristics during development.

maturational theory: Developmental theory that views development as a function of innate factors which proceed according to a maturational and developmental timetable.

mature group: Members take on all necessary roles, including leadership. The purpose is to balance task accomplishment with need satisfaction of all group members. The therapist is an equal member of this group.

maximal oxygen consumption (max V$_{O2}$, maximal oxygen uptake, aerobic capacity): The greatest volume of oxygen used by the cells of the body per unit time.

maximal voluntary ventilation (MVV): The greatest volume of air that can be exhaled in 15 seconds.

maximum heart rate (age predicted): Highest possible heart rate usually achieved during maximal exercise. Maximum heart rate decreases with age and can be estimated as 220 - age.

maximum voluntary contraction (MVC): Greatest amount of tension a muscle can generate and hold only for a moment, as in muscle testing.

Meals on Wheels: Program designed to deliver hot meals to the elderly, individuals with physical disabilities, or other people who lack the resources to provide for themselves with nutritionally adequate, warm meals on a daily basis.

mean (x): Arithmetic average. Measure of central tendency.

meaning: To make sense out of a situation using everything a person brings to it, including perception, attitudes, feelings, and social and cultural values.

meaningfulness: Amount of significance or value an individual associates with an experience after encountering it.

meatus: Passage or opening within the body.

mechanical advantage (MA): In kinesiology, the ratio of amount of effort expended to work performed. MA = length of force arm/length of resistance arm.

mechanical efficiency: Amount of external work performed in relation to the amount of energy required to perform the work; equal to force arm/resistance arm.

mechanical link: A gentle manual therapy that encourages the balance of tensions in the fascial system.

mechanical modalities: A broad group of agents that uses distraction, approximation, or compression to produce a therapeutic effect.

mechanical ventilation: The use of a respirator for external support of breathing and the use of an ambu bag for inflating the lungs mechanically.

mechanics: Study of physical forces.

mechanistic view (reductionism): Belief that a person is passive and that his/her behavior must be controlled or shaped by the society or environment in which he/she functions. Supports that the mind and body should be viewed as separate and that the human being, like a machine, can be taken apart and reassembled if its structure and function are sufficiently well understood.

medial: From anatomical position, located closer to the midline of the body.

median (Mdn): The value or score that most closely represents the middle of a range of scores.

mediastinum: The mass of tissues and organs separating the 2 lungs, between the sternum in front and the vertebral column behind, and from the thoracic inlet above to the diaphragm below. It contains the heart and its large vessels, the trachea, esophagus, thymus, lymph nodes, and other structures and tissues.

Medicaid: Federally funded, state-operated program funding medical assistance for people with low incomes, regardless of age.

medical gymnastics: A form of systematic body exercises with or without equipment designed to treat physical conditions.

medical skinfold caliper: Instrument used to measure body fat.

Medicare: Federally funded health insurance program for the elderly, certain people with disabilities, and most individuals with end-stage renal disease, funded by Title VIII of the Social Security Act.

Medicare Part A: Hospital Insurance Program of Medicare, which covers hospital inpatient care, care in skilled nursing facilities, and home health care.

Medicare Part B: Supplemental Medical Insurance Program of Medicare, which covers hospital outpatient care, physician fees, home health care, comprehensive outpatient rehabilitation facility fees, and other professional services.

medication: Treatment with remedies. Massage therapy may affect the dosage and effectiveness of various medication. For some medications massage therapy would be contraindicated. Consult with a physician if the effects of a medication are unknown.

medicine ball: Heavy exercise ball used to increase strength and coordination of a patient/client.

medium work: Exerting up to 20 to 50 pounds of force occasionally, or 10 to 25 pounds of force frequently, or greater than negligible up to 10 pounds of force constantly to move objects.

MEDLINE: National Library of Medicine computer database that covers approximately 600 000 references to biomedical journal articles published currently and in the previous 2 years.

megabyte: 1 000 kilobytes or 1 000 000 bytes of electronic information; measure of the capacity of memory, disk storage for a computer, and/or a computer disk.

melatonin: Hormone produced by the pineal gland; secreted into bloodstream.

memory: The mental process that involves registration and encoding, consolidation and storage, and recall and retrieval of information.

memory processes: Strategies for dealing with information that are under the individual's control.

memory structure: Unvarying physical or structural components of memory.

menarche: First menstrual period of a female; usually occurs between 9 and 17 years of age.

menopause: Period of life in women marking the end of the reproductive cycle; accompanied by cessation of menstruation for 1 year, decreases in hormonal levels, and alteration of the reproductive organs.

menstruation: Periodic discharge of a bloody fluid from the uterus through the vagina occurring at more or less regular intervals from puberty to menopause.

mental retardation: Significantly subaverage general intellectual functioning concurrent with deficits in adaptive behavior, and manifested during the developmental period.

mentastics: The phase of the Trager approach involving the client being taught self-care movements.

mesoderm: Middle layer of cells that develops from the inner cell mass of the blastocyst eventually becoming the muscles, the bones, the circulatory system, and the inner layer of the skin.

mesothelioma: A tumor developed from mesothelial tissue.

metabolic acidosis: Metabolic environment of acidity. A pathologic condition resulting from accumulation of acid or loss of base in the body, characterized by increase in hydrogen ion concentration (decrease in pH).

metabolic alkalosis: A pathologic condition resulting from the accumulation of base or loss of acid in the body, and characterized by decrease in hydrogen ion concentration (increase pH).

metabolic equivalent level (MET): Method used to measure endurance levels; represents the energy requirements needed to maintain metabolic functioning as well as perform varying activities. It is an abbreviation for oxygen consumption during activities. The greater the exertion, the greater the METs required for an activity.

metabolism: The sum of all physical and chemical processes by which living organized substance is produced and maintained, and the transformation by which energy is made available for the uses of the organism. Also, the term used to describe the process by which the body inactivates drugs. *Synonym*: biotransformation.

microcephalus: Condition in which an atypically small skull results in brain damage and mental retardation.

microchip: Electronic device that consists of thousands of electronic circuits, such as transistors on a small sliver or chip of plastic. Such devices are the building blocks of computers. *Synonym*: integrated circuit.

microcomputer: Medium-sized computer that usually serves as a central computer for many individuals. Used primarily in academic and research settings.

microneurography: A technique for the recording of action potentials from individual peripheral nerve fibers.

Middendorf breathwork: An artistic form of somatic therapy focusing on how our breath moves our bodies.

migraine: Headache associated with periodic instability of the cranial arteries; may be accompanied by nausea.

mind-body relationship: The effect of the mind (and mental disorders) on the body and the effect of the body (and physical disorders) on the mind.

mindfulness-based stress reduction: A program for people who want to learn to use their own internal resources to change their relationship to stress, chronic pain, or illness.

minimal brain damage (MBD): Superficial damage to the brain that cannot be detected using objective instruments. Such damage is usually assessed from deviations in behavior.

minimal risk: The probability and magnitude that harm and discomfort anticipated in the research are not greater in and of themselves than those ordinarily encountered in daily life or during the performance of routine physical or psychological examinations or tests.

minority group: Group differing, especially in race, religion, or ethnic background, from the majority of a population.

minute ventilation: The volume of air inspired and exhaled in 1 minute. The highest minute ventilation achieved during exercise is also called the maximum breathing capacity.

miscarriage: Spontaneous delivery/abortion of a fetus.

mission statement: Statement of purpose of an agency or organization.

mitogen: A substance that stimulates cell division (mitosis) in lymphocytes.

mitosis: Cell duplication and division that generates all of an individual's cells except for the sperm and ova.

mnemonics: Memory-enhancing learning techniques that link a new concept to an established one.

mobilization: A passive therapeutic movement at the end of the available range of motion at variable amplitudes and speed.

modality: A broad group of agents that may include thermal, acoustic, radiant, mechanical, or electrical energy to produce physiologic changes in tissues for therapeutic purposes.

mode (Mo): Value or score in a set of scores that occurs most frequently.

model: An approach, framework, or structure that organizes knowledge to guide reasonable decision making.

modeling: Process by which a behavior is learned through observation and imitation of others.

modem: Device that enables communication between 2 computers via telephone line signals.

modulation: A variation in levels of excitation and inhibition over sensory and motor neural pools.

molding: The shaping of the fetal head by the overlapping fetal skull bones to adjust to the size and shape of the birth canal.

molecular pharmacology: Study of interaction of drugs and subcellular entities.

monitoring: Determining a patient's/client's status on a periodic or ongoing basis.

monocular: Pertaining to 1 eye.

monocyte: A circulating phagocytic leukocyte which can differentiate into a macrophage upon migration into tissue.

mood: Pervasive and sustained emotion that, when extreme, can color one's whole view of life; generally refers to either elation or depression.

morbidity: Illness or abnormal condition.

mores: Very strong norms; often laws.

morphogenesis: The morphological transformation including growth, alterations of germinal layers, and differentiation of cells and tissues during development.

mortality: Being subject to death.

motivation: Individual drives toward the mastery of certain goals and skills; may be intrinsic or involve inducements and incentives.

motivational theory: Theory in which motivation is described as an arousal to action, initiating molding and sustaining specific action patterns. Certain reinforcers may be used to increase or decrease motivation. Internal rewards appear to be better motivators than extrinsic ones.

motor control: The ability of the central nervous system to control or direct the neuromotor system in purposeful movement and postural adjustment by selective allocation of muscle tension across appropriate joint segments.

motor coordination: Functions that are traditionally defined as motoric. Includes gross motor, fine motor, and motor planning functions.

motor deficit: Lack or deficiency of normal motor function that may be the result of pathology or other disorder. Weakness, paralysis, abnormal movement patterns, abnormal timing, coordination, clumsiness, involuntary movements, or abnormal postures may be manifestations of impaired motor function (motor control and motor learning).

motor development: Growth and change in the ability to do physical activities, such as walking, running, or riding a bike.

motor dysfunction/deficit/disorder/disturbance: Generic terms for any type of disorder found in any pathology leading to problems in movement in learning disabled children that have a motor component.

motor function: The ability to learn or demonstrate the skillful and efficient assumption, maintenance, modification, and control of voluntary postures and movement patterns.

motor lag: A prolonged latent period between the reception of a stimulus and the initiation of the motor response.

motor learning: The acquisition of skilled movement based on previous experience. A set of processes associated with practice or experience leading to relatively permanent changes in the capability for producing skilled action.

motor neuron: Nerve cell that sends signals from the brain to the muscles throughout the body.

motor planning: Ability to organize and execute movement patterns to accomplish a purposeful activity.

motor skill: The ability to execute coordinated motor actions with proficiency.

motor strip: Pre-central sulci in the brain that controls movement of all muscles.

motor time (MT): In a reaction time (RT) test, the time from onset of electromyographic activity to the initiation of the movement.

motor unit: One alpha motor neuron, its axon, and all muscle fibers attached to that axon.

mouse: Device that moves on a horizontal plane and controls the cursor on a computer monitor.

movement speed: The time elapsed between the initiation of a movement and its completion.

movement therapy: A variety of techniques that utilize movement re-education and proper body mechanics in combination with massage or soft tissue manipulation.

multiculturism: Awareness and knowledge about human diversity in ways that are translated into more respectful human interactions and effective interconnections.

multidimensional maps: Pictures of self and environment that are created within the central nervous system after receipt and analysis of multisensory input.

multidisciplinary team: Health care workers who are members of different disciplines, each one providing specific services to the patient/client.

multigenerational model: Model of family therapy that focuses on reciprocal role relationships over a period of time and thus takes a longitudinal approach.

multilingual: Speaking many languages fluently.

multiple myeloma: Primary malignant tumor of the plasma cells usually arising in bone marrow.

multiple regression: Making predictions of 1 variable (using the multiple R) based on measures of 2 or more others.

multiple sleep latency test: Test that measures the degree of daytime sleepiness and rapid eye movement (REM) sleep of an individual.

multiskilled practitioner: Person from one profession who has established competence in specific skills usually associated with another profession.

murmur: A gentle blowing auscultatory sound caused by friction between parts, a prolapse of a valve, or an aneurysm.

muscle: A type of tissue composed of contractile cells or fibers that effects movement of an organ or part of the body. Massage therapy is contraindicated for torn muscles. Vigorous massage could increase the tearing effect and postpone healing.

muscle endurance: Sustained muscular contraction, measured as repetitions of submaximal contraction (isotonic) or submaximal holding time (isometric).

muscle energy technique: A manual therapy technique that involves manipulation of the spinal segments and pelvis. A direct, non-invasive manual therapy used to normalize joint dysfunction and increase range of motion. The practitioner evaluates the primary areas of dysfunction in order to place the affected joints in precise positions that enable the client to perform gently isometric contractions.

muscle fiber types: Classification of muscle fibers based on anatomic, physiologic, and functional characteristics.

muscle performance: Execution or accomplishment of a movement resulting from muscle activity for effective, coordinated functioning.

muscle release technique: A combination of compression, extension, movement, and breath used to lengthen muscles, restore muscle memory, and provide relief from pain.

muscle spindles: Sensory receptors in the tendons of muscles which monitor tension of muscles.

muscle strength: Nonspecific term relating to muscle contraction, often referring to the force generated by a single maximal isometric contraction.

muscle testing: Method of evaluating the contractile unit, including the muscle, tendons, and associated tissues, of a moving part of the body by neurologic or resistance testing.

muscle tone: Amount of tension or contractibility among the motor units of a muscle; often defined as the resistance of a muscle to stretch or elongation.

muscle weakness: Lack of the full tension-producing capability of a muscle needed to maintain posture and create movement.

muscular atrophies: Diseases of unknown etiology that are caused by the breakdown of cells in the anterior horn of the spinal cord.

muscular system: Framework of voluntarily controlled skeletal muscles in the body.

musculoskeletal: System in the human body that is associated with the muscles and the bones to which they attach.

mutability: The muscle fiber's ability to change in response to a new demand.

mutation: Error in gene replication that results in a change in the molecular structure of genetic material.

myalgia: Pain in a muscle or muscles.

myelin: A fat-like substance forming the principle component of the sheath of nerve fibers in the CNS.

myelination: The process of forming the "white" lipid covering of nerve cell axons; myelin increases the conduction velocity of the neuronal impulse and forms the "white matter" of the brain and spinal cord.

myelitis: Inflammation of the spinal cord with associated motor and sensory dysfunction.

myoclonus: Sudden, quick spasms of a muscle or group of muscles.

myofascial release (MFR): Techniques used to release fascial tissue restrictions secondary to tonal dysfunction and decrease binding down of the fascia around a muscle. The 3-dimensional application of sustained pressure and movement into the fascial system in order to eliminate fascial restrictions and facilitate the emergence of emotional patterns and belief systems which are no longer relevant or are impeding progress.

myofascial trigger point therapy: Based on the discoveries of Drs. Janet Travell and David Simons. They found the causal relationship between chronic pain and its source. Myofascial trigger point therapy is used to relieve muscular pain and dysfunction through applied pressure to trigger points of referred pain and through stretching exercises.

myofascial web: The tough, continuous sheath of connective tissue that spreads around the body from head to toe.

myokymia: Continual, irregular twitching of a muscle often seen around the eye in the facial region.

myoma: Benign tumor consisting of muscle tissue.

myomassology: A comprehensive wellness program that includes training in Swedish massage, aromatherapy, reflexology, ear candling, craniosacral therapy, iridology, herbology, energy balancing, nutrition, meditation, yoga, tai-chi, and qi-gong.

myopathic muscular therapy: A system of muscular manipulation designed to accomplish relaxation in muscles in which there is progressive and residual tension from strains of various sorts.

myopathy: Abnormal muscle function.

myopractic muscle therapy: A body therapy that uses deep muscle therapy and structural integration techniques to achieve deep relaxation and relief from chronic pain.

myorrhaphy: Suture of a muscle.

myosin: A protein in muscles.

myoskeletal alignment technique: A technique combining deep-tissue work with assisted stretching and non-force spinal aligment.

myotasis: Stretching of muscle.

myotherapy: *See* Bonnie Prudden Myotherapy.

Nambudripad's allergy elimination technique: Muscle testing is used to diagnose an allergy or sensitivity followed by treatment consisting of a combination of spinal stimulation, acupressure, and abstinence.

naprapathy: A system of treatment using soft tissue manipulation to release tension and balance energy flows in the body. Repetitive rhythmic thrusts are used to gently stretch contracted connective tissues.

narcissism: Egocentricity; dominant interest in one's self.

narcolepsy: Chronic sleep disorder manifested by excessive and overwhelming daytime sleepiness.

narrative: The interpretation of events through stories.

narrative documentation: System of documentation that uses summary paragraphs to describe evaluation data and treatment progress.

narrative reasoning: An aspect of clinical reasoning requiring understanding of "life stories" of patients/clients.

national health insurance: Form of insurance sponsored by a national government intended to pay for health services used by its citizens.

natural environments: All integrated community settings.

naturalistic observation: Technical term that refers to a qualitative research technique of observing an individual in his or her natural environment.

natural killer cell (NK): A large granular lymphocyte capable of killing certain tumor and virally infected cells.

nature/nurture controversy: Debate over the extent to which inborn, hereditary characteristics, as compared to life experiences and environmental factors, determine a person's identity and psychological makeup.

naturopathic medicine: An integration of a wide range of natural healing techniques based on belief in the body's innate self-healing properties.

nausea: The sensation of having a queasy stomach, often preceding vomiting. Massage is contraindicated as it may exacerbate the sensation and cause vomiting; refer to a physician.

nebulizer: An atomizer; a device for throwing a spray or mist.

necrosis: Death of tissue usually resulting in gangrene.

needs assessment: Systematic gathering of information about strengths, problems, resources, and barriers in a given population or community. Results of needs assessment are the basis of program planning.

negative reinforcement: Removing an aversive stimulus following an inappropriate response.

negligence: Commission of an act that a prudent person would not have done or the omission of a duty that a prudent person would have fulfilled, resulting in injury or harm to another person. May be basis for malpractice suit.

nerve conduction tests: Measurement of electrical conductivity of motor and sensory nerves by application of an external electrical stimulus to the nerve and evaluation of parameters such as nerve conduction time, velocity, amplitude, and shape of the resulting response as recorded from another site on the nerve or from a muscle supplied by the nerve.

nervous system: The network of neural tissues in the body comprised of the central and peripheral divisions, which are responsible for the processing of impulses.

network: Communication link between computers, communication between a central computer and users, or any group of computers that are connected in order to send messages to each other.

networking: Process that links people and information in order to accomplish objectives; often informal.

neural kinesiology: A diagnostic technique used to determine therapeutic need in 4 categories: neurological, structural, biochemical, and psychological.

neuralgia: Attacks of pain along the entire course or branch of a peripheral sensory nerve.

neurapraxia: Interruption of nerve conduction without loss of continuity of the axon.

neuritic plaques: Normative age-related change in the brain involving amyloid protein collecting on dying or dead neurons. A discrete structure found outside the neuron that is composed of degenerating small axons, some dendrites, astrocytes, and amyloid. *Synonym:* senile plaque.

neuritis: Condition causing a dysfunction of cranial or spinal nerve; in sensory nerves, paresthesia is present.

neuroanatomy: Structures within the central, peripheral, and autonomic nervous systems.

neuroblastoma: A malignant tumor of the nervous system composed chiefly of neuroblasts.

neurodevelopment: The progressive growth and development of the nervous system.

neurogenic pain: Pain in the limbs caused by neurologic lesions.

neurography: Study of the action potentials of nerves.

neurohypophysis: Posterior lobe of the pituitary gland.

neurologic impairment: Any disability caused by damage to the central nervous system (brain, spinal cord, ganglia, and nerves).

neurologist: Specialist who diagnoses and treats diseases of the nervous system.

neuroma: Tumor or growth along the course of a nerve or at the end of a lacerated nerve, which is often very painful.

neuromechanism: A neurologic system whose component parts work together to produce central nervous system function.

neuromuscular: Pertaining to the nerves and the muscles.

neuromuscular facilitation: Increasing the activity of the muscles through sensory stimuli.

neuromuscular inhibition: Decreasing the activity of the muscles through the specific application of sensory stimuli.

neuromuscular integrative action: A fitness program consisting of a combination of tai chi, yoga, martial arts, and modern ethnic dancing.

neuromuscular re-education: Specific treatment regimens carried out by occupational and physical therapists to improve motor strength and coordination in persons with brain or spinal cord injuries.

neuromuscular reprogramming: A comprehensive program of soft tissue manipulation, which balances the body's central nervous system with the musculoskeletal system.

neuromuscular therapy: The comprehensive program of soft tissue manipulation, balancing the body's central nervous system with the musculoskeletal system. Based on neurological laws that explain how the central nervous system initiates and maintains pain. The goal is to help relieve the pain and dysfunction by understanding and alleviating the underlying cause.

neuron: Nerve cell.

neuropathy: Any disease or dysfunction of the nerves.

neuropharmacology: Study of the effects of drugs on the brain.

neurosis: Mental disorder in which reality testing is not seriously disturbed, but individual is fearful or overly anxious about various elements of his or her life.

neurostructural bodywork: A combination of fascial release, neuromuscular re-education, craniosacral adjustment, and breathwork.

neurotic: Analytic concept that reflects psychodynamic conflicts that cause difficulty for an individual to remain in contact with reality.

neurotransmitters: Chemical substances that are released from presynaptic cells and travel across the synapse to stimulate or inhibit postsynaptic cells, thereby facilitating or inhibiting neural transmission.

Nikon restorative massage/Okazaki restorative massage: A blending of Japanese, Hawaiian, and Chinese techniques, applied mostly with the elbow.

nociceptor: A peripheral nerve ending that appreciates and transmits painful or injurious stimuli.

nominal (or categorical) data: Numbers are utilized to name mutually exclusive categories.

nominal scales: Measurement scales that contain information that is categorical and mutually exclusive (ie, it can only be contained in 1 category).

nonhuman environment: Everything that is not human.

nonjudgmental acceptance: Therapist or group therapist lets the patient/client know that his/her ideas and thoughts will be valued and not rejected.

nonrapid eye movements (NREM): Sleep state when brain waves become slower and less regular.

norepinephrine: A hormone secreted by the adrenal medulla in response to splanchnic stimulation, and stored in the chromaffin granules, being released predominantly in response to hypotension. Stimulates the sympathetic nervous system.

normal curve: When scores and frequency of occurrence are plotted on the x and y axes, respectively, this frequency distribution curve ensues.

normality: Range of behavior considered acceptable by a social group or culture.

normative ethics: Examination of daily debates between group members about what is right and what is wrong.

norm-referenced test: Any instrument that uses the typical scores of members of a comparison group as a standard for determining individual performance.

norms: Standards of comparison derived from measuring an attribute across many individuals to determine typical score ranges.

noticing: Act of knowing; awareness of critical issues.

novitiate: Beginning stages or apprenticeship within a professional career.

noxious: Harmful to health; injurious (eg, noxious gas, noxious stimuli).

Nuad Bo Rarn: *See* Thai massage.

Nuat Thai: Thai medical massage. It is a type of Vajrayana yoga.

nuchal rigidity: Reflex spasm of the neck extensor muscles resulting in resistance to cervical flexion.

null hypothesis: In research, a hypothesis that predicts that no difference or relationship exists among the variables studied that could not have occurred by chance alone.

objective measure: Method of assessment that is not influenced by the emotions or personal opinion of the assessor.

obligatory reflexive response: Reflex that is consciously present in a motor pattern; this reflex may dominate all other movement components.

observer bias: When the previous experiences of the individual influence his/her observations and interpretations of behaviors being assessed or evaluated.

obsession: Irresistible thought pattern, usually anxiety provoking, which intrudes on normal thought processes.

obsessive-compulsive disorder: Anxiety disorder characterized by recurrent uncontrollable thoughts, irresistible urges to engage repetitively in an act, or both, such that they cause significant anxiety or interfere with daily functioning.

occupational therapy (OT): Therapeutic use of self-care, work, and play activities to increase independent function, enhance development, and prevent disability. May include adaptation of task or environment to achieve maximum independence and to enhance the quality of life. Definition by American Occupational Therapy Association can be found on Web page www.aota.org. From the AOTA's Position Paper—*Occupational Performance: Occupational Therapy's Definition of Function*, health profession that helps people address challenges or difficulties that threaten or impair their ability to perform activities and tasks that are basic to the fulfillment of their roles as worker, parent, spouse or partner, sibling, and friend to self or others.

oculomotor: Pertains to movements of the eyeballs.

Ohashiatsu: A hands-on technique using gentle exercises, stretch, and meditation.

ointment: A medicated substance (salve) intended for application to the skin.

old age: Arbitrary or societally defined period of life; specifically, over 65 years of age in the United States.

older person: Term used to refer to individuals in the later years of the life span. Arbitrarily set between 65 and 70 years old in American society for the purpose of age-related entitlements.

olfactory: Pertaining to the sense of smell.

oligodendroglia: Myelin-producing cells in the CNS.

ombudsman: An official appointed to receive and investigate complaints made by individuals against public officials and institutions.

on-line: Monitor linked to an off-site computer.

Onsen technique: Onsen is a Japanese word meaning "at rest" or "at peace". It is a state of mind and a state of body. Three components are included—muscle energy technique, post-isometric relaxation, and transverse friction.

on-site massage: *See* chair massage.

open-ended question: Question that may have multiple correct responses rather than a finite correct answer.

open enrollment period: Period of time in which new subscribers may elect to enroll in a health insurance plan.

open system: System of structures that function as a whole and maintains itself by means of input from the environment and organismic change occurring as needed.

operant conditioning: A form of conditioning in which positive or negative reinforcement is contingent upon the occurrence of the desired response.

ophthalmoplegia: Paralysis of ocular muscles.

opioid: Terminology used to refer to synthetic drugs that have pharmacological properties similar to opium or morphine.

opposition: The movement in which the thumb is brought across to meet the little finger.

optical character recognition: Technology used in scanning to convert the images of typed text into a computer code (ie, translating the analog signal from the voltage of reflected light to a digital value readable by the computer).

oral-motor control: Coordinated ability of opening and closing the mouth and being able to manage chewing, swallowing, and speaking.

order: The desired state of affairs, which is an absence of disease in medicine and competence in the performance of work, play, or self-care. Disorder is defined as disease in medicine and performance dysfunction.

ordinal data: Rank-ordered data.

ordinal scales: Measurement scales that contain information that can be rank ordered.

organic brain syndrome: Cluster of mental disorders characterized by impaired cerebral function resulting from damage to or changes in the brain.

organization: Group of individuals organized for the attainment of a common goal.

organizational patterns: Hierarchic patterns of personnel ranking that indicate the underlying chain of command in an organization.

Oriental bodywork: A term encompassing a set of bodyworking practices that base their practice on the monitoring and manipulation of the body's energy system.

orientation: Initial stage of group development that includes a search for structure, goals, and dependency on the leader.

origin: Proximal attachment of a muscle that remains relatively fixed during normal muscular contraction.

ortho-bionomy: A gentle, non-invasive, osteopathically-based form of body therapy which uses gentle movements and positions of the body to facilitate a change in stress and pain patterns. A strong focus is placed on the comfort of the individual, no forceful manipulations are used.

orthopedic: Branch of medical science that deals with the prevention or correction of disorders involving locomotor structures of the body.

orthopedic impairment: Any disability caused by disorders to the musculoskeletal system.

orthostatic hypotension: A dramatic fall in the blood pressure when a patient/client assumes an upright position, usually caused by a disturbance of vasomotor control decreasing the blood supply returning to the heart.

orthopedic massage: A comprehensive treatment approach that emphasizes assessment, matching the mode of treatment to the condition being treated, adaptability of treatment, and understanding the rehabilitative protocol.

orthotic: An external device utilized to apply forces to a body part to limit movement, increase the velocity or power of a movement, stop movement, or hold the body part in a particular position. Previously called braces.

orthotics: External devices used to support and correct deformities or add stability to enhance control and function.

oscilloscope: Instrument that displays a visual representation of an electrical wave such as a muscle contraction.

osmosis: The passage of pure solvent from the lesser to the greater concentration when 2 solutions are separated by a membrane that selectively prevents the passage of solute molecules, but is permeable to the solvent. An attempt to equalize concentrations on both sides of a membrane.

osteoblast: Any cell that develops into bone or secretes substances producing bony tissue.

osteochondrosis: A disease of 1 or more of the growth or ossifications centers in children, which begins as a degeneration or necrosis followed by regeneration or recalcification.

osteoclast: Any of the large multinucleate cells in bone that absorb or break down bony tissue.

osteokinetics: A combination of techniques (dialogue, coached breathing, qi gong) with lengthening, stretching and manipulating the body results in clearing of emotional and psychological restrictions.

osteopathic medicine: Traditional medicine augmented by musculoskeletal therapy and wellness training.

osteoplasty: Plastic surgery of the bones; bone grafting.

osteoporosis: A general term for any disease that results in a reduction of the mass of a bone. Massage therapy is contraindicated without physician supervision due to the possibility of breaking a bone.

osteotomy: Operation to cut across a bone.

otitis media: Inflammation of the inner ear, which usually causes dizziness.

otosclerosis: Hardening of the bony tissue of the ear resulting in conductive hearing loss.

outcome: The way something turns out; result; consequence. Outcomes are the result of patient/client management. They relate to remediation of functional limitation and disability, primary or secondary prevention, and optimization of patient/client satisfaction.

outcome measure: Instrument designed to gather information on the efficacy of service programs; a means for determining if goals or objectives have been met.

out-of-pocket payment or costs: Costs borne solely by an individual without the benefit of insurance.

outpatient services: Ambulatory care provided in outpatient departments of health facilities.

outreach services: Services that seek out and identify hard-to-reach individuals and assist them in gaining access to needed services.

overuse syndrome: Musculoskeletal disorder manifested from repetitive upper extremity movements occurring during activities. Symptoms include persistent pain in joints, muscles, tendons, or other soft tissues of the upper extremities. *Synonyms*: cumulative trauma disorder, repetitive strain disorder.

oxygen consumption (V_{O2}): The amount of oxygen used by the tissues of the body, usually measured in oxygen uptake in the lung; normally about 250 mL/min and it increases with increased metabolic rate. The difference between the oxygen inspired and the oxygen exhaled is the amount of oxygen used. Maximum oxygen consumption is the highest amount of oxygen used during exercise (V_{O2MAX}). The oxygen consumption will not increase even if the exercise intensity increases. This value is often used to measure maximal exercise capacity.

oxygen saturation: The degree to which oxygen is present in a particular cell, tissue, organ, or system.

pacemaker: Electrical device implanted to control the beating of the heart.

pacing: Accommodating for time in a test or treatment session; the rate at which instruction is given or practice is provided.

pain: A sensation of hurting, or strong discomfort in some part of the body caused by an injury, disease, or functional disorder, and transmitted through the nervous system.

pain character measurements: Any of the tools used to define the character of a patient's/client's pain.

pain estimates: A pain intensity measurement in which patient's/client's pain is rated on pain scale of 0 to 10.

pain intensity measurements: Any of the scales used to quantify pain intensity.

pain management: Use of treatment to control chronic pain, including the use of behavioral modification, relaxation training, physical modalities and agents, medication, and surgery.

pain modulation: Variation in the intensity and appreciation of pain secondary to CNS and ANS effects on the nociceptors and along the pain pathways, as well as secondary to external factors such as distraction and suggestion.

pain pathway: The route along which nerve impulses arising from painful stimuli are transmitted from the nociceptor to the brain, including transmission within the brain itself.

pain quality: A description of the nature, type, or character of pain (eg, burning, dull, sharp, throbbing, etc).

pain response: Physical or emotional response to the presence of pain.

pain-spasm-pain cycle: When the body's reaction to a stimulus results in pain the body adjusts to eliminate the pain. That adjustment becomes a stimulus causing more pain. The body then adjusts again and so on until therapy breaks the cycle of pain-spasm-pain.

palliative: Relieving but not curing.

palliative care: Care rendered to temporarily reduce or moderate the intensity of an otherwise chronic medical condition.

pallor: Paleness; absence of the skin coloration.

palmar: Palm of the hand.

palpate: To examine by touching or feeling.

palpation: Examination using the hands (eg, palpation of muscle spasm, palpation of the thoracic cage, etc).

palpitation: Rapid, violent, or throbbing pulsation in a body part.

palsy: The loss of movement or ability to control movement.

pancreatitis: Inflammation of the pancreas, with pain and tenderness of the abdomen, tympanities (gaseous pockets), and vomiting.

pandiculation: Coordinated, slowly performed, full-body muscular contractions and elongations to reawaken the mind's sense and control of your muscles and movement. *See* somatic education.

panic attack: State of extreme anxiety, usually including sweating, shortness of breath, chest pains, and fear. May come on unpredictably or as a result of a particular stimulus.

paradigm: Refers to the organization of knowledge, as well as the changes in scientific thought over time; an organizing interaction. A pattern, example, or model.

paradox: A statement to the contrary of belief. A statement that is self-contradictory and, hence, false.

paraffin bath: A superficial thermal modality using paraffin wax and mineral oil.

parallel processing: Learning or solving a problem through a global approach integrating data into a whole experience.

paralysis: Condition in which one loses voluntary motor control over a section of the body due to trauma or injury.

paranoia: Thought pattern that reflects a belief that others are persecuting or attempting to harm one, in the absence of a realistic basis for such fears.

paraplegia (PARA): Paralysis of the spine affecting the lower portion of the trunk and legs. The impairment or loss of motor and/or sensory function in the thoracic, lumbar, or sacral (but not cervical) segments of the spinal cord, secondary to damage of neural elements within the spinal canal.

parasomnia: Abnormal sleep behavior, including sleepwalking and bruxism (grinding the teeth).

parasympathetic nervous system: Autonomic nervous system that serves to relax the body's responses and is the opposite of the sympathetic nervous system.

paraxial: Lying near the axis of the body.

parenchyma: Essential parts of an organ, which are concerned with its function rather than its framework.

paresis: Weakness in voluntary muscle with slight paralysis.

paresthesia: Abnormal sensation, such as burning or pricking, tickling, or tingling.

parity: A condition of having produced viable offspring. The state or condition of being the same in power, value, and rank. Equality.

paroxysm: Sudden, periodic attack or recurrence or intensification of symptoms of a disease (eg, paroxysmal atrial tachycardia).

participant-observer: Descriptor that can be applied when a therapist observes and evaluates an individual's performance while engaged in an activity with the person.

passive-aggressive personality disorder: Disorder that is characterized by resistance to social and occupational performance demands through procrastination, dawdling, stubbornness, inefficiency, and forgetfulness that appears to border on the intentional.

passive range of motion (PROM): Amount of motion at a given joint when the joint is moved by the therapist.

passive joint movements: Joint movements performed by the therapist.

passive stretch: Stretch applied with external force.

paternalism: Acting or making decisions on behalf of others without their consent.

pathology: The study of the characteristics, causes, and effects of disease, as observed in the structure and function of the body.

pathophysiology: An interruption or interference of normal physiological and developmental processes or structures.

patient/client: A person receiving care or treatment. An individual who is a recipient of physical therapy and direct intervention.

patient management interview: Interview used by multiple professionals to identify the type of intervention or treatment needed.

patient's rights: The rights of patients/clients to be informed about their conditions and prognoses and to make decisions concerning their treatment.

peer culture: Stable set of activities or routines, artifacts, values, and concerns that a group of individuals produce or share.

peer review: Appraisal by professional co-workers of equal status of the way health practitioners conduct practice, education, or research.

pelvic floor: A sling arrangement of ligaments and muscles that supports the reproductive organs.

percent body fat: Percent of body weight that is fat; includes storage fat (expendable), essential fat, and sex-specific fat reserve.

perception: Ability to organize and interpret incoming sensory information.

perceptual-motor: The interaction of the various channels of perception with motor activity, including visual, auditory, tactual, and kinesthetic channels.

perceptual-motor skill: Ability to integrate perceptual (sensory) input with motor output in order to accomplish purposeful activities.

perceptual processing: Ability to integrate and understand perceptual (sensory) input in order to respond appropriately with motor output.

perceptual trace: Memory for past movement; the internal reference of correctness.

percussion: Blows to the body delivered with varying degrees of force.

percussion (diagnostic): A procedure in which the clinician taps a body part manually or with an instrument to estimate its density.

per diem rate: Fixed all-inclusive price for 1 day of hospital or nursing facility care, including all supplies and services provided to the patient/client during a day, excluding the professional fees of nonstaff physicians.

performance components: Sensorimotor, cognitive, integration, psychosocial, and psychological skills and abilities.

perfusion: The act of pouring over or through, especially the passage of a fluid through the vessels of a specific organ or body part.

peripheral nerve: Any nerve that supplies the peripheral parts and is a branch of the central nervous system (eg, the spinal cord).

peripheral nerve injuries: Loss of precision pinch and grip due to crushing, severance, or inflammation/degeneration of the peripheral nerve fibers.

peripheral nervous system (PNS): Consists of all of the nerve cells outside the central nervous system, including motor and sensory nerves.

peripheral neuropathy: Any functional or organic disorder of the peripheral nervous system; degeneration of peripheral nerves supplying the extremities, causing loss of sensation, muscle weakness, and atrophy.

peripheral pain: Pain arising from injury to a peripheral structure.

peristalsis: Movement by which a tube in the body (primarily the alimentary canal) sends contents within it to another part of the body. This is accomplished through alternative contractions and relaxations which resemble a wave- or worm-like movement.

peritonitis: Inflammation of the peritoneum; a condition marked by exudations in the peritoneum of serum, fibrin, cells, and pus. It is attended by abdominal pain and tenderness, constipation, vomiting, and moderate fever.

perseveration: Inability to shift from thought to thought, persistence of an idea even when the subject changes.

personal boundaries: The sense of self which limits interaction physically, mentally, and spiritually with others.

personal factors: The background of a person's life and living that is composed of features of him/herself that are not parts of a health condition or disablement, including age, gender, educational background, experiences, personality, character style, aptitudes, other health conditions, fitness, lifestyle, habits, upbringing, coping styles, social background, profession, and past and current experience.

personality: Individual's unique, relatively consistent, and enduring methods of behaving in relation to others and the environment.

personality trait: Distinguishing feature that reflects one's characteristic way of thinking, feeling, and/or adapting.

persons with disabilities: Individuals who experience substantial limitations in 1 or more major life activities, including, but not limited to, such functions as performing manual tasks, walking, seeing, hearing, speaking, breathing, learning, and working.

petit mal: Type of seizure characterized by a momentary lapse of consciousness that starts and ends abruptly.

petrissage: Slow, gentle kneading of the soft tissues.

Pfrimmer technique: Deep cross-fiber strokes applied with the thumbs and fingers.

phagocytosis: A process by which a leukocyte (monocyte, neutrophil) engulfs, ingests, and degrades a foreign particle or organism.

phalanges: Bones of the fingers and toes.

phantom limb pain: Paresthesia or severe pain felt in the amputated part of a limb.

phenol block: An injection of phenol (hydroxybenzene) into individual nerves. Used as a topical anesthetic and produces a selective block of these nerves. Sometimes used to control severe spasticity in specific muscle groups.

phenotype: Observable characteristics of an organism that result from the interaction of the genotype with the organism's environment.

phlebitis: Inflammation of a vein resulting in pain and swelling. Massage therapy is contraindicated due to the potential for loosening blood clots.

phlebotomy: Opening or piercing the vein.

phobia: Characterized by an extreme fear of a person, place, or thing when the situation is not hazardous.

Phoenix Rising yoga therapy: A combination of assisted yoga postures, non-directive dialogue, and directed breathing used to foster personal growth and healing.

phototherapy: Intervention using the application of light.

physical: Pertaining to the body.

physical agent: A form of thermal, acoustic, or radiant energy that is applied to tissues in a systematic manner to achieve a therapeutic effect; a therapeutic modality used to treat physical impairments.

physical agent modalities (PAMs): Modalities such as hot packs, paraffin, electrical stimulation, and ultrasound, used by qualified practitioners to prepare for, or as an adjunct to, purposeful activity.

physical environment: Part of the environment that can be perceived directly through the senses. The physical environment includes observable space, objects and their arrangement, light, noise, and other ambient characteristics that can be objectively determined.

physical function: Fundamental component of health status describing the state of those sensory and motor skills necessary for mobility, work, and recreation.

physical therapist (PT): A person who is a graduate of an accredited physical therapist education program and is licensed to practice physical therapy, whose primary purpose is the promotion of optimal human health and function through the application of scientific principles to prevent, identify, assess, correct, or alleviate acute or prolonged movement dysfunction.

physical therapy: Treatment of injury and disease by mechanical means, such as heat, light, exercise, massage, and mobilization.

physician assistant: Health professional licensed or, in the case of those employed by the Federal government, credentialed, to practice medicine with physician supervision.

***Physicians' Desk Reference* (PDR):** Provides a listing of medications, including both the trade and generic names, the manufacturing company, the side effects and/or adverse reactions and their appropriate interventions, and any incompatible medications.

physiohelanics: A healing treatment; the body's own energy system to clean, balance, and repairing the etheric energy field which surrounds the body. The healer channels energy. Touch is very light and focused on areas that need cleansing and clearing

physiology: Area of study concerned with the functions of the structures of the body.

phytotherapy: A form of herbal therapy that uses a wide variety of treatments including massage, mud packs, wraps, baths, water and steam treatments, and inhalation treatments using herbs and essential oils.

pica: Compulsive eating of nonnutritive substances like dirt. A bizarre appetite.

pilates method: An exercise program for the entire body focused on improving flexibility and strength but not bulk.

piriformis syndrome: A condition characterized by over activity of the piriformis muscle, causing external rotation of the leg and buttock pain.

planes of motion: Imaginary lines that divide the body into right and left, front and back, and top and bottom portions.

plan of care: Statements that specify the anticipated long-term and short-term goals and the desired outcomes, predicted level of optimal improvement, specific interventions to be used, duration, and frequency of the intervention required to reach the goals, outcomes, and criteria for discharge.

plaque: A lesion characterized by loss of myelin and hardening of tissue in diseases such as multiple sclerosis (peripherally) or Alzheimer's disease (in the brain).

plasma cell: Mature antibody secreting cell derived from the B cell.

plasticity: *Neuroscience*: Ability of the central nervous system to adapt structurally or functionally in response to environmental demands. Anatomical and electrophysiological changes in the central nervous system. *Biomechanics*: Defined as continued elongation of a tissue without an increase in resistance from within the tissue.

play: Choosing, performing, and engaging in an intrinsically motivated activity (attitude or process) that is experienced as pleasurable.

pleura: The serous membrane investing the lungs and lining the thoracic cavity, completely enclosing a potential space known as the pleural cavity. There are 2 pleurae, right and left, entirely distinct from each other.

pleurisy: Inflammation of the pleural membrane surrounding the lungs. *Synonym*: pleuritis.

pneumopathology: Any disease involving the respiratory system.

pneumothorax: An accumulation of air or gas in the pleural cavity, which may occur spontaneously or as a result of trauma or a pathological process. Prevents the lung from expanding.

point holding: Acupressure points are held by multiple practitioners for time periods of up to 2 hours. Point holding removes blockages from the meridians and stimulates emotional release.

point stimulation: The stimulation of sensitive areas of skin using electricity, pressure, laser, or ice for the purpose of relieving pain.

polarity therapy: A comprehensive health system involving energy-based bodywork, diet, exercise, and self-awareness.

policy: A principle, law, or decision that guides actions (eg, the sources and distribution of services and funds).

poliomyelitis: Viral infection of the motor cells in the spinal cord.

polymyositis: Systemic connective tissue disease characterized by inflammatory and degenerative changes in the muscles. Leads to symmetric weakness and some degree of muscle atrophy; etiology unknown.

polyneuropathy: A disease involving several nerves such as that seen in diabetes mellitus.

polyp: Tumor with a stem (pedicle) that projects from a mucous membrane surface.

population at-risk: Group of people who share a characteristic that causes each member to be vulnerable to a particular event (eg, nonimmunized children exposed to the polio virus).

position in space: Person's awareness of the place of his/her body in space.

positive reinforcement: Providing a desired reinforcer following an appropriate response.

positron emission tomography (PET): Dynamic brain imaging technique that produces a very detailed image of the brain that can reflect changes in brain activity.

posterior: Toward the back of the body.

postpartum: The period following birth.

post-polio syndrome: Collection of impairments occurring in persons who have had poliomyelitis many years ago; related to chronic mechanical strain of weakened musculature and ligaments.

posttraumatic amnesia: The time elapsed between a brain injury and the point at which the functions concerned with memory are determined to have been restored.

posttraumatic stress disorder (PTSD): Characterized by intense negative feelings or terror in re-experiencing a traumatic or disastrous event either in thoughts, nightmares, or dreams experienced over time. May also include physiological responses such as excessive alertness, inability to concentrate or follow through on tasks, or difficulty sleeping.

postural alignment: The relationship of all the body parts around the center of gravity. Relationship of one body segment to another in standing or sitting or any other position. *See* posture.

postural control: The ability to effectively correct for perturbation of the center of gravity and regain postural alignment without falling.

postural integration: *See* Rolfing structural integration.

postural integration and energetic integration: With a focus on the unity of tissue, feeling and awareness breathwork, deep fascia manipulation, emotional expression, and meditation are used to achieve body-mind balance.

postural tremor: A pathological tremor of 3 to 5 Hz that appears in a limb or the trunk when either is working against the pull of gravity.

posture: The attitude of the body. The position maintained by the body in standing or in sitting. The alignment and positioning of the body in relation to gravity, center of mass, and base of support. In the strictest sense, the position of the body or body part in relation to space and/or to other body parts. Functionally, the anticipation of, and response to, displacement of the body's center of mass.

power: Ability to impose one's will upon the behavior of other persons. The ability to perform work over time.

powered wheelchair: Motorized wheelchair that allows a person to control speed and direction by pushing a button or using a joystick. It enables those without the use of their arms to move their wheelchairs without assistance.

power of attorney: Document authorizing one person to take legal actions on behalf of another who acts as an agent for the grantor.

pragmatics: The study of language as it is used in context.

pragmatism: Practical way of solving problems.

prana: A vital life force energy.

pranic healing: A kind of bioenergetic healing in which practitioners use their hands to evaluate the energetic condition of the aura, clean and correct the aura, and re-energize it with fresh prana.

preferred provider organization (PPO): Acts as a broker between the purchaser of health care and the provider.

prefix: Word element of 1 or more syllables placed in front of a combining form in order to change its meaning.

pregnancy: Condition of carrying a fertilized ovum (zygote) in the uterus.

pregnancy (prenatal) massage: The prenatal use of massage therapy to support the physiologic, structural, and emotional well being of both mother and fetus. Specific pregnancy massage training is needed before performing massage on pregnant patients. Inappropriate massage techniques could induce delivery.

prejudice: Unreasonable feelings, opinions, or attitudes directed against a race, religion, or national group.

premature: Child born before the 37th week of gestation; birth or infant.

premenstrual syndrome (PMS): A set of symptoms that occurs monthly after ovulation and usually ceases at menstruation or shortly thereafter.

premium: Amount paid to an insurer or third party for insurance coverage under an insurance policy.

prenatal massage: Massage performed by a trained perinatal specialist, and includes many methods of massage and somatic therapies that are both effective and safe prenatally, during labor and postpartum. *See* pregnancy massage.

prepaid health plan: An insurance plan provided by health maintenance organizations (HMOs) and competitive medical plans. Preventive and wellness services are available in addition to care for illnesses.

prepared learning: Form of learning to which an individual is biologically predisposed.

presbyastasis: Age-related disequillibrium in the absence of known pathology.

presbycusis: Age-related hearing loss in the absence of pathology.

presbyopia: Age-related farsightedness with a loss in the ability to focus on objects that are near.

presenile: Pertaining to a condition in which a person manifests signs of aging early or in mid-life.

pressure point: Point over an artery where the pulse may be felt.

prevalence: The total number of persons with a disease in a given population at a given point in time. Prevalence is usually expressed as the percentage of the population that has the disease.

prevention: The act of preventing. Decreasing the risk of disease or disability. Activities that are directed toward slowing or stopping the occurrence of both mental and physical illness and disease, minimizing the effects of a disease or impairment on disability, or reducing the severity or duration of an illness. *Primary*: Prevention of the development of disease in a susceptible or potentially susceptible population through such specific measures as general health promotion efforts. *Secondary*: Efforts to decrease the duration of illness, reduce severity of diseases, and limit sequelae through early diagnosis and prompt intervention. *Tertiary*: Efforts to limit the degree of disability and promote rehabilitation and restoration of function in patients/clients with chronic and irreversible diseases.

preventive intervention: Occurs when therapists use their expertise to anticipate problems in the future, and design interventions to keep negative outcomes from occurring.

preventive medicine: Care designed to deter disease and maintain optimal health.

primary care: Ongoing monitoring of health status to prevent disease and sequelae of disease. First encounter in time or order of care giving.

primary care provider: Clinician who assumes ongoing responsibility for a patient's/client's overall health care needs.

primary health care: Basic level of health care that includes programs directed at health promotion, early diagnosis, and prevention of disease.

primary intracerebral hemorrhage: Syndrome in which bleeding occurs spontaneously in the brain.

primary prevention: Efforts that support or protect the health and well being of the general population.

prime mover: Muscle with the principal responsibility for a given action. For example, the biceps brachii is the prime mover for flexing the arm at the elbow.

primitive reflex (reaction): Any reflex normal in an infant or fetus. Its presence in an adult usually indicates serious neurologic disease (eg, grasp reflex, Moro reflex, sucking reflex, etc).

principle: A general truth or rule that emerges from the testing of assumptions and hypotheses; generally proven or tested.

problem solving: Ability to manipulate knowledge and apply the information to new or unfamiliar situations.

procedures: The sequence of steps to be followed in performing an action; criteria for the way in which things are done.

process acupressure: A combination of acupressure, zero balancing, and psychological processing used to enhance well being.

productivity: It is viewed as a controlling mechanism for top-level management. It is the ratio between the output and the resources expended to obtain the desired output.

product line: Services that are labeled to ensure that consumers understand what they are purchasing.

professional boundaries: The limiting of therapist-client relationships to the interaction necessary to achieve the established goals of the therapy session.

prognosis: Prediction of the probable outcome. The determination of the level of optimal improvement that might be attained by the patient/client and the amount of time needed to reach that level.

program evaluation: Measuring the effectiveness or goal attainment of programs.

programmed cell death: Physiological process in that cells die in the body, thought to be involved in the aging process.

programming: Creating a set of instructions which a computer is able to follow; also a term used to refer to the structuring of activity or influencing of behavior through environmental design, organization, or manipulation.

progressive: Compilation of stages which increase in complexity toward maturity (eg, course of a disease or condition in which signs and symptoms become more prominent and severe over time).

prolapsed: Any organ that descends and protrudes through an external cavity due to weakness of the supporting structures (eg, prolapsed uterus, prolapsed bladder, etc).

pronation: The act of assuming the prone position. Rotation of the forearm medially so the palm is facing down towards the floor. Applied to the foot, a combination of eversion and abduction movements taking place in the tarsal and metatarsal joints and resulting in lowering of the medial margin of the foot, hence of the longitudinal arch, so that the plantar surface of the foot turns outward.

prone: Lying with face down.

prophylactic: Preventive.

proprietary (commercial) facilities: Refers to private profit-making institutions or facilities (eg, nursing homes).

proprioception: Awareness of posture, movement, and changes in equilibrium and the knowledge of position, weight, and resistance of objects in relation to the body. The reception of stimuli from within the body (eg, from muscles and tendons); includes position sense (the awareness of the joints at rest) and kinesthesia (the awareness of movement).

proprioceptive: The state of proprioception.

proprioceptive neuromuscular facilitation (PNF): A form of therapeutic exercise in which accommodating resistance is manually applied to various patterns of movement for the purpose of strengthening and restraining the muscles guiding joint motion using proprioceptive input.

prostaglandins: Lipid-soluble, hormone-like acetic compounds occurring in nearly all tissues, used for inducing labor.

prostaglandin-synthetase inhibitors: Substances that inhibit the synthesis of prostaglandins.

prosthesis: Artificial substitutes, often mechanical or electrical, used to replace missing body parts.

protective devices: External supports to protect weak or ineffective joints or muscles including braces, protective taping, cushions, and helmets.

protective extension response: Reflexive act consisting of extending one's arms in front of the head to protect the face and head during forward falling.

proteinemia: Excess protein in the blood.

proteinuria: The presence of protein in the urine.

protopathic sensation: Gross sensory abilities in the extremities, allowing one to detect light moving touch, pain, and temperature, but without the ability to make fine discrimination of extent. Pertaining to the somatic sensations of fast, localized pain, slow, poorly localized pain, and temperature.

provider: Person or organization who actually provides the health care.

proximal: From anatomical position, located nearer to the trunk; near the attachment of an extremity to the trunk.

prudence: The ability to govern and discipline oneself through the use of reason.

psychoanalysis: Branch of psychiatry founded by Sigmund Freud, using the techniques of free association, interpretation, and dream analysis.

psychoanalytic theory: Approach to the treatment of neuroses that emphasizes unlocking long-repressed feelings and past experiences in order to allow the patient/client to better understand his/her behavior.

psychodynamic: Any therapy that examines the forces motivating behavior.

psychogenic: Having an emotional or psychological origin.

psychological age: Definition of age based on the functional level of psychological processes rather than on calendar time.

psychological constructs: Psychological concepts; terms (without universal definitions) commonly used to describe mental states.

psychometric instruments: Apparatus and paper-and-pencil techniques for measuring general intelligence, achievement, abilities, and related characteristics.

psychometric techniques (tests): Methods for measuring personality, interest, and attitude (frequently used in psychology).

psychoneuroimmunology: Field of study that links psychological, neural, and immunological processes.

psychosis: A major mental disorder of organic or emotional origin which can cause extreme personality disorganization, loss of reality orientation, and inability to function appropriately in society. Because massage can be used to stimulate or sedate, massage therapy for psychosis needs to be done with the supervision of a qualified health professional.

psychosocial: Pertaining to interpersonal and social interactions that influence behavior and development.

psychosocial development: Erik Erikson's theory of human development throughout the lifespan as a progression of stages named according to the possible outcome.

psychosocial disability: Disorder, impairment, or handicap relating to interpersonal relationships and social interactions that influence behavior and development.

psychosomatic: Psychological foundation for physiological symptoms.

psychotic: Psychological state characterized by hallucinations and delusions.

puberty: Period in life when the individual becomes functionally capable of reproduction.

public good: General welfare or benefit to the majority or large contingent of citizens.

pulmonary embolism: An obstruction of the pulmonary artery or 1 of its branches, usually caused by an embolus from a lower extremity thrombosis.

pulmonary postural drainage: Placing the body in a position that uses gravity to drain fluid from the lungs.

pulse rate: Number of beats per minute as measured on the radial, carotid, femoral, and pedal arteries.

punctuation: A form of tapotement in which the tips of the fingers are used, principally around the heart and the head.

punishment: Providing an aversive stimulus following an appropriate response.

Purkinje cells: Large neurons found in the cerebral cortex, which provide the only output from the cerebellar cortex after the cortex processes sensory and motor signals from the rest of the nervous system.

purpose: The desire to engage in behavior to accomplish a goal.

purposeful activity: Actions that are goal directed.

purposefulness: An individual's plan of action to achieve a goal.

purpura: Hemorrhagic disease which leaves red to purple spots on the skin.

purulent: Consisting of or containing pus.

pyrosis: Burning sensation in the epigastric and sternal region with raising of acid liquid from the stomach; heartburn.

Q

qi gong: *See* chi gong.

qi gong meridian therapy: A natural healing system derived from traditional Chinese medicine that is based on the concept of qi, the vital energy that is an unseen life force that courses through the body enabling the body to perform its functions. Qi permeates all of nature.

quadriplegia (QUAD): Paralysis of all 4 extremities.

qualification: A qualifying or being qualified with the skill, knowledge, and experience that fits a person for a position, office, or profession.

qualitative: Subjective elements.

qualitative research: Methods for knowing that consider the unique properties of a natural setting without a reliance on quantitative data.

quality assurance (QA): Maintenance of quality by constant measuring and comparison to set standards. Quality maintenance problems may be identified and corrected through this procedure.

quality improvement (QI): Continuous improvement of performance; sometimes referred to as continuous quality improvement, or CQI.

quality of care: Providing the optimal care in any practice setting.

quality of life: The degree of satisfaction that an individual has regarding a particular style of life. Concept defined by an individual's perceptions of overall satisfaction with his/her living circumstances, including physical status and abilities, psychological well being, social interactions, and economic conditions; the degree of satisfaction that an individual has regarding a particular style of life.

quantitative: Measurable.

quantum: As in the quantum theory, a fixed elemental unit, as of energy, angular momentum, and other physical properties of physics.

quantum energetics: An energy healing system that utilizes numerical codes that correspond to the vibrational frequencies of the body and also applied kinesiology.

quantum touch: An energy focusing system that uses the practitioners high vibrational field to elevate the client's field to match it and promote healing.

R

race: Group of people united or classified together on the basis of common history, nationality, or geographical distribution.

radiance technique: A science of universal energy. Students of radiance technique learn a basic 12 step program of hands-on self treatment.

radical mastectomy: Removal of the entire breast and lymph nodes.

radiography: Commonly referred to as an "x-ray."

radix: A form of psychotherapeutic bodywork that deepens the experience of living.

raindrop technique: An application technique originally developed for the treatment of scoliosis that uses essential oils and massage.

ramus: A branch; used in anatomical nomenclature as a general term to designate a smaller structure given off by a larger one, such as a blood vessel or a nerve.

randomization: Process of assigning participants or objects to a control or experimental group on a random basis.

random practice: Tasks practiced in a mixed order.

range of motion (ROM): Path of motion a joint can move in any one direction, measured in degrees. The space, distance, or angle through which movement occurs at a joint or a series of joints.

rapid eye movement (REM): Sleep state where brain waves show an active pattern; dreaming is occurring. This state is thought to be important for adequate rest, repair, immunity, and health.

rapport: Harmonious relationship between people.

raw score: Unadjusted score derived from observations of performance; frequently, the arithmetic sum of a subject's responses.

rayid method: A system of interpretation of the patterns in the iris of the eye.

reaction time (RT): The interval between the application of a stimulus and the detection of a response. The time required to initiate a movement following stimulus presentation.

reactivity: Characteristic of assessment instruments whereby the act of administering the assessment changes the behavior of the person being evaluated, thus distorting the representatives of the findings.

reality orientation: Therapeutic technique often used with confused or disoriented patients/clients. Includes both group techniques to remind the patient/client of facts, and patterned environment which provides memory cues.

reappraisal: In coping, reconsideration of a harm, threat, or loss episode after an initial appraisal has taken place. It is thought that during coping, individuals constantly reassess the stressful episode and their resources and alternatives for dealing with it.

reasonable accommodations (RA): In order to allow equal opportunity to a worker with a disability, a company may modify the work environment by doing things such as job restructuring, providing adaptable equipment, or making other such adjustments for modification.

reasoning: The use of one's ability to think and draw conclusions, motives, causes, or justifications that will form the basis of actions.

rebalancing: A combination of energy balancing, joint release, deep tissue massage, and dialogue to relieve pain and induce emotional healing and relaxation. A combination of the best of several therapies: Rolfing, Trager, pulsation therapy, psychotherapy, and craniosacral therapy.

rebound phenomenon: Inability to stop a resisted muscle contraction, such that movement of the limb occurs when the resistance is unexpectedly withdrawn from the limb.

reciprocal: Present or existing on both sides expressing mutual, corresponding, or complementary action.

reciprocal innervation: Excitatory innervation of synergists and inhibitory innervation of antagonists. The function is to permit the action of the group of synergists to reinforce one another while eliminating the action of the antagonistic muscles that would oppose the particular movement, either slowing the movement or preventing it.

reciprocity: Mutual exchange between entities. For instance, reciprocity between states for licensing of therapists whereby one state accepts the licensing qualifications of another state.

recognition: A recognizing or being recognized as an object, person, accomplishment, or place. Identification of a person, place, or object.

reduction: Realignment of a dislocated bone to its original position.

reductionistic: An approach to understanding wherein the problem is broken into parts, and the parts are viewed and managed separately.

re-entry programs: Rehabilitation programs designed to maximize independence; usually the final rehabilitation program after hospitalization and rehabilitation programs are completed. Re-entry programs are often outpatient or community programs.

reexamination: The process by which patient/client status is updated following the initial examination, due to new clinical indications, failure to respond to interventions, or failure to establish progress from baseline data.

referral: A recommendation that a patient/client seek service from another health care provider or resource.

referred pain: Visceral pain felt in a somatic area away from the actual source of pain.

reflective healing: A form of energy healing utilizing a combination of guided imagery and energy body manipulations to heal a specific joint or body organ.

reflex: Subconscious, involuntary reaction to an external stimulus.

reflexognosy: The application of appropriate pressure to the legs and feet to bring about physiological and psychological changes in the body.

reflux: Back flow of any substance (eg, urine from bladder to ureters or food returning to the esophagus from the stomach).

refractive error: Nearsightedness (myopia), farsightedness (hyperopia), astigmatism, or presbyopia. All conditions are improved with corrective lenses.

regression: A retreat or backward movement in conditions, signs, and symptoms (eg, returning to behavior patterns that were characteristic of a previous stage of development).

rehabilitation: Helping individuals regain skills and abilities that have been lost as a result of illness, injury or disease, disorder or incarceration. The restoration of a disabled individual to maximum independence commensurate with his/her limitations.

Reichian release: Manipulation of the musculoskeletal system is used to release emotional blockages from the body.

reiki: The combining of universal energy with individual energy to open pathways for healing. This energy healing method involves placing the hands on or just above the body in order to align chakras and bring healing energy to organs and glands.

reiki-alchemia: A union of reiki and alchemia.

reinforcement: Desired outcome of behavior. In behavior therapy, reinforcement is provided to encourage specific activities, strengthened by fear of punishment or anticipation of reward.

relative value unit (RVU): An index of measure for Medicare resource-based relative value scale.

relaxation: Techniques that increase relaxation by reducing tension (eg, biofeedback, systematic relaxation exercises).

relaxation techniques: A cognitive treatment technique that addresses muscle tension accompanying pain.

release phenomenon: Ongoing action of one part of the central nervous system without modulation from a complementary functional component.

reliability: Predictability of an outcome, regardless of observer. In diagnosis, refers to the probability that several therapists will apply the same label to a given individual.

remission: Lessening in severity or abatement of symptoms of a disease.

repetition maximum (RM): Maximum weight that can be lifted in isotonic contraction. One RM = maximum that can be lifted 1 time; two RM = maximum weight that can be lifted twice, etc.

reposturing dynamics: A system of stretches and massage techniques designed to restore balance and flexibility to the body.

reprimand: Expression of disapproval of conduct.

reprivatize: Return responsibility to the private sector as opposed to public responsibility.

research: Systematic investigation, including development, testing, and evaluation design.

resistance: Amount of weight to be moved.

resistance exercise training: Exercise that applies sufficient force to muscle groups to improve muscle strength.

resonance: The prolongation and intensification of sound produced by the transmission of its vibrations to a cavity, especially a sound elicited by percussion. Decrease in resonance is called dullness; absence of resonance is called flatness.

resonant kinesiology: A meditative form of educational bodywork utilizing sound, movement, and touch to promote health.

resource-based relative value system (RBRVS): A system of reimbursement being developed by Medicare for outpatient service based on assessing the intensity and complexity of a service and assigning a numerical value and dollar amount related to that value.

respiration: The act or process of breathing; inhaling and exhaling air. The processes by which a living organism or cell takes in oxygen from the air or water, distributes and utilizes it in oxidation, and gives off products of oxidation, esp. carbon dioxide.

respiratory failure: Failure of the pulmonary system in which inadequate exchange of carbon dioxide and oxygen occurs between an organism and its environment.

respite care: Short-term health services to the dependent adult, either at home or in an institutional setting.

response speed: The time elapsed between presentation of a stimulus and the patient's/client's initiation of movement.

responsivity: Level that the sensory input facilitates reaction or noticing.

restoration therapy: A full body treatment performed mostly with the elbow. It is a combination of amma, acupressure, shiatsu, lomi lomi, herbology, reflexology, and Western massage.

restraints: Devices used to aid in immobilization of patients/clients.

rest/relaxation: Performance during time not devoted to other activity and during time devoted to sleep.

retention: Resistance to movement or displacement.

retirement planning: Preparing for retirement financially, considering leisure and instrumental activities, and planning for residence and travel prior to retiring from a job or career.

retrograde amnesia: The inability to recall events that have occurred during the period immediately preceding a brain injury.

retrospective memory: Remembering information that occurred in the past.

retrospective recording: Waiting until the evaluation is completed to record observations of patient/client function.

retroviruses: A group of RNA viruses causing a variety of diseases in humans. This group of viruses have RNA as their genetic code, and are capable of copying RNA and DNA and incorporating them into an infected cell.

Rh factor: Hereditary blood factor found in red blood cells determined by specialized blood tests; when present, a person is Rh positive; when absent, a person is Rh negative.

rheumatism: A general term for acute and chronic conditions of soreness and stiffness of joints, muscles, and associated structures.

ribonucleic acid (RNA): Basic genetic material in which a nucleic acid is associated with the control of chemical activities within a cell.

righting reactions: Stimuli go through the labyrinths and to tactile receptors in the trunk, neck, and ears and function to keep the upper part of the body upright and to maintain the head and trunk in their proper relationship.

right-left discrimination: The ability to distinguish right- from left-sidedness.

right to die: A person's right to die on his/her terms.

right-to-know law: Law that dictates that employers must inform their employees of any chemical hazards or health effects caused by toxic substances used in each workplace.

rigidity: Hypertonicity of agonist and antagonist that offers a constant, uniform resistance to passive movement. The affected muscles seem unable to relax and are in a state of contraction even at rest.

risk factors: Factors that cause a person or group of people to be particularly vulnerable to an unwanted, unpleasant, or unhealthy event.

risky shift: Type of group polarization of which the post discussion behaviors of individuals are less safe than before the group discussion.

robotics: Science of mechanical devices that work automatically or by remote control.

roentgenogram: An x-ray. A film produced by roentgenography.

Ro-Hun transformation therapy: A form of energy healing in which the practitioner manipulates the client's energy bodies near each chakra.

role: Set of behaviors that have some socially agreed-upon functions and for which there is an accepted code of norms.

role competence: Achievement of the behaviors which have some socially agreed-upon function and for which there is an accepted code of behavioral norms or expectations.

role conflict: Occurs when a person encounters pressures within an important role that are in opposition to another valued role.

Rolfing structural integration: Founded by American biochemist Dr. Ida Rolf in the 1940s, Rolfing utilizes physical manipulation and movement awareness to bring head, shoulders, thorax, pelvis, and legs into vertical alignment.

Romberg's sign: Inability to maintain body balance when the eyes open and then eyes closed with the feet close together; unsteadiness when eyes are closed indicates a loss of proprioceptive control.

Rosen method bodywork: Physical and emotional awareness is brought about by gentle, non-invasive touch. Focusing on the changes in the breath leads to awareness of the client's inner process.

rotation: Movement around the long axis of a limb.

rotator cuff: The muscle complex of the shoulder that provides stability of the glenohumeral joint inclusive of the suprispinatus, infraspinatue, teres minor, and subscapularis muscles.

rote: Habit performance without meaning.

routines: Occupations with established sequences.

routine supervision: Direct contact at least every 2 weeks at the site of work, with interim supervision occurring by other methods, such as telephone or written communication.

rubefacient: A medicine for external application that produces redness of the skin.

rules-oriented style: Main assumption in this style is that people require reinforcement from the manager to function. This manager does things by the book; enforcing policies, rules, and procedures with employees ensures motivation and achievement.

Rubenfeld synergy method: Founded by Ilana Rubenfeld, this method integrated elements of the body/mind teachers—FM Alexander and Moshe Feldenkrais, together with the Gestalt theory and practice of Fritz and Milton Erickson. The method uses many avenues, including verbal expression, movement, breathing patterns, body posture, kinesthetic awareness, imagination, sound, and caring touch to access reservoirs of feeling.

rumination: Repetitive chewing of food; regurgitated after ingestion.

rupture: A bursting or the state of being broken apart.

Russian massage: A combination of shiatsu, acupressure, classic Swedish massage, sports medicine, reflexology, Upledger cranial sacral, and various neuromuscular disciplines.

safety grab bars: Bars mounted on bath tub walls that provide a person with a secure fixture to hold and prevent falling.

sagittal plane: Runs from front to back, dividing the body into left and right segments.

St. John's neuromuscular therapy: A form of bodywork developed by Paul St. John that focuses on 5 basic principles—biomechanics, ischemias, trigger points, postural distortion, and nerve entrapment and compression. Attention is also given to hormonal balance, nutrition, and the elimination of toxins.

salt rubs/salt glows: Salt is added to oil and used to scrub the skin to remove dead surface cells and dirt. It also lubricates the skin.

sample of behavior: Selected test items chosen because they constitute a subset of the behaviors that need to be assessed.

sarcoidosis: A disorder that may affect any part of the body but most frequently involving the lymph nodes, liver, spleen, lungs, eyes, and small bones of the hands and feet; characterized by the presence in all affected organs or tissues of epitheloid cell tubercles, without caseation, and with little or no round-cell reaction, becoming converted, in the older lesions, into a rather hyaline featureless fibrous tissue.

sarcoma: Malignant tissue that originates in connective tissue and spreads through the bloodstream, often attacking bones.

satellite trigger point: A trigger point created by another distant trigger point.

scanning: Technique for making selections on a device such as a communication aid, computer, or environmental control system. Scanning involves moving sequentially through a given set of choices and making a selection when the desired position is reached. Types of scanning include automatic, manual, row-and-column, and directed.

scapegoat: A symbolic person or thing blamed for other problems.

scapula: Flattened, triangular bone found on the posterior aspect of the body. It is part of the pectoral girdle, which joins the clavicle and humerus.

schemata: Basic units of all knowledge. Each simple organization of experience and knowledge by the mind make up the original "schema" or framework that represents our everyday experiences. Each experience, thought, and idea is a structural element in an organizational matrix that integrates each person's experiences and history into a meaningful set of categories, each filled with data from one's memory of prior events.

schema theory: Notion that standard routine performances occur in given situations in a typical sequence and with typical kinds of participants; within the general framework or structure the details of a given performance may vary but the basic structure remains consistent.

schemes: Structural elements of cognition; plans, designs, or programs to be followed.

schizophrenia (Sz): Pervasive psychosis that affects a variety of psychological processes involving cognition, affect, and behavior, and is characterized by hallucinations, delusions, bizarre behavior, and illogical thinking.

school professionals: School principals, program directors, and directors of special education are committee members who interpret local administrative policies in special education.

sciatica: Nerve inflammation characterized by sharp pains along the sciatic nerve and its branches; area extends from the hip down the back of the thigh and surrounding parts.

scissors gait: Gait in which the legs cross the midline upon advancement.

scleroderma: Disease characterized by chronic hardening and shrinking of the connective tissue of any organ in the body.

scoliosis: Abnormal lateral curvature of the spine. This usually consists of 2 curves, the original abnormal curve and a compensatory curve in the opposite direction. Consult with the patient's physician before applying massage therapy. Massage techniques could increase the severity of scoliosis.

scope of practice: Encompassing all of the skills, knowledge, and expertise required to practice a profession, such as massage therapy.

screening: Review of a patient's/client's case to determine if services are necessary. Determining the need for further examination or consultation by a therapist or for referral to another health professional.

screening instrument: Assessment device used for purposes of identifying potential problem areas for further in-depth evaluation.

script: General sequence of events about a common routine or scenario, usually with a common goal.

seasonal affective disorder (SAD): Mood disorder associated with shorter days and longer nights of autumn and winter. Symptoms include lethargy, depression, social withdrawal, and work difficulties.

seated massage: Techniques that provide fully-clothed seated bodywork and somatic therapies to clients generally in corporate or business settings. Practitioners use shiatsu, amma, and/or Swedish techniques.

seborrhea: Disease of the sebaceous glands marked by the increase in amount and quality of their secretions.

secondary aging: Changes in physical functioning as a result of aging, that are not universal or inevitable, but are commonly shared by humans as a result of environmental conditions or circumstances.

secondary care: Intervention provided once a disease state has been identified (eg, treating hypertension).

secondary conditions: Also called secondary disabilities. Pathology, impairment, or functional limitations derived from the primary condition.

secondary prevention: Efforts directed at populations who are considered "at risk" by early detection of potential health problems, followed by the interventions to halt, reverse, or at least slow the progression of that condition.

secretion: The process of elaborating a specific product as a result of the activity of a gland. This activity may range from separating a specific substance of the blood to the elaboration of a new chemical substance.

sedative effect: To experience soothing or quieting influences.

sedentary work: Exerting up to 10 pounds of force occasionally or a negligible amount of force frequently to lift, carry, push, pull, or otherwise move objects.

seizure disorders: Presence of abrupt, irrepressible episodes of electrical hyperactivity in the brain.

selective abstraction: Focusing on one insignificant detail while ignoring the more important features of a situation.

self-actualization: Process of striving to achieve one's ultimate potential in life with accompanying feelings of accomplishment and personal growth.

self-care: The set of activities that comprise daily living, such as bed mobility, transfers, ambulation, dressing, grooming, bathing, eating, and toileting.

self-care activities: Personal activities an individual performs to prepare for and maintain a daily routine.

self-concept: View one has of oneself (eg, ideas, feelings, attitudes, identity, worth, capabilities, and limitations).

self-control: Ability to control one's behaviors.

self-deprecator: Type of person who seeks praise by devaluing him/herself; successful attention-getter initially, but fails over the longer term when other group members become aware of circumstances.

self-efficacy: An individual's belief that he/she is capable of successfully performing a certain set of behaviors.

self-esteem: An individual's overall feeling of worth.

self-expression: An individual's ability to make his/her thoughts and feelings known.

self-fulfilling prophecy: A principle that refers to a belief in or the expectation of a particular outcome as a factor that contributes to its fulfillment.

self-help: Various methods by which individuals attempt to remedy their difficulties without making use of formal care providers (eg, Alcoholics Anonymous).

self-identity skill: Ability to perceive oneself as holistic and autonomous, and to have permanence and continuity over time.

self-image: Internalized view a person holds of him/herself which usually varies with changing social situations over one's lifespan.

self-monitoring: Process whereby the patient/client records specific behaviors or thoughts as they occur.

self-report: Type of assessment approach where the individual reports on his/her level of function or performance.

semantic memory: Memory for general knowledge.

semantics: The study of language with special attention to the meanings of words and other symbols.

semi-autonomous: Individual is partially dependent upon another for the satisfaction of needs.

semicircular canals: Organ in the inner ear that transmits information about head position.

senile dementia: An organic mental disorder resulting from generalized atrophy of the brain with no evidence of cerebrovascular disease.

sensation: Receiving conscious sensory impressions through direct stimulation of the body, such as hearing, seeing, touching, etc.

sense of control: Perception of being able to direct and regulate.

sense of security: Feeling of comfort in being able to trust, in knowing that there is predictability in the environment.

sensitivity: Capacity to feel, transmit, and react to a stimulus; rating of how well changes will be measured on subsequent tests to show improvement.

sensitivity to stimuli: Due to low thresholds, persons who act in accordance with those thresholds tend to seem hyperactive or distractible. They have a hard time staying on tasks to complete them or to learn from their experiences, because their low neurological thresholds keep directing their attention from one stimulus to the next, whether it is part of the ongoing task or not.

sensitization: An acquired reaction; the process of a receptor becoming more susceptible to a given stimulus.

sensorimotor therapy: Therapy planned to enhance the integration of reflex phenomena and the emergence of voluntary motor behaviors concerned with posture and locomotion.

sensory: Having to do with sensations or the senses; including peripheral sensory processing (eg, sensitivity to touch) and cortical sensory processing (eg, two-point and sharp/dull discrimination).

sensory awareness: Understanding of sensory signals.

sensory conflict: Situations in which sensory signals that are expected to match do not match, either between systems (vision, somatosensory, or vestibular) or within a system (left versus right sides).

sensory defensiveness: Constellation of symptoms that are the result of adversive or defensive reactions to non-noxious stimuli across 1 or more sensory modalities.

sensory deprivation: An involuntary loss of physical awareness caused by detachment from external sensory stimuli, which can result in psychological disturbances. An enforced absence of the usual repertoire of sensory stimuli producing sever mental changes, including hallucinations, anxiety, depression, and insanity.

sensory environment: The conditions which exist in the real world around us that impact balance (ie, darkness, visual movement, complaint surfaces, etc).

sensory integration (SI): Ability of the central nervous system to process sensory information to make an adaptive response to the environment; also refers to a therapeutic intervention that uses strong kinesthetic and proprioceptive stimulation to attempt to better organize the central nervous system. The ability to integrate information from the environment to produce normal movement. The organization of sensory input for use, a perception of the body or environment, an adaptive response, a learning process, or the development of some neural function.

sensory integrative dysfunction: A disorder or irregularity in brain function that makes sensory integration difficult. Many, but not all, learning disorders stem from sensory integrative dysfunctions.

sensory integrative therapy: Therapy involving sensory stimulation and adaptive responses to it according to a patient's/client's neurological needs. Treatment usually involves full body movements that provide vestibular, proprioceptive, and tactile stimulation. The goal is to improve the brain's ability to process and organize sensations.

sensory memory: Memory store that holds sensory input in its uninterpreted sensory form for a very brief period of time.

sensory neuron: Nerve cell that sends signals to the spinal cord or brain.

sensory processing: Brain's ability to receive information and respond appropriately.

sensory registration: Brain's ability to receive input and select what will receive attention and what will be inhibited from consciousness.

sensory stimulation: Therapeutic intervention that makes use of patterned sensory input.

sensory testing: Evaluation of sensory system.

sensory training: General term for therapy aimed at enabling a person to regain contact with his/her environment; usually offered in groups, sensory training includes social introductions among the group, body-awareness exercises, and sensory activities utilizing objects.

sepsis: Poisoning that is caused by the products of a putrefractive process. Infection.

septicemia: Systemic disease associated with the presence and persistence of pathogenic microorganisms or toxins in the blood.

sequencing: Putting things in order. Ability to accomplish a task in a logistical order.

serial speech: Overlearned speech involving a series of words, such as counting and reciting the days of the week.

serology: Study of blood serum.

set: A belief or expectation one has about a person, place, or thing.

severe retardation: Within an IQ range of 20 to 34.

sex identification: Assigning of a masculine or feminine connotation to a given activity.

sexuality: The behaviors that relate psychological, cultural, emotional, and physical responses to the need to reproduce.

sexually transmitted disease (STD): A contagious disease usually acquired by sexual intercourse or genital contact.

shadow integration: Self-examination based upon Carl Jung's theory of the shadow self. This is the part of us where we place our negative thoughts and feelings.

shaken baby syndrome: A condition of whiplash-type injuries, ranging from bruises on the arms and trunk to retinal hemorrhages or convulsions, as observed in infants and children who have been violently shaken; a form of child abuse which often results in intracrancial bleeding from tearing of cerebral blood vessels.

shaman: An individual who changes his or her state of consciousness to contact or travel to another reality to obtain power and knowledge. He or she then returns home to use that power and knowledge to help him- or herself or others.

shearing: Pressure exerted against the surface and layers of the skin as tissues slide in opposite but parallel planes.

sheltered housing: Living arrangements (eg, group homes) that provide structure and supervision for individuals who do not require institutionalization but are not fully capable of independent living.

SHEN therapy: An acronym for specific human energy nexus. SHEN therapy is an energy therapy that discharges debilitating emotions.

shiatsu: A finger-pressure technique utilizing the traditional acupuncture points of Oriental healing.

shingles: Viral disease of the peripheral nerves with the eruption of skin vesicles along the path of the nerve.

shinkiko: The study of the non-physical world in relation to the physical world. A kind of medical qi gong.

shock therapy: Induced by delivering an electric current through the brain; a procedure used for treating depression.

short-term memory: Limited capacity memory store that holds information for a brief period of time; the so-called "working memory."

shoulder separation: Separation of the acromioclavicular joint due to trauma, injury, or disease.

shoulder subluxation: Incomplete downward, usually partial, dislocation of the humerus out of the glenohumeral joint caused by weakness, stretch, or abnormal tone in the scapulohumeral and/or scapular muscles.

shunt: Passage between 2 natural channels, especially blood vessels.

side effect: Other than the desired action (eg, effect produced by a drug).

signage: Displayed verbal, symbolic, tactile, or pictorial information.

signal risk factors: Workers exposed to these factors are at greater risk for developing work-related musculoskeletal disorders. The factors are: fixed or awkward work posture for more than 2 hours; performance of the same motion or motion pattern every few seconds for more than a total of 2 hours; use of vibrating or impact tools or equipment for more than a total of 1 hour; and unassisted frequent or forceful manual handling for more than 1 hour.

sign of behavior: Patient's/client's responses that are viewed as "indirect manifestations" (or signs) of one's underlying personality.

simple fracture: Bone is broken internally but does not pierce the skin so that it can be seen.

simple reflex: Reflex with a motor nerve component that involves only 1 muscle.

single trait sample: Evaluation that focuses on the assessment of a single worker trait.

situational assessment: Assesses the person's performance under each circumstance of a realistic work situation by systematically altering variables such as production demands and stress factors.

situation-specific: In psychosocial assessment, those behaviors and tasks that must be mastered to function every day in a particular environment.

skeletal demineralization: The loss of bone mass due to loss of minerals from the bone, as seen in conditions like osteoporosis.

skeletal system: Supporting framework for the body that is comprised of the axial and appendicular divisions.

skilled nursing facility (SNF): Institution or part of an institution that meets criteria for accreditation established by the sections of the Social Security Act that determine the basis for Medicaid and Medicare reimbursement. Provides care that must be rendered by or under the supervision of professional personnel such as a registered nurse. The care must be required daily and must be a continuation of the care begun in the hospital.

skin fold measurement: Method for estimating percent body fat by measuring subcutaneous fat with skin fold calipers.

skin sensitivity, abnormal: When a condition is present that results in abnormal levels of pain when the skin is contacted by another. Massage therapy is contraindicated due to the increased pain levels experienced by the client.

slapping: A type of tapotement using the flat open palms of each hand in an alternating rhythmic pattern.

sleep apnea: Disorder characterized by periods of an absence of attempts to breathe; person is momentarily unable to move respiratory muscles or maintain air flow through nose and mouth.

sleep paralysis: Temporary inability to talk or move when falling asleep or waking up.

SOAP (subjective, objective, assessment, plan): The 4 parts of a written account of a health problem.

social: Having to do with human beings living together as a group in a situation in which their dealings with one another affect their common welfare.

social age: Definition of age emphasizing the functional level of social interaction skills rather than calendar time.

social climate: Combined variables in the social environment that directly or indirectly influence individual behavior, and that are influenced by individual behavior.

social clock: Set of internalized beliefs that forms the standards that individuals use in assessing their conformity to age-appropriate expectations.

social conduct: Behavior in a group.

social disadvantage or handicap: Results when an individual is not able to fulfill a role that he/she expects or is required to fill.

social environment: Those social systems or networks within which a given person operates; the collective human relationships of individuals, whether familial, communal, or organizational in nature, constitute the social environment of that individual.

socialization: Development of the individual as a social being and a participant in society that results from a continuing, changing interaction between a person and those who attempt to influence him/her.

social modeling theory: Maintains that learning is accomplished through observing others. A person may learn a behavior or its consequences by watching another person experience that behavior.

social systems: Organized interactions among individuals, as within marriages, families, communities, and organizations, both formal and informal.

socket: The part of a prosthesis into which a stump of the remaining limb fits.

soft tissue integrity: Health of the connective tissue of the body.

soft tissue release (Taws technique): A coordinated and very precise movement is applied in a systematic compression and extension of a muscle resulting in relief from pain in as little as one treatment.

software: Programs that run on computers.

solitary play: Play in which a child is completely involved in the activity and blocks out the surroundings both physically and psychologically.

soma: Cell body of a nerve that contains the nucleus. A 10 session series that structurally balances the body in gravity and integrates the nervous system through manipulation of the fascia.

soma neuromuscular integration: A system of bodywork that works by way of the fascial network to release chronic, stored structural aberrations, and effectively realign the entire body.

somatic education: A technique that uses posture and movement, monitored by the practitioner, to guide the client through specific, slow, gentle movements. The movement explorations remind the brain how to efficiently use the muscles.

somatic experiencing: A naturalistic approach to the healing of trauma.

somatic nervous system: Portion of the nervous system composed of a motor division that excites skeletal muscles and a sensory division that receives and processes sensory input from the sense organs.

somatic psychology: A body-based psychological treatment that brings the client to an awareness of their own experience of sensation, tension, relaxation, breath, response, and evoked thoughts.

somato-emotional release: A therapeutic technique that uses and expands on the principles of cranial-sacral therapy to help rid the mind and body of the residual effects of trauma.

somatoform disorders: Group of mental disorders characterized by (a) loss or alteration in physical functioning, for which there is no physiological explanation, (b) evidence that psychological factors have caused the physical symptoms, (c) lack of voluntary control over physical symptoms, and (d) indifference by the patient/client to the physical loss.

sores: Any type of tender or painful ulcer or lesion of the skin or mucous membrane. Massage of wounded area is contraindicated to prevent further damage; nearby healthy tissues may be massaged.

sound therapy: The use of sound in its various forms as a tool for healing.

spasm: An involuntary muscle contraction.

spastic diplegia: An increase in postural tonus that is distributed primarily in the lower extremities and the pelvic area.

spastic gait: Stiff movement, toes drag, legs held together, hip and knee joints are slightly flexed.

spasticity: Increase in the muscle tone and stretch reflex of a muscle resulting in increased resistance to passive stretch of the muscle and hyper-responsivity of the muscle to sensory stimulation.

spastic quadriplegia: An increase in postural tonus that is distributed throughout all 4 extremities. These findings are often coexistent with relatively lower tone in the trunk and severe difficulty in controlling posture.

spatial awareness: Ability to orient oneself in space, to visualize what an object looks like from all angles, to know where sounds are coming from, and to know where body parts are in space.

spatial relations: Ability to perceive the self in relation to other objects.

special interest groups: Collectives of individuals and organizations who are bound by beliefs about specific issues or populations, and who seek to influence decisions about the allocation of resources.

specialized battery: Tests that measure a specific component (eg, cognitive functioning, such as attention or language).

specificity: Instrument's ability to accurately identify subjects possessing a specific trait.

speech: The meaningful production and sequencing of sounds by the speech sensorimotor system (eg, lips, tongue, etc) for the transmission of spoken language.

sphygmomanometer: Instrument used to measure arterial blood pressure indirectly.

spinal: An injection of anesthesia into the spinal fluid to produce numbness.

spinal fusion: Joining together spinal vertebrae to prevent damage to the bones or spinal cord from disease processes.

spinal nerve: Nerve extending from the spinal cord.

spinal release: A technique that allows the therapist to correct distortions of the central nervous system and restore the body's center of gravity.

spinocerebellar tracts: Dorsal tract consisting of the afferent ipsilateral ascending tract to cerebellum serving mostly lower extremities for touch, pressure, and proprioception. The ventral tract consisting of the afferent contralateral ascending tract to cerebellum serving lower extremities for proprioception.

spinothalamic tract: Afferent contralateral and ipsilateral ascending tract to thalamus for sensation of pain, temperature, and light (erude) touch. *Synonym*: anterolateral system (ALS).

spiritual: Having to do with the vital principle believed to give life to physical organisms.

spiritual meaning: Meaning, usually symbolic, related to one's concerns with matters that transcend physical life.

spirometry: The measurement of air inspired and expired.

splint: Supportive device used to immobilize, fix, or prevent deformities or assist in motion. Support of a body segment through application of an external device. *Static*: Customized and prefabricated splints, inhibitory casts, and spinal and other braces that are designed to maintain joints in a desired position. *Dynamic*: Customized and prefabricated supports that allow for or control motion while providing support.

spondylitis: Inflammation of the vertebrae.

spondylolisthesis: Forward displacement of one vertebra over another, usually of the fifth lumbar vertebra over the body of the sacrum, or the fourth lumbar over the fifth.

spontaneous remission: Unusual occurrence (eg, when cancer cells revert back to normal without aid or apparent cause).

sports massage: A type of massage therapy designed specifically for those involved in athletic activities. Before applying massage, pay close attention to any physical conditions or medications that could be contraindicated for massage therapy.

sprain: Injury to a joint that causes pain and disability, with the severity depending on the degree of injury to ligaments or tendons. An injury to a joint resulting in tearing or stretching of the ligaments. Massage therapy is contraindicated until the injury reaches the subacute stage; massage with caution thereafter.

spreadsheet: Type of computer software organized in section or table format used in financial management and accounting systems.

sputum: Substance expelled by coughing or clearing the throat. Matter ejected from the lungs, bronchi, and trachea through the mouth.

stabilizer: Any muscle that acts to fix one attachment of a prime mover or hold a bone steady to provide a foundation for movement; equipment or device used to maintain a particular position.

staff development: Various educational resources for professionals that are used to attain new skills and knowledge.

staging: Classification of tumors by their spread through the body.

standard assessment: Tests and evaluation approaches with specific norms, standards, and protocol.

standard deviation: Mathematically determined value used to derive standard scores and compare raw scores to a unit normal distribution.

standard error: Possible range in the variability of a person's "true" score in a test; a number that recognizes the amount by which a score might vary on different days or in different situations.

standard error of the mean: Standard deviation of the entire distribution of random sample means, successively selected from a single population.

standardization: Method by which test scores of a typical population are derived, thus allowing subsequent test scores to be analyzed in light of that broad population; standardization requires a rigorous process of data collection and comparison.

standardized battery: A battery of tests in which the testing and scoring procedures are well defined and fixed, and the interpretation involves the use of standardized norms.

standard scores: Raw scores mathematically converted to a scale that facilitates comparison.

state dependent memory: Learning that takes place under a certain set of circumstances is then recalled when that set of circumstances is re-experienced or approximated.

static equilibrium: Ability of an individual to adjust to displacements of his/her center of gravity while maintaining a constant base of support.

static flexibility: Range of motion, in degrees, that a joint will allow.

static stretching: Stretching to the farthest point and then holding that position.

statics: Study of objects at rest.

step test: Graded exercise test in which a person is required to rhythmically step up and down steps of gradually increasing heights.

stereognosis: Ability to identify common objects by touch with vision occluded.

stereopsis: Quality of visual fusion.

stereotypic behavior: Repeated, persistent postures or movements, including vocalizations.

stereotyping: Applying generalized and oversimplified labels of characteristics, actions, or attitudes to a specific socioeconomic, cultural, religious, or ethnic group. Often used to belittle or discount a particular group.

stethoscope: Instrument used to listen to heart and lung sounds.

stigma: An undesirable difference that becomes a basis for separating an individual bearing such traits from the rest of society.

stimulation: Arousal of attention, interest, or tension.

stimulus-arousal properties: Alerting potential of various sensory stimuli, generally thought to be related to their intensity, pace, and novelty.

storage fat: Adipose tissue found primarily subcutaneously that surrounds the major organs.

strabismus: Oculomotor misalignment of one eye.

strain: Usually a muscular injury caused by the excessive physical effort that leads to a forcible stretch. Refers to the percent change in original length of a deformed tissue.

strain/counterstrain: A non-invasive treatment that helps decrease protective muscle spasms and alleviate somatic dysfunction in the musculosketal system through the use of palpation and passive positional procedures.

strain counterstrain techniques: Therapy techniques that assist the elongation of the muscle by using the force of the contracting muscle.

strategy: A plan of action.

strength: Nonspecific term relating to muscle contraction, often referring to the force generated by a single maximal isometric contraction. Force-generating capacity of muscle.

strengthening: *Active*: A form of strength-building exercise in which the therapist applies resistance through the range of motion of active movement. *Assistive*: A form of strength-building exercise in which the therapist assists the patient/client through the available range of motion. *Resistive*: Any form of active exercise in which a dynamic or static muscular contraction is resisted by an outside force. The external force may be applied manually or mechanically.

stress: Individual's general reaction to external demands or stressors. Stress results in psychological as well as physiological reactions. *Biomechanical*: The force developed in a deformed tissue divided by the tissue's cross-sectional area.

stress incontinence: A type of urinary incontinence which occurs when the bladder pressure exceeds urethral resistance and sphincter activity is weak or absent.

stress management techniques: Methods of relieving or controlling chronic stress by interrupting reflexive neurologic stress reactions.

stressors: External events that place demands on an individual above the ordinary.

stretch: Temporary lengthening of tissues that is not maintained for a sufficient period of time to encourage collagen remodeling.

stretching: Drawing out or extending to full length.

stripping and ligation: Removal and tying off of a vein.

stroke: Syndrome characterized by a sudden onset in which blood vessels in the brain have become narrowed or blocked. *Synonym*: cerebrovascular accident.

stroke volume (SV): The amount of blood ejected from the left ventricle on one beat. *Maximum stroke volume* is the highest volume of blood expelled from the heart during a single beat. This value is usually reached when exercise is only about 40% to 50% of maximum exercise capacity.

structural energetic therapy: A combination of cranial/structural techniques, myofascial unwinding, myofascial restructuring, emotional energy release, kinesiology, and postural analysis.

structural integration: Based on the work of Dr. Ida P. Rolf, structural integration centers on the idea the entire structural order of the body needs to be realigned and balanced with the gravitational forces around a central vertical line representing gravity's influence. *See* Rolfing structural integration.

structural theory: Dividing of the mind into 3 structures: the id, the ego, and the superego.

structured activities: Activities that have rules and can be broken down into manageable steps that have been preplanned and preorganized.

sty, stye: Localized circumscribed inflammatory swelling of one of the sebaceous glands of the eyelid. *Synonym*: hordeolum.

subacute: Between acute and chronic.

subacute care: Short-term, comprehensive inpatient level of care.

subacute patient: Medically complex cases requiring a longer period of rehabilitation and recovery, usually 1 to 6 weeks.

subcortical: Region beneath the cerebral cortex.

subculture: Ethnic, regional, economic, or social group exhibiting characteristic patterns of behavior sufficient to distinguish it from others within an embracing culture or society. Does not usually include rejection of the larger culture. Most people are members of several subcultures.

subjective measure: Assessment designed to identify the patient's/client's own view of problems and performance.

sublingual: Under the tongue.

subluxation: Partial or incomplete dislocation (eg, shoulder of patient/client with cerebrovascular accident).

sudomotor: Stimulating the sweat glands.

suffix: Word element of 1 or more syllables added to the end of a combining form in order to change its meaning.

superego: In psychoanalytic theory, 1 of 3 personality components. It houses one's values, ethics, standards, and conscience; an analytic concept that equates roughly to the conscience.

superficial: Area of the body that is located closest to the surface.

superior: Toward the head or upper portion of a part or structure. *Synonym*: cephalad.

supervisor: Any person having authority in the interests of the employer to hire, transfer, lay off, recall, promote, assign, reward, or discipline other employees.

supination (Sup): The act of assuming the supine position. Rotation of the forearm laterally so the palm is facing up toward the ceiling. Applied to the foot, it implies movement resulting in raising of the medial margin of the foot, hence of the longitudinal arch, so that the plantar surface of the foot is facing inward.

supine: Lying on the spine with the face up.

supported employment: Paid employment for people with disabilities without employment or for those whose employment has been interrupted as a result of a severe disability and need support services to perform job-related tasks.

supportive devices: External supports to protect weak or ineffective joints or muscles. Supportive devices include supportive taping, compression garments, corsets, slings, neck collars, serial casts, elastic wraps, and oxygen.

supportive services: Those that enable and empower an individual to function more independently within a community or facility.

suppression: Ability of the central nervous system to screen out certain stimuli so that others may be attended to more carefully.

surfactant: A surface agent.

surgery: The branch of medicine dealing with manual and operative procedures for the correction of deformities and defects, repair of injuries, and diagnosis and cure of certain diseases. Massage therapy is contraindicated both pre and post surgical unless performed under the supervision of a physician.

surrogate: Person or thing that replaces another (eg, substitute parental figure).

swan neck deformity: Condition of the hand characterized by hyperextension of the proximal interphalangeal joint and flexion of the distal interphalangeal joint.

Swedish massage: A vigorous system of treatment designed to energize the body by stimulating circulation. Five basic strokes, all flowing toward the heart, are used to manipulate the soft tissues of the body.

Swedish gymnastics: A form of treatment by movements and exercises in which systematized movements of the body and limbs are regulated by the resistance made by an attendant.

swollen: An abnormal transient enlargement of a surface of the body. Massage of swollen area is contraindicated to prevent damage to the inflamed tissues. Nearby healthy tissue may be massaged.

symbols: Abstract representations of perceived reality.

symmetrical: Equal in size and shape; very similar in relative placement or arrangement about an axis.

sympathetic nervous system: Autonomic nervous system that mobilizes the body's resources during stressful situations.

symptom (Sx): Subjective indication of a disease or a change in condition as perceived by the individual.

synapse: Minuscule space that exists between the end of the axon of one nerve cell and the cell body or dendrites of another.

synaptogenesis: The process of forming "synaptic connections" between nerve cells, or between nerve cells and muscle fibers; the basis of neuronal communication.

syndrome: Combination of symptoms resulting from a single course, or commonly occurring together so that they constitute a distinct clinical picture.

synergism: Action of 2 or more substances, organs, or organisms to achieve an effect of which each is not individually capable.

synergist: Any muscle that functions to inhibit extraneous action from a muscle that would interfere with the action of prime mover.

synergy: Fixed set of muscles contracting with a present sequence and time of contraction.

synovectomy: Excision of the synovial membrane (eg, as in the knee joint).

syntropy insight bodywork: A combination of neuromuscular re-education, hands-on application, qi gong, Taoism, and meditation.

systematic desensitization: Behavioral procedure that uses relaxation paired with an anxiety-provoking stimulus in an attempt to reduce the anxiety response.

systemic: Involving the whole system, such as in systemic rheumatoid arthritis.

systems interactions: The ways the various CNS systems affect or interact with each other in order to provide a more integrative and functional nervous system.

systems model: A conceptual representation which incorporates a set of major functional divisions or systems within the CNS that interlock and interrelate to create the functional whole. Although each division may be considered a whole in and of itself, with multiple subsystems interlocking to form its entire division, each major component or division influences and is influenced by all others, and thus the totality of the CNS is based on the summation of interactions, not individual function.

systems model/approach: A cyclical framework for understanding postural control which includes 1) environmental stimuli, 2) sensory reception, perception, and organization, and 3) motor planning, execution, and modification.

systems theory: A theory describing movements emerging as a result of an interaction among many peripheral and central nervous system components with influence changing depending on the task.

systole: Contraction of the heart, especially of the ventricles, during which blood is forced into the aorta and pulmonary artery. Systolic blood pressure occurs during systole.

tai chi chih: Meditation in motion. It consists of 19 movements and 1 posture.

tai chi chuan: A blend of healing, martial arts, and meditative art. Originally developed for self-defense.

table mechanics: Synonymous with body mechanics; referring to a proper matching of the table characteristics with the physical attributes of the therapist including weight, height, strength, and the modality of work practiced.

tachycardia: Rapid heartbeat.

tachypnea: Excessively rapid respiration marked by quick, shallow breathing.

tacit: Implied understanding that is not verbalized.

tactile defensiveness: Adverse reaction to being touched. A sensory integrative dysfunction characterized by tactile sensations that cause excessive emotional reactions, hyperactivity, or other behavioral problems.

tactile discrimination: Ability to discriminate among objects by the sense of touch.

tactile cues: Perceptible touch stimuli.

taikyo shiatsu: A Japanese form of bodywork that uses compression, point work, stretching, and energy work to balance chi.

tantsu tantric shiatsu: *See* watsu acquatic shiatsu. Tantsu is performed on land.

tapotement: Percussion, including beating, clapping, hacking, and punctuation.

Tara approach: A holistic system for the critical transformation of psychological, physical, and emotional shock and trauma. This work combines the ancient oriental healing art of jin shin with therapeutic dialogues.

target site: Desired site for a drug's action within the body.

task: Work assigned to, selected by, or required of a person related to development of occupational performance skills; collection of activities related to accomplishment of a specific goal.

taxonomy: Laws and principles for classification of living things and organisms; also used for learning objectives.

T cell: A heterogeneous population of lymphocytes comprising helper/inducer T cells and cytotoxic/suppressor T cells.

technology: *See* low-technology.

telecommunication device for the deaf (TDD) or teletypewriter (TTY): Device connected to a telephone by a special adapter, which allows telephone communication between a hearing person and a person with impaired hearing.

telereceptive: The exteroceptors of hearing, sight, and smell that are sensitive to distant stimuli.

tender point: A specific locus of pain or sensitivity.

tendon: Bands of strong fibrous tissue that attach muscles to bones.

tendon injuries: Lacerations, avulsion-type injuries, and crash injuries to the flexor or extensor tendons of the hand; frequently work- or sports-related. Massage therapy is contraindicated for tendon injuries due to the potential for increased injury to tissues.

TENS (transcutaneous electrical nerve stimulation): Application of mild electric stimulation to skin electrodes placed over region of pain to cause interference with the transmission of painful stimuli.

tensile force: Resistive force generated within a tissue in response to elongation or stretch.

tensiometer: Device used to measure force produced from an isometric contraction.

Tera-Mai Seichem: A complete energy system, incorporating all the basic elements of life—air, water, spirit, earth, and fire. Tera-Mai Seichem focuses on the patient's mental, physical, emotional, and spiritual well being.

test protocol: Specific procedures that must be followed when assessing a patient; formal testing procedures.

test-retest reliability: Extent to which repeated administrations of a test to the same people produce the same results.

tests and measures: Specific standardized methods and techniques used to gather data about the patient/client after the history and systems review has been performed.

test sensitivity: An instrument's ability to detect change within a measured variable.

tetany: A syndrome manifested by sharp flexion of joints, especially the wrist and ankle joints, muscle twitching, cramps, and convulsions, sometimes with attacks of difficult breathing.

tetraplegia: Impairment or loss of motor and/or sensory function in the cervical segments of the spinal cord due to damage of neural elements within the spinal cord.

Thai massage (Nuad Bo Rarn): A form of complimentary and integrative medicine based on ancient yoga and ayurvedic sciences. It utilizes yoga positions, yoga therapeutic practices, reflexology, and Thai foot massage.

thalamic pain: CNS pain caused by injury to the thalamus and characterized by contralateral and sometimes migratory pain brought on by peripheral stimulation.

thalassotherapy: A therapy that uses the therapeutic benefits of the sea and seawater products to restore health and vitality to the skin and hair.

theoretical rationale: Reason, based on theory or empirical evidence, for using a particular intervention for a specific person.

theory: Set of interrelated concepts used to describe, explain, or predict phenomena.

therapeutic activities: Activities within the limits of the patient's/client's physical, social, or cognitive capacity.

therapeutic community: Structured inpatient environment designed to provide a rehabilitative experience.

therapeutic effects: The numerous beneficial results of the application of massage techniques to the human body.

therapeutic environment: Organizing all aspects of the environment in a systematic way so that they enhance a patient's/client's abilities to perform desired tasks and activities (mental, emotional, functional).

therapeutic exercise: Exercise interventions directing towards maximizing functional capabilities. A broad range of activities intended to improve strength, range of motion (including muscle length), cardiovascular fitness, or flexibility or to otherwise increase a person's functional capacity.

therapeutic touch: Based on ancient energy healing methods. Practitioners feel or sense energy imbalances in the client and use laying on of hands to disperse blocks and channel healing forces to the client's body.

thermotherapy: Intervention through the application of heat, causing vasodilitation to enhance the healing process. The use of heat or cold for therapeutic purposes.

third-party payment: Payment for services by someone other than the person receiving them.

thoracic: Pertaining to the chest.

thought disorder: Disturbance in thinking, including distorted content (eg, ideas, beliefs, sensory interpretation) and distorted written and spoken language (eg, word salad, loose associations, echolalia).

three-point pressure splints: Type of splint in which the middle force is directed opposite to the 2 distal or end forces. These splints operate through a series of reciprocal forces. Most splints incorporate the three-point pressure design.

threshold: Level at which a stimulus is recognized by sensory receptors.

thrombin: The enzyme derived from prothrombin that converts fibrinogen to fibrin.

thromboplastin: Enzyme that assists in the process of blood clotting.

thrombosis: Coagulation of the blood in the heart or a blood vessel forming a clot. Massage therapy is contraindicated due to the potential for loosening blood clots.

thumping: A form of tapotement; a pounding of the soft tissues of the body.

thyrotropin-releasing hormone: A hormone of the anterior pituitary gland having an affinity for and specifically stimulating the thyroid gland.

Tibetan point holding: As many as 5 practitioners are used to hold points for up to 2 hours. The long period of holding allows time for the client to address internal thoughts as they arise.

tibial torsion: Rotation occurring inherently in the shaft of the tibia from proximal to distal ends.

tic: Spasmodic muscular contraction, usually involving the face, head, and neck.

tinnitus: Subjective ringing or tinkling sound in the ear.

titer: The required quantity of a substance needed to produce a reaction to a given amount of another substance. Titer is synonymous with level.

titration: Volumetric determinations by means of standard solutions of known strength.

tolerance: Physiological and psychological accommodation or adaptation to a chemical agent over time.

tone: State of muscle contraction at rest, may be determined by resistance to stretch.

tonus: A partial, steady contraction of a muscle.

top-down processing: When processing starts with higher order stored knowledge and depends upon contextual information or is "conceptually driven."

torque: Rotating tendency of force; equals the product of force and the perpendicular distance from the axis of a lever to the point of application of the same force.

torsion dystonia: A condition in which twisting occurs in the alignment of body parts due to a lack of normal muscle tone secondary to infection or disease of the nervous system.

torticollis: Irresistible turning of the head that becomes more persistent, so that eventually the head is held continually to one side. The spasm of the muscles is often painful and this condition may be caused by a birth injury to the sternocleidomastoid muscle. *Synonym*: wryneck.

total hip arthroplasty: Type of hip surgery involving the removal of the head and neck of the femur and replacement with a prosthetic appliance.

total lymphoid irradiation (TLI): Radiation therapy targeted to the body's lymph nodes; the goal is to suppress immune system functioning (reduce the number of lymphocytes in the blood).

total quality management (TQM): Paradigm for management developed by Deming; emphasizes 3 themes: continuous quality improvement, empowerment of workers at all levels, and having a standard to do things right the first time.

touch for health: Combines methods and techniques that include acupuncture principles, acupressure, muscle testing, massage, and dietary guidelines. The method of treatment requires a second person who performs muscle testing.

Touch Research Institute: A facility at Miami University in Florida dedicated to studying the effects of touch therapy.

toxicology: Branch of pharmacology that examines harmful chemicals and their effects on the body.

tracheotomy: Incision of the trachea through the skin and muscles of the neck, for establishment of an airway, exploration, removal of a foreign body, or for obtaining a biopsy specimen or removal of a local lesion.

trackball: Control device used to move and operate the cursor on the computer screen.

traction: The therapeutic use of manual or mechanical tension created by a pulling force to produce a combination of distraction and gliding to relieve pain and increase tissue flexibility.

Trager: An approach to bodywork developed in the 1920s by American medical practitioner Dr. Milton Trager. It makes extensive use of touch-contact and encourages the client to experience the freeing-up of different parts of the body.

training effect: As a result of exercise, heart rate and blood pressure become less than previously required for the same amount of work.

tranquilizer: Drug that produces a calming effect, relieving tension and anxiety.

transcutaneous electrical nerve stimulation (TENS): The use of electrical energy to stimulate cutaneous and peripheral nerves via electrodes on the skin's surface. A procedure in which electrodes are placed on the surface of the skin over specific nerves and electrical stimulation is done in a manner that is thought to improve CNS function, reduce spasticity, and control pain.

transfer: The process of relocating a body from one object or surface to another (eg, getting into or out of bed, moving from a wheelchair to a chair).

transfer of learning: Practice and learning of one task can influence the learning of another task.

transient ischemic attack (TIA): Episode of temporary cerebral dysfunction caused by impaired blood flow to the brain. TIAs have many symptoms, such as dizziness, weakness, numbness, or paralysis of a limb or half of the body. TIA may last only a few minutes or up to 24 hours, but does not have any persistent neurologic deficits.

transudate: A fluid substance that has passed through a membrane or been extruded from a tissue, sometimes as a result of inflammation. A transudate, in contrast to an exudate, is characterized by high fluidity and a low content of protein, cells, or solid materials derived from cells.

trauma touch therapy: A 10 session program using therapeutic movement, breath work, and psychotherapeutic elements to relearn healthy touch.

traumatic brain injury (TBI): Injury caused by impact to the head. An insult to the brain caused by an external physical force, that may produce a diminished or altered state of consciousness, which results in impairment of cognitive abilities or physical functioning.

treatment: The sum of all interventions provided by the physical therapist to a patient/client during an episode of care. Application of or involvement in activities/stimulation to effect improvement in abilities for self-directed activities, self-care, or maintenance of the home.

tremor: Involuntary shaking or trembling.

treppe: Type of muscle contraction in which the first few contractions increase in strength when a rested muscle receives repeated stimuli.

trigeminal neuralgia: A neurologic condition of the trigemial facial nerve, characterized by brief but frequent flashing, stab-like pain radiating usually throughout mandibular and maxillary regions. Caused by degeneration of the nerve or pressure on it. *Synonym*: tic doulourex.

trigger point: A focus of hyperirritability in a tissue that, when compressed, is locally tender. If sufficiently hypersensitive the trigger point causes referred pain and sensitivity.

trigger point myotherapy: Another name for neuromuscular therapy. *See* Bonnie Prudden Myotherapy.

triglyceride: Any of a group of esters, derived from glycerol and 3 fatty acid radicals; the chief component of fats and oils.

trophotropic: Combination of parasympathetic nervous system activity, somatic muscle relaxation, and cortical beta rhythm synchronization. Resting or sleep state.

truncal ataxia: Uncoordinated movement of the trunk.

truth: Faithful to facts and reality.

tuberosity: Medium-sized protrusion on a bone.

tui na: A 2 000-year-old Chinese modality that uses massage and manipulation to release the flow of qi.

tunnel vision: The visual field is limited to one side; the peripheral fields are lost, usually due to damage to the optic chiasm.

turaya touch system: A practitioner touches areas of the head, neck, shoulders, and abdomen using the body's system of light energy to release the energy blocks that cause physical and mental distress.

Type A behavior: A cluster of personality traits that includes high achievement motivation, drive, and a fast-paced lifestyle. Associated with stress-related diseases, such as heart disease.

Type B behavior: A cluster of personality traits that include low achievement motivation, laziness, and a laid-back sort of lifestyle. Associated with inactivity, lack of exercise, and sedentary-related diseases, such as heart disease.

ulcer: An open sore on the skin or some mucous membrane characterized by the disintegration of tissue and, often, the discharge of serous drainage.

ultrasound: A diagnostic or therapeutic technique using high-frequency sound waves to produce heat. *Pulsed ultrasound:* The application of therapeutic ultrasound using predetermined interrupted frequencies.

ultraviolet: A form of radiant energy using light rays with wavelengths beyond the violet end of the visible spectrum.

universal: Pertaining to any group, need, or environment.

Universal Calibration Matrix (UCL): The UCL forms part of the energy anatomy of a human being. *See* EMF balancing technique.

universal goniometer: Instrument used to measure joint motion. It consists of a protractor, an axis, and 2 arms.

universal precautions: An approach to infection control designed to prevent transmission of blood-borne diseases such as AIDS and hepatitis B; includes specific recommendations for use of gloves, protective eyewear, and masks.

untie: A therapy based upon attention being given to the sensitivity of the client, working with the practitioner, to identify the patterns of soft tissue dysfunction. The practitioner uses their hand and finger sensitivity to react to the changes created by their presence thus having a lasting effect on even the deepest tissues.

upper motor neuron (UMN): Neurons of the cerebral cortex that conduct stimuli from the motor cortex of the brain to motor nuclei of cerebral nerves of the ventral gray columns of the spinal cord.

ealing massage therapy: A synthesis of apy, massage, dance, tai chi, aikido, and ixteen basic techniques that align, loosen, the body restoring the body to the liquid opriate to it.

forcement: Idea that one person's obser- other person experiencing a positive con- a result of a particular behavior increases ity that the observer will exhibit that

opy: Radiological study that allows visu- he pharyngeal and esophageal phases of

Alternative measurement of hand strength the person to squeeze a rubber bulb.
: Term describing any optical or sensory something real, to the point of confound- s into accepting that simulation.

ulation: The visceral organs are returned al state of flexibility and position enhanc- ity to function normally and in compati- e other organ systems of the body.
ribes the extent to which a tissue's resist- rmation is dependent on the rate of the rce.

g: Can include distance and near visual omotilities, eye alignment or posture, ion, and visual fields.
ted with or used in seeing. Interpreting h the eyes, including peripheral vision

Measure of visual discrimination of fine contrast.
An effective means of deepening relax- nsitizing a real-life situation that is gen- h stress and tension.

oordination: The ability to coordinate e movements of the body or parts of the

unction: The ability to draw or copy rform constructive tasks.

urbanization: Fundamental belief and societal attitude that men were to provide financial support and women were to care for their families. This is a 19th century concept.

uremia: Toxic condition associated with renal insuffi- ciency in which urine is present in the blood.

urgency: Need to excrete urine immediately.

uterine dysfunction: The inability of the uterus to con- tract and relax in a coordinated fashion.

uterine inversion: When the uterus loses its shape and comes out toward its opening.

uterus: The pear-shaped organ in which the fetus grows. *Synonym:* womb.

utilization review: Assessment of the appropriateness and economy of an admission to a health care facility or continued hospitalization.

V

valgus: A limb deformity in which the extremity is moved away (laterally) from the midline.

validity: Degree to which a test measures what it is intended to measure.

values: Operational beliefs that one accepts as one's own; determines behavior.

variance: Measure that demonstrates how scores in a distribution deviate from the mean.

varicocele: Enlargement of the veins in the spermatic cord.

varicose veins: Enlarged, twisted superficial veins. Massage therapy is contraindicated over varicose veins due to the possibility of breaking loose a blood clot.

vasomotor center: A regulatory center in the lower pons and medulla oblongata that regulates the diameter of blood vessels, especially the arterioles.

vasopneumatic compression device: A device to decrease edema by using compressive forces that are applied to the body part.

vasopressor: Stimulating contraction of the muscular tissue of the capillaries and arteries. An agent that stimulates the contraction of the muscular tissue of the capillaries and arteries.

vector: Arrow that indicates direction and magnitude of a force.

ventilation: The circulation of air; to aerate (blood); oxygenate. Mechanical ventilation is the use of equipment to circulate oxygen to the respiratory system.

ventilatory pump cles and their in The muscles inc scalene, and ste muscles of venti and quadratus lu

ventilatory pump thoracic skeleto lungs that inter breathing or ven

ventral: From an front or the belly

veracity: Obligati pist to tell the tr

verbal communic words and expre through words.

verbal rating sc which patients/c subdivided from pain intensities.

verbal therapies sion are the prir

vertigo: One's se ing objects mov

vestibular: Perta the entrance o Describing the ear. Interpretin movement base receptors.

vestibular funct

vestibulocochlea eighth cranial r

vestibuloocular position comp induced by exc

vibration: A ma are shaken wit to accomplish

vibrational polarity the meditation. and connec process app

vicarious rei vation of a sequence as the probab behavior.

videofluorosc alization of swallowing.

vigorometer: that requires

virtual realit simulation c ing the sens

visceral mani to their norr ing their ab bility with t

viscosity: Des ance to def deforming fc

vision screeni acuities, oc depth percer

visual: Conne stimuli thro and acuity.

visual acuity: details of hig

visualization: ation and de erally met w

visual motor vision with t body.

visual motor forms or to p

visual motor integration: The ability to integrate vision with movements of the body or parts of the body by coordinating the interaction of information from the eyes with body movement during activity.

visual neglect: Inattention to visual stimuli occurring in the space on the involved side of the body.

visual orientation: Awareness and location of objects in the environment and their relationship to each other and to oneself.

visual perception: Brain's ability to understand sensory input to determine size, shape, distance, and form of objects.

visual perceptual dysfunction: May include deficits in any of the areas of visual perception: figure-ground, form constancy, or size discrimination. Distinct from deficits in functional visual skills and tested separately.

vital capacity (VC): Measurement of the amount of air that can be expelled at the normal rate of exhalation after a maximum inspiration, representing the greatest possible breathing capacity.

vital signs: Measurements of pulse rate, respiration rate, and body temperature.

vocational activities: Participating in tasks associated with performance of work-related activities and skills.

vocational maturity: Scale along which people are placed during their working lives. Maturity is reached when occupational activities are aligned with what is expected of the corresponding age group.

volar: Palm of the hand or the sole of the foot.

volar splint: Splint that runs from the lower third of the forearm to the individual's fingertips, with the thumb extended and abducted. The phalangeal joint should be slightly flexed, thus enabling this type of splint construction to prevent stiffening of the phalangeal joints in extension. This splint is often used as a night splint for inpatients.

volitional postural movements: Movement patterns under volitional control that relate specifically to controlling the center of gravity, as in skating, ballet, gymnastics, etc.

Volkmann's contracture: Permanent contracture of a muscle due to replacement of destroyed muscle cells with fibrous tissue that lacks the ability to stretch. Destruction of muscle cells may occur from interference with circulation caused by a tight bandage, splint, or cast.

volume measurement: The amount of fluid that has been displaced from a container (of any size) following the introduction of part or all of the body.

voluntary muscle: Type of muscle tissue that can be controlled by the brain to produce movement.

volvulus: Twisting of the bowel upon itself.

vomiting: The forceful dispelling of stomach contents through the mouth. Massage is contraindicated as it may over stimulate the digestive system.

vortex healing energetic therapy: A realm (whose whole purpose is to help us heal) is created by the combined energies of 7 divine beings and connects us with their transformational energies as well as their divine consciousness.

waddling gait: Gait pattern in which the feet are wide apart, resembling the gait of a duck.

warm-up: Exercise that prepares the person for the experience to follow.

watsu aquatic shiatsu: A form of zen shiatsu performed in water.

wear-and-tear theory: Theory that describes the biological effects of aging as the body deteriorates.

weight: Measure of matter that incorporates the effect of gravity on an object; a kinematic measurement.

weight shift: Bearing the body's weight from one leg to another; shifting the center of gravity.

wellness: Dynamic state of health in which an individual progresses toward a higher level of functioning, achieving an optimum balance between internal and external environments. Concepts that embrace positive health behaviors (eg, exercise, nutrition, stress reduction).

wheeze: A whistling sound made in breathing resulting from constriction and/or partial obstruction of the airways. Heard on auscultation; however, in severe cases of asthma and COPD, can often be audible without the use of a stethoscope.

whiplash injury: Caused by sudden hyperextension and flexion of the neck traumatizing cervical ligaments; common in rear end car accidents or falls.

white matter: Area of the central nervous system that contains the axons of the cells.

wholistic: A model or approach to health care that takes into account all internal and external influences during the process.

within normal limits (WNL): The normal range of motion at a given joint.

Wolff's law: States that bone is formed in areas of stress and reabsorbed in areas of nonstress.

word processing: Type of application software that is used to enter, edit, manipulate, and format text.

work behaviors: Behaviors that are necessary for successful participation in a job or independent living (eg, cooperative behavior). *Synonyms*: prevocational readiness, personal skills.

work capacity evaluation: Comprehensive process that systematically uses work, real or simulated, to access and measure an individual's physical abilities to work.

work setting: Any environment in which an individual performs productive activity.

work space: Physical area in which one performs work.

work tolerance: Refers to how a person deals with his/her work environment. This includes being able to handle the stress and pressures that are part of the job and to maintain one's productivity, quality, and effort, time after time.

work-up: The process of performing a complete evaluation of an individual including history, physical examination, laboratory test, and x-ray or other diagnostic procedures to acquire an accurate database on which a diagnosis and treatment plan may be established.

wounds: Any type of tender or painful ulcer or lesion of the skin or mucous membrane. Massage of wounded area is contraindicated to prevent re-injury or further injury to affected tissues; nearby healthy tissues may be massaged.

wound care: Procedures used to achieve a clean wound bed, promote a moist environment or facilitate autolytic debridement, and absorb excessive exudation from a wound complex.

xeroderma: Condition of rough and dry skin.

yoga: A series of Hindu practices designed to enable people to begin from their present state of consciousness and move forward day by day into a state of wholeness, well being, and enlightenment.

yogassage: A combination of a deep stretch for surface muscles (yoga positions) and a deep massage for the internal systems.

Z

z score (standard score): Numerical value from the transformation of a raw score into units of standard deviation.

zen body therapy: A combination of zen training with Eastern teachings of the circulation of vital energy.

zen shiatsu: A system of bodywork whose purpose is to restores the proper flow of energy to optimum levels.

zero balancing: A simple method of aligning body energy with body structure. It integrates fundamental principles of Western science with Eastern concepts of body, mind, and spirit.

zip disk: Disk that stores 100 megabytes of data.

zone: An area or belt, such as reflex zones, pain referral zones, dermatones.

Bibliography

American Occupational Therapy Association. Occupational performance: occupational therapy's definition of function. Available at: www.aota.org. Accessed December 27, 2004.

Anderson DL. *Muscle Pain Relief in 90 Seconds: The Fold and Hold Method*. Minneapolis, Minn: Chronimed Publishing; 1995.

Andrade, Clifford. *Outcome-Based Massage*. Baltimore, Md: Lippincott Williams & Wilkins; 2001.

Ashley M. *Massage: A Career at Your Fingertips*. Barrytown, NY: Station Hill Press; 1992.

Associated Bodywork & Massage Professionals. *Successful Business Handbook*. Evergreen, Colo: 2002

Beck MF. *Theory and Practice of Therapeutic Massage*. Albany, NY: Milady Publishing; 1999.

Business of Massage. Evanston, Ill: American Massage Therapy Association; 2002.

Capellini S. *Massage Therapy Career Guide for Hands-On Success*. New York, NY: Milady Press; 1999.

Clay, Pounds. *Basic Clinical Massage Therapy: Integrating Anatomy and Treatment*. Baltimore, Md: Lippincott Williams & Wilkins; 2002.

Greene E. Massage therapy for health and fitness. American Massage Therapy Association. Available at: http://www.amtamassage.org/publications/massage.html. Accessed December 27, 2004.

treppe: Type of muscle contraction in which the first few contractions increase in strength when a rested muscle receives repeated stimuli.

trigeminal neuralgia: A neurologic condition of the trigemial facial nerve, characterized by brief but frequent flashing, stab-like pain radiating usually throughout mandibular and maxillary regions. Caused by degeneration of the nerve or pressure on it. *Synonym*: tic douylourex.

trigger point: A focus of hyperirritability in a tissue that, when compressed, is locally tender. If sufficiently hypersensitive the trigger point causes referred pain and sensitivity.

trigger point myotherapy: Another name for neuro-muscular therapy. *See* Bonnie Prudden Myotherapy.

triglyceride: Any of a group of esters, derived from glycerol and 3 fatty acid radicals; the chief component of fats and oils.

trophotropic: Combination of parasympathetic nervous system activity, somatic muscle relaxation, and cortical beta rhythm synchronization. Resting or sleep state.

truncal ataxia: Uncoordinated movement of the trunk.

truth: Faithful to facts and reality.

tuberosity: Medium-sized protrusion on a bone.

tui na: A 2 000-year-old Chinese modality that uses massage and manipulation to release the flow of qi.

tunnel vision: The visual field is limited to one side; the peripheral fields are lost, usually due to damage to the optic chiasm.

turaya touch system: A practitioner touches areas of the head, neck, shoulders, and abdomen using the body's system of light energy to release the energy blocks that cause physical and mental distress.

Type A behavior: A cluster of personality traits that includes high achievement motivation, drive, and a fast-paced lifestyle. Associated with stress-related diseases, such as heart disease.

Type B behavior: A cluster of personality traits that include low achievement motivation, laziness, and a laid-back sort of lifestyle. Associated with inactivity, lack of exercise, and sedentary-related diseases, such as heart disease.

ulcer: An open sore on the skin or some mucous membrane characterized by the disintegration of tissue and, often, the discharge of serous drainage.

ultrasound: A diagnostic or therapeutic technique using high-frequency sound waves to produce heat. *Pulsed ultrasound:* The application of therapeutic ultrasound using predetermined interrupted frequencies.

ultraviolet: A form of radiant energy using light rays with wavelengths beyond the violet end of the visible spectrum.

universal: Pertaining to any group, need, or environment.

Universal Calibration Matrix (UCL): The UCL forms part of the energy anatomy of a human being. *See* EMF balancing technique.

universal goniometer: Instrument used to measure joint motion. It consists of a protractor, an axis, and 2 arms.

universal precautions: An approach to infection control designed to prevent transmission of blood-borne diseases such as AIDS and hepatitis B; includes specific recommendations for use of gloves, protective eyewear, and masks.

untie: A therapy based upon attention being given to the sensitivity of the client, working with the practitioner, to identify the patterns of soft tissue dysfunction. The practitioner uses their hand and finger sensitivity to react to the changes created by their presence thus having a lasting effect on even the deepest tissues.

upper motor neuron (UMN): Neurons of the cerebral cortex that conduct stimuli from the motor cortex of the brain to motor nuclei of cerebral nerves of the ventral gray columns of the spinal cord.

urbanization: Fundamental belief and societal attitude that men were to provide financial support and women were to care for their families. This is a 19th century concept.

uremia: Toxic condition associated with renal insufficiency in which urine is present in the blood.

urgency: Need to excrete urine immediately.

uterine dysfunction: The inability of the uterus to contract and relax in a coordinated fashion.

uterine inversion: When the uterus loses its shape and comes out toward its opening.

uterus: The pear-shaped organ in which the fetus grows. *Synonym*: womb.

utilization review: Assessment of the appropriateness and economy of an admission to a health care facility or continued hospitalization.

valgus: A limb deformity in which the extremity is moved away (laterally) from the midline.

validity: Degree to which a test measures what it is intended to measure.

values: Operational beliefs that one accepts as one's own; determines behavior.

variance: Measure that demonstrates how scores in a distribution deviate from the mean.

varicocele: Enlargement of the veins in the spermatic cord.

varicose veins: Enlarged, twisted superficial veins. Massage therapy is contraindicated over varicose veins due to the possibility of breaking loose a blood clot.

vasomotor center: A regulatory center in the lower pons and medulla oblongata that regulates the diameter of blood vessels, especially the arterioles.

vasopneumatic compression device: A device to decrease edema by using compressive forces that are applied to the body part.

vasopressor: Stimulating contraction of the muscular tissue of the capillaries and arteries. An agent that stimulates the contraction of the muscular tissue of the capillaries and arteries.

vector: Arrow that indicates direction and magnitude of a force.

ventilation: The circulation of air; to aerate (blood); oxygenate. Mechanical ventilation is the use of equipment to circulate oxygen to the respiratory system.

ventilatory pump: Thoracic skeleton and skeletal muscles and their innervation responsible for ventilation. The muscles include the diaphragm; the intercostal, scalene, and sternocleidomastoid muscles; accessory muscles of ventilation; and the abdominal, triangular, and quadratus lumborum muscles.

ventilatory pump dysfunction: Abnormalities of the thoracic skeleton, respiratory muscles, airways, or lungs that interrupt or interfere with the work of breathing or ventilation.

ventral: From anatomical position, located toward the front or the belly.

veracity: Obligation of the patient/client and the therapist to tell the truth at all times.

verbal communication: Process of interpreting another's words and expressing one's own thoughts and emotions through words.

verbal rating scale: A pain intensity measurement in which patients/clients rate pain on a continuum that is subdivided from left to right into gradually increasing pain intensities.

verbal therapies: Any therapy in which talk and discussion are the primary modes of intervention.

vertigo: One's sensation of revolving in space or of having objects move around him/her.

vestibular: Pertaining to a vestibule, cavity, or space at the entrance of a canal, such as in the inner ear. Describing the sense of balance located in the inner ear. Interpreting stimuli regarding head position and movement based on the shift of fluid and inner ear receptors.

vestibular function: Pertaining to the sense of balance.

vestibulocochlear nerve: Combined portions of the eighth cranial nerve.

vestibuloocular reflex: A normal reflex in which eye position compensates for movement of the head, induced by excitation of vestibular apparatus.

vibration: A massage technique in which the soft tissues are shaken with varying degrees of vigor and pressure to accomplish therapeutic effects.

vibrational healing massage therapy: A synthesis of polarity therapy, massage, dance, tai chi, aikido, and meditation. Sixteen basic techniques that align, loosen, and connect the body restoring the body to the liquid process appropriate to it.

vicarious reinforcement: Idea that one person's observation of another person experiencing a positive consequence as a result of a particular behavior increases the probability that the observer will exhibit that behavior.

videofluoroscopy: Radiological study that allows visualization of the pharyngeal and esophageal phases of swallowing.

vigorometer: Alternative measurement of hand strength that requires the person to squeeze a rubber bulb.

virtual reality: Term describing any optical or sensory simulation of something real, to the point of confounding the senses into accepting that simulation.

visceral manipulation: The visceral organs are returned to their normal state of flexibility and position enhancing their ability to function normally and in compatibility with the other organ systems of the body.

viscosity: Describes the extent to which a tissue's resistance to deformation is dependent on the rate of the deforming force.

vision screening: Can include distance and near visual acuities, oculomotilities, eye alignment or posture, depth perception, and visual fields.

visual: Connected with or used in seeing. Interpreting stimuli through the eyes, including peripheral vision and acuity.

visual acuity: Measure of visual discrimination of fine details of high contrast.

visualization: An effective means of deepening relaxation and desensitizing a real-life situation that is generally met with stress and tension.

visual motor coordination: The ability to coordinate vision with the movements of the body or parts of the body.

visual motor function: The ability to draw or copy forms or to perform constructive tasks.

visual motor integration: The ability to integrate vision with movements of the body or parts of the body by coordinating the interaction of information from the eyes with body movement during activity.

visual neglect: Inattention to visual stimuli occurring in the space on the involved side of the body.

visual orientation: Awareness and location of objects in the environment and their relationship to each other and to oneself.

visual perception: Brain's ability to understand sensory input to determine size, shape, distance, and form of objects.

visual perceptual dysfunction: May include deficits in any of the areas of visual perception: figure-ground, form constancy, or size discrimination. Distinct from deficits in functional visual skills and tested separately.

vital capacity (VC): Measurement of the amount of air that can be expelled at the normal rate of exhalation after a maximum inspiration, representing the greatest possible breathing capacity.

vital signs: Measurements of pulse rate, respiration rate, and body temperature.

vocational activities: Participating in tasks associated with performance of work-related activities and skills.

vocational maturity: Scale along which people are placed during their working lives. Maturity is reached when occupational activities are aligned with what is expected of the corresponding age group.

volar: Palm of the hand or the sole of the foot.

volar splint: Splint that runs from the lower third of the forearm to the individual's fingertips, with the thumb extended and abducted. The phalangeal joint should be slightly flexed, thus enabling this type of splint construction to prevent stiffening of the phalangeal joints in extension. This splint is often used as a night splint for inpatients.

volitional postural movements: Movement patterns under volitional control that relate specifically to controlling the center of gravity, as in skating, ballet, gymnastics, etc.

Volkmann's contracture: Permanent contracture of a muscle due to replacement of destroyed muscle cells with fibrous tissue that lacks the ability to stretch. Destruction of muscle cells may occur from interference with circulation caused by a tight bandage, splint, or cast.

volume measurement: The amount of fluid that has been displaced from a container (of any size) following the introduction of part or all of the body.

voluntary muscle: Type of muscle tissue that can be controlled by the brain to produce movement.

volvulus: Twisting of the bowel upon itself.

vomiting: The forceful dispelling of stomach contents through the mouth. Massage is contraindicated as it may over stimulate the digestive system.

vortex healing energetic therapy: A realm (whose whole purpose is to help us heal) is created by the combined energies of 7 divine beings and connects us with their transformational energies as well as their divine consciousness.

W

waddling gait: Gait pattern in which the feet are wide apart, resembling the gait of a duck.

warm-up: Exercise that prepares the person for the experience to follow.

watsu aquatic shiatsu: A form of zen shiatsu performed in water.

wear-and-tear theory: Theory that describes the biological effects of aging as the body deteriorates.

weight: Measure of matter that incorporates the effect of gravity on an object; a kinematic measurement.

weight shift: Bearing the body's weight from one leg to another; shifting the center of gravity.

wellness: Dynamic state of health in which an individual progresses toward a higher level of functioning, achieving an optimum balance between internal and external environments. Concepts that embrace positive health behaviors (eg, exercise, nutrition, stress reduction).

wheeze: A whistling sound made in breathing resulting from constriction and/or partial obstruction of the airways. Heard on auscultation; however, in severe cases of asthma and COPD, can often be audible without the use of a stethoscope.

whiplash injury: Caused by sudden hyperextension and flexion of the neck traumatizing cervical ligaments; common in rear end car accidents or falls.

white matter: Area of the central nervous system that contains the axons of the cells.

wholistic: A model or approach to health care that takes into account all internal and external influences during the process.

within normal limits (WNL): The normal range of motion at a given joint.

Wolff's law: States that bone is formed in areas of stress and reabsorbed in areas of nonstress.

word processing: Type of application software that is used to enter, edit, manipulate, and format text.

work behaviors: Behaviors that are necessary for successful participation in a job or independent living (eg, cooperative behavior). *Synonyms*: prevocational readiness, personal skills.

work capacity evaluation: Comprehensive process that systematically uses work, real or simulated, to access and measure an individual's physical abilities to work.

work setting: Any environment in which an individual performs productive activity.

work space: Physical area in which one performs work.

work tolerance: Refers to how a person deals with his/her work environment. This includes being able to handle the stress and pressures that are part of the job and to maintain one's productivity, quality, and effort, time after time.

work-up: The process of performing a complete evaluation of an individual including history, physical examination, laboratory test, and x-ray or other diagnostic procedures to acquire an accurate database on which a diagnosis and treatment plan may be established.

wounds: Any type of tender or painful ulcer or lesion of the skin or mucous membrane. Massage of wounded area is contraindicated to prevent re-injury or further injury to affected tissues; nearby healthy tissues may be massaged.

wound care: Procedures used to achieve a clean wound bed, promote a moist environment or facilitate autolytic debridement, and absorb excessive exudation from a wound complex.

xeroderma: Condition of rough and dry skin.

yoga: A series of Hindu practices designed to enable people to begin from their present state of consciousness and move forward day by day into a state of wholeness, well being, and enlightenment.

yogassage: A combination of a deep stretch for surface muscles (yoga positions) and a deep massage for the internal systems.

Z

z score (standard score): Numerical value from the transformation of a raw score into units of standard deviation.

zen body therapy: A combination of zen training with Eastern teachings of the circulation of vital energy.

zen shiatsu: A system of bodywork whose purpose is to restores the proper flow of energy to optimum levels.

zero balancing: A simple method of aligning body energy with body structure. It integrates fundamental principles of Western science with Eastern concepts of body, mind, and spirit.

zip disk: Disk that stores 100 megabytes of data.

zone: An area or belt, such as reflex zones, pain referral zones, dermatones.

Bibliography

American Occupational Therapy Association. Occupational performance: occupational therapy's definition of function. Available at: www.aota.org. Accessed December 27, 2004.

Anderson DL. *Muscle Pain Relief in 90 Seconds: The Fold and Hold Method*. Minneapolis, Minn: Chronimed Publishing; 1995.

Andrade, Clifford. *Outcome-Based Massage*. Baltimore, Md: Lippincott Williams & Wilkins; 2001.

Ashley M. *Massage: A Career at Your Fingertips*. Barrytown, NY: Station Hill Press; 1992.

Associated Bodywork & Massage Professionals. *Successful Business Handbook*. Evergreen, Colo: 2002

Beck MF. *Theory and Practice of Therapeutic Massage*. Albany, NY: Milady Publishing; 1999.

Business of Massage. Evanston, Ill: American Massage Therapy Association; 2002.

Capellini S. *Massage Therapy Career Guide for Hands-On Success*. New York, NY: Milady Press; 1999.

Clay, Pounds. *Basic Clinical Massage Therapy: Integrating Anatomy and Treatment*. Baltimore, Md: Lippincott Williams & Wilkins; 2002.

Greene E. Massage therapy for health and fitness. American Massage Therapy Association. Available at: http://www.amtamassage.org/publications/massage.html. Accessed December 27, 2004.

Kellogg JH. *The Art of Massage*. Battle Creek, Mich: Modern Medicine Publishing; 1929.

National Institutes of Health. Universal precautions. Available at: http://www.niehs.nih.gov/odhsb/biosafe/univers.htm. Accessed December 27, 2004.

Netter FH. *Atlas of Human Anatomy*. Summit, NJ: CIBA-GEIGA Corporation; 1989.

Rich GJ. *Massage Therapy: The Evidence for Practice.* New York, NY: Mosby; 2002.

Simons D, Travell J, Simons L. *Myofascial Pain and Dysfunction: The Trigger Point Manual, Vol. I Upper Half of Body.* Baltimore, Md: Lippincott Williams & Wilkins; 1999.

Simons D, Travell J, Simons L. *Myofascial Pain and Dysfunction: The Trigger Point Manual, Vol. I Lower Half of Body*. Baltimore, Md: Lippincott Williams & Wilkins; 1999.

Tappan FM, Benjamin PJ. *Tappan's Handbook of Healing Massage Techniques: Classis, Holistic, and Emerging Methods*. Stanford, Conn: Appleton & Lange; 1998.

Thompson DL. *Hands Heal: Communication, Documentation, and Insurance Billing for Manual Therapists.* Baltimore, Md: Lippincott Williams & Wilkins; 2002.

Touch Research Institute. The benefits of massage. Available at: http://www.miami.edu/touch-research. Accessed December 27, 2004.

List of Appendices

Appendix 1:   AMTA Code of Ethics 191
Appendix 2:   ABMP Professional
              Code of Ethics 196
Appendix 3:   IMA Group Code of Ethics 200
Appendix 4:   The Benefits of Massage 202
Appendix 5:   Safety and Hygiene 204
Appendix 6:   Suggested Reading 209
Appendix 7:   General Acronyms and
              Abbreviations. 215
Appendix 8:   Organization Acronyms 242
Appendix 9:   Selected National and International
              Massage Associations 254
Appendix 10: Medical Roots: Etymology 257
Appendix 11: Massage Techniques and Modalities
              Contact Information 284
Appendix 12: Range of Motion 330
Appendix 13: Bones of the Body 332
Appendix 14: Muscles of the Body 333
Appendix 15: Metric System 363
Appendix 16: Weight and Measure
              Conversions 365
Appendix 17: Peripheral Nerve Innervations:
              Upper Extremity 369
Appendix 18: Peripheral Nerve Innervations:
              Lower Extremity 372
Appendix 19: Diseases, Pathologies, and
              Syndromes Defined 378
Appendix 20: Licensure by State 451
Appendix 21: Canada Licensure by Province . . . 463
Appendix 22: Medical Codes for Massage
              Therapy 466

American Massage Therapy Association Code of Ethics

This **Code of Ethics** *is a summary statement of the standards by which massage therapists agree to conduct their practices and is a declaration of the general principles of acceptable, ethical, professional behavior.*

MASSAGE THERAPISTS SHALL:

1. Demonstrate commitment to provide the highest quality massage therapy/bodywork to those who seek their professional service.
2. Acknowledge the inherent worth and individuality of each person by not discriminating or behaving in any prejudicial manner with clients and/or colleagues.
3. Demonstrate professional excellence through regular self-assessment of strengths, limitations, and effectiveness by continued education and training.
4. Acknowledge the confidential nature of the professional relationship with clients and respect each client's right to privacy.
5. Conduct all business and professional activities within their scope of practice, the law of the land, and project a professional image.
6. Refrain from engaging in any sexual conduct or sexual activities involving their clients.
7. Accept responsibility to do no harm to the physical, mental and emotional well being of self, clients, and associates.

STANDARDS OF PRACTICE

Purpose Statement: These American Massage Therapy Association (AMTA) Standards of Practice were developed to assist the professional massage therapist to:

- Provide safe, consistent care
- Determine the quality of care provided
- Provide a common base to develop a practice
- Support/preserve the basic rights of the client and professional massage therapist
- Assist the public to understand what to expect from a professional massage therapist

This document allows the professional massage therapist to evaluate and adapt performance in his/her massage/bodywork practice. The professional massage therapist can evaluate the quality of his/her practice by utilizing the *Standards of Practice* in conjunction with the *Code of Ethics*, the *Bylaws and Policies* of AMTA, and precedents set by the AMTA Grievance, Standards, and Bylaws Committees.

CONDUCT OF THE PROFESSIONAL MASSAGE THERAPIST OR PRACTITIONER, HEREINAFTER REFERRED TO AS "PRACTITIONER."

- AMTA members must meet and maintain appropriate membership requirements.
- Individual AMTA members, who engage in the practice of professional massage/bodywork, shall adhere to standards of professional conduct, including the AMTA *Code of Ethics*.
- The Practitioner follows consistent standards in all settings.

- The Practitioner seeks professional supervision/consultation consistent with promoting and maintaining appropriate application of skills and knowledge.

SANITATION, HYGIENE AND SAFETY

- The Practitioner provides an environment consistent with accepted standards of sanitation, hygiene, safety, and universal precautions.
- The Practitioner maintains current knowledge and skills of pathophysiology and the appropriate application of massage/bodywork.
- The Practitioner monitors feedback from the client throughout a session.
- The Practitioner makes appropriate referrals to other reputable health care providers.

PROFESSIONAL RELATIONSHIPS WITH CLIENTS

- The Practitioner relates to the client in a manner consistent with accepted standards and ethics.
- The Practitioner maintains appropriate professional standards of confidentiality.
- The Practitioner relates to the client in a manner that respects the integrity of the client and practitioner.
- The Practitioner ensures that representations of his/her professional services, policies, and procedures are accurately communicated to the client prior to the initial application of massage/bodywork.
- The Practitioner elicits participation and feedback from the client.

PROFESSIONAL   RELATIONSHIPS   WITH   OTHER
PROFESSIONALS

- The Practitioner relates to other reputable professionals with appropriate respect and within the parameters of accepted ethical standards.
- The Practitioner's referrals to other professionals are only made in the interest of the client.
- The Practitioner's communication with other professionals regarding clients is in compliance with accepted standards and ethics.
- A Practitioner possessing knowledge that another practitioner: (1) committed a criminal act that reflects adversely on the Practitioner's competence in massage therapy, trustworthiness, or fitness to practice massage therapy in other respects; (2) engaged in an act or practice that significantly undermines the massage therapy profession; or (3) engaged in conduct that creates a risk of serious harm for the physical or emotional well being of a recipient of massage therapy; shall report such knowledge to the appropriate AMTA committee if such information is not protected or restricted by a confidentiality law.

RECORDS

- The Practitioner establishes and maintains appropriate client records.
- The Practitioner establishes and maintains client financial accounts that follow accepted accounting practices.

MARKETING

- Marketing consists of, but is not limited to, advertising, public relations, promotion, and publicity.
- The Practitioner markets his/her practice in an accurate, truthful, and ethical manner.

LEGAL PRACTICE

- American Massage Therapy Association members practice or collaborate with all others practicing professional massage/bodywork in a manner that is in compliance with national, state, or local municipal law(s) pertaining to the practice of professional massage/bodywork.

RESEARCH

- The Practitioner engaged in study and/or research is guided by the conventions and ethics of scholarly inquiry.
- The Practitioner doing research avoids financial or political relationships that may limit objectivity or create conflict of interest.

Associated Bodywork and Massage Professionals Professional Code of Ethics

As a member of Associated Bodywork & Massage Professionals, I hereby pledge to abide by the ABMP **Code of Ethics** *as outlined below.*

CLIENT RELATIONSHIPS

- I shall endeavor to serve the best interests of my clients at all times and to provide the highest quality service possible.
- I shall maintain clear and honest communcations with my clients and shall keep client communications confidential.
- I shall acknowledge the limitations of my skills and, when necessary, refer clients to the appropriate qualified health care professional.
- I shall in no way instigate or tolerate any kind of sexual advance while acting in the capacity of a massage, bodywork, somatic therapy, or esthetic practitioner.

PROFESSIONALISM

- I shall maintain the highest standards of professional conduct, providing services in an ethical and professional manner in relation to my clientele, business associates, health care professionals, and the general public.

- I shall respect the rights of all ethical practitioners and will cooperate with all health care professionals in a friendly and professional manner.
- I shall refrain from the use of any mind-altering drugs, alcohol, or intoxicants prior to or during professional sessions.
- I shall always dress in a professional manner, proper dress being defined as attire suitable and consistent with accepted business and professional practice.
- I shall not be affiliated with or employed by any business that utilizes any sexual suggestiveness or explicit sexuality in its advertising or promotion of services, or in the actual practice of its services.

SCOPE OF PRACTICE/APPROPRIATE TECHNIQUES

- I shall provide services within the scope of the ABMP definition of massage, bodywork, somatic therapies, and skin care, and the limits of my training. I will not employ those massage, bodywork, or skin care techniques for which I have not had adequate training and shall represent my education, training qualifications, and abilities honestly.
- I shall be conscious of the intent of the services that I am providing and shall be aware of and practice good judgment regarding the application of massage, bodywork, or somatic techniques utilized.

- I shall not perform manipulations or adjustments of the human skeletal structure, diagnose, prescribe, or provide any other service, procedure, or therapy which requires a license to practice chiropractic, osteopathy, physical therapy, podiatry, orthopedics, psychotherapy, acupuncture, dermatology, cosmetology, or any other profession or branch of medicine unless specifically licensed to do so.

- I shall be thoroughly educated and understand the physiological effects of the specific massage, bodywork, somatic, or skin care techniques utilized in order to determine whether such application is contraindicated and/or to determine the most beneficial techniques to apply to a given individual. I shall not apply massage, bodywork, somatic, or skin care techniques in those cases where they may be contraindicated without a written referral from the client's primary care provider.

IMAGE/ADVERTISING CLAIMS

- I shall strive to project a professional image for myself, my business or place of employment, and the profession in general.

- I shall actively participate in educating the public regarding the actual benefits of massage, bodywork, somatic therapies, and skin care.

- I shall practice honesty in advertising, promote my services ethically and in good taste, and practice and/or advertise only those techniques for which I have received adequate training and/or certification. I shall not make false claims regarding the potential benefits of the techniques rendered.

International Massage Association (IMA) Group Code of Ethics

As an IMA Group member, you agree to abide by the following standards of professional and ethical behavior in your field:

- To put my clients' well being first and foremost.
- To conduct myself professionally and responsibly.
- To uphold the integrity of my profession.
- To acknowledge, respect, and cooperate with my colleagues and peers in order to advance our profession and ensure that the highest level of excellence is available to the consuming public.
- I shall promote myself, The IMA Group, and my profession honestly, tactfully, and with the aim of educating both my peers and the public, so that they may be empowered to demand and receive all the benefits that my profession provides.
- To acknowledge the limitations of my skills and scope of practice and refer clients, when necessary, to other health professionals to provide the most appropriate care.
- To maintain a safe and comfortable working environment, paying particular attention to avoidable hazards and respecting personal boundaries.

- To ascertain and comply with the requirements of all governing laws and abide by them to the best of my ability. Where laws are unjust, I will labor with my association to change them.
- To communicate responsibly, truthfully, and respectfully with clients and to hold their communications in strict confidence.

Any member failing to abide by the Code of Ethics shall be answerable to the board of directors for "peer review."

The Benefits of Massage

The following benefits of massage items are selected items from an article written by Elliot Greene (*Massage Therapy For Health and Fitness*) featured on the American Massage Therapy Association's Web site and from the benefits of massage section of the Touch Research Institute Web site.

The opinions of massage therapists regarding the benefits of massage are increasingly being supported by research. No attempt has been made to cite research evidence to support each listed benefit.

MASSAGE THERAPY SKILLFULLY APPLIED RESULTS IN THESE BENEFICIAL EFFECTS:

- Causes changes in the blood
- Increases oxygen capacity
- Reduces blood pressure
- Affects muscles throughout the body by:
  ○ Loosening tight muscles
  ○ Speeding recovery from fatigue
  ○ Stretching muscles and connecting tissue
  ○ Reducing muscle spasms
- Increasing the body's secretions and excretions—possibly increasing metabolic rate
- Affects the nervous system—soothes or stimulates according to the effect needed
- Enhances skin condition—increases the

function of the sebaceous and sweat glands
- Affects the internal organs—through an increased blood flow
- Boosts the immune system—increases the activity level of "killer cells"
- Reduces pain
- Alters EEG in the direction of heightened awareness
- Reduces stress hormones

BENEFITS IN SPECIFIC CASES
- Office workers—decreases tension while increasing performance
- Burn patients—decreased anxiety, tension, depression, pain, and itching
- Abdominal surgery patients—recover more quickly after surgery
- Premature infants—gain weight faster and fare better than those not massaged
- Autistic children—show less erratic behavior

Safety and Hygiene

PHYSICAL SAFETY

The physical safety of the client is one aspect involved in the selection of a place in which to practice. The following are a few physical safety considerations:

- Consider the location of the office. Is it in a safe neighborhood?
- Is the parking lot maintained? Salted and plowed, if applicable, in winter?
- Are ramps available for the handicapped?
- Are entranceway steps hazardous? Cracked or broken, icy in winter?
- Are all walking surfaces slip resistant?
- Is carpeting securely fastened to floor? Are throw rugs used that might trip a client?
- Do extension cords cross or lay close to walking areas?
- Is there anything inside the treatment room that might tip over or fall on a client?
- Are sources of heat or cold placed a safe distance from the client disrobing/dressing area?
- Are all of the surfaces a client is likely to come into contact with hypoallergenic?
- Does the client intake form include information regarding allergies?

- The containers that house spoilable oils and lotions need to be clearly labeled to facilitate timely disposal.
- All massage equipment needs to be safety inspected at least once a year.
- All office furniture needs to be inspected for safety at least once a year.

Hygiene

A standard reference for hygiene in any setting is the Web site "Universal Precautions" available at www.niehs.nih.gov/odhsb/biosafe/univers.htm. Additional sources of sanitation and hygiene information for massage therapy are found at the end of this appendix.

Personal Hygiene and Dress

Clean clothes, appearance, and shoes are required. Avoid perfumes or lotions. Hair must be cared for and groomed in such a manner that it does not contact client during the massage session. The therapist's body should be odor free. Blue jeans and shorts are not appropriate attire for a practitioner of a limited medical practice. Clean hands and fingernails, healthy skin and scalp (no dandruff) provide the appearance of good health, which we want our clients to emulate.

A cheerful countenance and smile are part of a good business plan. Jewelry can contact the client's skin or get caught in his or her hair. Don't wear jewelry.

SANITATION

The primary precaution in infection control for massage therapists is hand washing. Hand washing with hot water using an antibacterial/antiviral agent should be thorough, extending up onto the forearms. Hand washing must be done before and after each client. Paper towels can be used to dry hands and then used to open/close doors to avoid recontamination.

Touching items around the office between massage sessions could result in contaminating organisms being transmitted to the next client. That's why washing needs to be done thoroughly and often.

AREAS OF TRAFFIC

Areas of traffic need to be cleaned regularly. Sweepers with HEPA filters are helpful in keeping dust and similar agents from being propelled into the air.

Door knobs are handled by everyone and can be a major source of infectious material. They need to be washed with a disinfectant solution often.

MASSAGE TOOLS

Massage tools that come into contact with clients regularly, such as wooden or plastic massage tools or vibrators, must be disinfected after each use.

The oil bottles and lotion containers used by massage therapists need to be cleaned frequently with an antibacterial/antiviral agent.

LINENS

All linens are single-service items. After use they need to be stored in a container specified for that purpose.

Soiled linens should be washed at 140°F or more. Drying should also be at a high temperature. Storage of the clean laundry should be in a closed container designated for that purpose at least 4 inches off of the floor.

INTERPERSONAL TOUCH

The therapist needs to be especially aware of the client's skin condition. Avoidance of skin rashes and other skin abnormalities will help to prevent spread of the condition on the clients body and to the bodies of others.

MASSAGE SPECIALTIES

Massage specialties such as infant massage, prenatal massage, geriatric massage, hospice care, massage for specific diseases, and massage in hospitals, clinics, nursing homes, assisted living facilities, and day care facilities may have rules for safety and hygiene specific to the nature of health care or disease involved. Entering into such practices requires attention to the details of those specialties or locations.

REFERENCES

Fritz S. *Mosby's Fundamentals of Therapeutic Massage.* Mosby Lifeline, 1995.

American Massage Therapy Association. *The Business of Massage.* 2002.

Beck MF. *Milady's Theory and Practice of Therapeutic Massage.* Milady Publishing; 1999.

*Although this appendix covers many aspects of safety and hygiene, it is not possible to cover every possible safety and hygiene issue in massage therapy in the space available.

Suggested Reading

American Massage Therapy Association. *The Business of Massage*. Evanston, Ill; 2002. Available at: www.amtamassage.org.

Anderson DL. *Muscle Pain Relief in 90 Seconds, The Fold and Hold Method*. Minneapolis, Minn: Chronimed Publishing; 1995. Available at: www.chronimed.com.

Andrade, Clifford. *Outcome Based Massage*. Baltimore, Md: Lippincott Williams & Wilkins; 2001. Available at: www.lww.com.

Ashley M. *Massage: A Career at Your Fingertips*. Barrytown, NY: Station Hill Press; 1992. Available at: info@stationhill.org.

Beck MF. *Theory and Practice of Therapeutic Massage*. Albany, NY: Milady Publishing Co; 1999. Available at: www.milady.com.

Benjamin, Sohnen-Moe. *The Ethics of Touch*. Tucson, Ariz: Sohnen-Moe Publishers; 2003. Available at: www.sohnen-moe.com.

Brown Menard M. *Making Sense of Research*. Toronto, Ontario, Canada: Curties-Overzet Publications; 2003. Available at: www.sutherland-chan.com /copi.

Burch S. Holistic pathology for body-centered therapists. In: Lawrence, KS, ed. *Health Positive*. Available at: www.healthpositive.com.

Burch S. Recognizing health and illness: pathology for massage therapy and bodywork students. In: Lawrence, KS, ed. *Health Positive*. Available at: www.healthpositive.com.

Calvert RN. *The History of Massage.* Rochester, Vt: Healing Arts Press; 2002. Available at: www.massagemag.com.

Capellini S. *Massage Therapy Career Guide for Hands On Success.* New York, NY: Milady Press; 1999. Available at: www.milady.com.

Carlson, J. *Complementary Therapies and Wellness.* Saddle River, NJ: Prentice Hall; 2003. Available at: www.prenhall.com.

Chaitow L, Walker DeLaney, J. *Clinical Application of Neuromuscular Techniques; V-I, The Upper Body.* NY: Mosby; 2000. Available at: www.elsevierhealth.com.

Chaitow L, Walker DeLaney, J. *Clinical Application of Neuromuscular Techniques; V-II, The Lower Body.* NY: Mosby; 2000. Available at: www.elsevierhealth.com.

Chaitow L. *Fibromyalgia Syndrome.* Edinburgh, London, NY: Mosby; 2000. Available at: www.elsevierhealth.com.

Chaitow L. *Muscle Energy Techniques: Advanced Soft Tissue Techniques.* London, England: Churchill Livingstone; 2001. Available at: www.harcourt. com.

Clarkson H. *Musculoskeletal Assessment.* Baltimore, Md: Lippincott Williams & Wilkins; 2000. Available at: www.lww.com.

Clay, Pounds. *Basic Clinical Massage Therapy: Integrating Anatomy and Treatment.* Baltimore, Md: Lippincott Williams & Wilkins; 2002. Available at: www.lww.com.

Curties D. *Breast Massage.* Toronto, Ontario, Canada: Curties-Overzet Publications; 2003. Available at: www.sutherland-chan.com/copi.

Curties D. *Massage Therapy & Cancer*. Toronto, Ontario, Canada: Curties-Overzet Publications; 2003. Available at: www.sutherland-chan.com/copi.

Ebner M. *Connective Tissue Manipulations*. Malabar, Fla: Krieger Publishing Co; 1985. Available at: www.krieger-publishing.com.

Goodman S. *The Book of Shiatsu: The Healing Art of Finger Pressure*. Garden City, NY: Avery Publishing Group Inc; 1990. Available at: www.averypublishing.com.

Greenman P. *Principles of Manual Medicine.* Baltimore, Md: Lippincott Williams & Wilkins; 2001. Available at: www.lww.com.

Hendrickson T. *Massage for Orthopedic Conditions*. Baltimore, Md: Lippincott Williams & Wilkins; 2002. Available at: www.lww.com.

Hess M, Mochizuki S. *Japanese Hot Stone Massage*. Boulder, Colo: Kotobuki Publications; 2002. Available at: www.japanesemassage.com.

Hoppenfeld S. *Physical Examination of the Spine and Extremities*. East Norwalk, Conn: Appleton-Century-Crofts Publishers; 1976. Available at: www.prenhall.com.

Jewell Rich G, ed. *Massage Therapy: The Evidence for Practice*. NY: Mosby. Available at: www.elsevierhealth.com.

Jones LH. *Strain and Counterstrain*. Newark, Ohio: American Academy of Osteopathy; 1992. Available at: www.academyofosteopathy.org.

Juhan D. *Job's Body: A Handbook for Bodywork*. Barrytown, NY: Station Hill Press; 1998. Available at: info@stationhill.org.

Kellogg JH. *The Art of Massage*. Battle Creek, Mich: Modern Medicine Publishing Company; 1929. Available at: www.meridianinstitute.com/eamt/files/kellogg/kelcont.html.

Kendall, McCreary, Provance. *Muscles: Testing and Function with Posture and Pain.* Baltimore, Md: Lippincott Williams & Wilkins; 2001. Available at: www.lww.com.

Lowe W. *Functional Assessment in Massage Therapy.* Bend, Ore: Orthopedic Massage Education Research Institute; 1997. Available at: www.omeri.com.

Lowe W. *Orthopedic Massage.* NY: Mosby. Available at: www.elsevierhealth.com.

Mattes AL. *Flexibility: Active and Assisted Stretching.* Sarasota, Fla: Aaron L. Mattes Publisher; 1990. Available at: www.stretchingusa.com.

Mense, Simons. *Muscle Pain: Understanding Its Nature, Diagnosis and Treatment.* Baltimore, Md: Lippincott Williams & Wilkins; 2001. Available at: www.lww.com.

Miller E. *Shiatsu Massage.* Albany, NY: Milady Publishing Co; 1996. Available at: www.milady.com.

Mochizuki S. *Hand Maintenance Guide for Massage Therapists.* Boulder, Colo: Kotobuki Publications; 1999. Available at: www.japanesemassage.com.

Mochizuki S. *Zoku Shin Do: The Art of Asian Foot Reflexology, Vol I.* Boulder, Colo: Kotobuki Publications; 1999. Available at: www.japanese-massage.com.

Myers T. *Anatomy Trains, Myofascial Meridians for Manual and Movement Therapists.* Edinburgh, London, NY: Mosby. Available at: www.elsevierhealth.com.

Netter FH. *Atlas of Human Anatomy.* Summit, NJ: CIBA-GEIGA Corp.;1989.

Palmer D. *The Bodywork Entrepreneur.* San Francisco, Calif: Thumb Press; 1990. Available at: www.touchpro.com.

Persad RS. *Massage Therapy & Medications.* Toronto, Ontario, Canada: Curties-Overzet Publications; 2003. Available at: www.sutherland-chan.com/copi.

Petty NJ, Moore AP. *Neuromusculoskeletal Examination and Assessment: A Handbook for Therapists.* NY: Mosby. Available at: www.elsevierhealth.com.

Premkumar K. *Pathology A to Z: Handbook for Massage Therapists.* Baltimore, Md: Lippincott Williams & Wilkins; 2001. Available at: www.lww.com.

Premkumar K. *The Massage Connection: Anatomy, Physiology & Pathology.* Baltimore, Md: Lippincott Williams & Wilkins; 2002. Available at: www.lww.com.

Scheumann DW. *The Balanced Body, A Guide to Deep Tissue and Neuromuscular Therapy.* Philadelphia, Pa: Lippincott, Williams & Wilkins; 2002. Available at: www.lww.com.

Simons D, Travell J, Simons L. *Myofascial Pain and Dysfunction: The Trigger Point Manual, Vol. I, Upper Half of Body.* Baltimore, Md: Lippincott Williams & Wilkins; 1999. Available at: www.lww.com.

Simons D, Travell J, Simons L. *Myofascial Pain and Dysfunction: The Trigger Point Manual, Vol. II, Lower Half of Body.* Baltimore, Md: Lippincott Williams & Wilkins; 1999. Available at: www.lww.com.

Sohnen-Moe CM. *Business Mastery.* Tucson, Ariz: Sohnen-Moe Associates, Inc; 1997. Available at: www.sohnen-moe.com.

Stone R, Stone J. *Atlas of Skeletal Muscles.* Dubuque, Iowa: McGraw Hill Publishers; 2000. Available at: www.mhhe.com.

Successful Business Handbook. Evergreen, Colo: Associated Bodywork & Massage Professionals; 2002. Available at: www.abmp.com.

Tappan FM, Benjamin PJ. *Tappan's Handbook of Healing Massage Techniques: Classis, Holistic, and Emerging Methods.* Stamford, Conn: Appleton & Lange; 1998. Available at: www.prenhall.com.

Thompson D. *Hands Heal: Communication, Documentation, and Insurance Billing For Manual Therapists.* Baltimore, Md: Lippincott Williams & Wilkins; 2002. Available at: www.lww.com.

Werner R. *A Massage Therapist's Guide to Pathology.* Baltimore, Md: Lippincott Williams & Wilkins; 2002. Available at: www.lww.com.

General Acronyms and Abbreviations

(A): assisted, assistance

A: accommodation

a.: artery

AAROM: active assistive range of motion

ABD: abduction

ABNORM: abnormal

ABR: absolute bedrest

AC: acromioclavicular

ACCE: Academic Coordinator of Clinical Education

ACLF: adult congregate living facility

ACT: adaptive control of thoughts

ACTH: adrenocorticotrophic hormone

AD: admitting diagnosis

AD: Alzheimer's disease

AD: autogenic drainage

ADA: Americans with Disabilities Act

ADD: adduction

ADD: attention deficit disorder

ADH: antidiuretic hormone

ADHD: attention deficit hyperactivity disorder

ADL: activities of daily living

ad lib: as desired

ADM: administration

ADP: adenosine diphosphate

ADS: alternative delivery system

AE: above elbow

AFDC: Aid to Families with Dependent Children

AFO: ankle foot orthosis

AI: autistic impaired

AIDS: acquired immmunodeficiency syndrome

AJPT: *American Journal of Physical Therapy*

AK: above knee

ALOS: average length of stay

ALS: amyotrophic lateral sclerosis

AMA: against medical advice

Am't: amount

ANCOVA: analysis of covariance

ANOVA: analysis of variance

ANS: autonomic nervous system

Ant: anterior

AP: anterior-posterior

APG: Ambulatory Patient (Payment) Group

Approx: approximately

AROM: active range of motion

ART: active resistive training

ASA: aspirin

ASAP: as soon as possible

ASCII: American Standard Code for Information Interchange

ASHD: arterial sclerotic heart disease

ASO: arteriosclerosis obliterans

ASROM: assistive range of motion

AT: assistive technology

ATNR: asymmetrical tonic neck reflex

ATP: adenosine triphosphate

(B): both, bilateral

BADL: basic activities of daily living

Ba Enema: barium enema

BBA: Balanced Budget Act

BBS: bulletin board system

BE: base equivalent

BE: below elbow

BG: blood glucose

bid: twice a day

Bilat: bilateral

BK: below knee

BKA: below-knee amputee

Bl: blood

BLT: bilateral lung transplant

bm: body mechanics

BM: bowel movement

BMD: bone mineral density

BMI: body mass index

BMR: basal metabolic rate

BOS: base of support

BP: blood pressure

BPM: beats per minute

BR: bedrest

BRP: bathroom privileges

BS: blood sugar

BSA: body surface area

BSF: benign senescent forgetfulness

BT: brain tumor

BUN: blood urea nitrogen

C: centigrade, Celsius

C: cervical

Ca: calcium

CA: cancer

Cal: calorie

CART: classification and regression trees

CAT: computer-assisted tomography

CBC: complete blood count

CBI: closed brain injury

CBR: complete bedrest

CBS: chronic brain syndrome

CC: chief complaint

cc: cubic centimeter(s)

CCCE: Clinical Coordinator of Clinical Education

CCS: Certified Cardiopulmonary Specialist

CCU: coronary care unit

CDC: Centers for Disease Control and Prevention

CDM: Charge Description Master (HCFA)

CE: continuing education

CEO: chief executive officer

CF: cystic fibrosis

CFR: code of federal regulations

CHAMPUS: Civilian Health and Medical Program of the Uniformed Services

CHD: coronary heart disease

CHF: congestive heart failure

CHI: closed head injury

CHT: certified hand therapist

CI: cardiac index

CI: clinical instructor

CICU: coronary intermediate care unit

CK: creatine kinase

Cl: chloride; chlorine

cm: centimeter(s)

CMP: competitive medical plan

CNS: central nervous system

CO: carbon monoxide

CO_2: carbon dioxide

c/o: complains of

COB: coordination of benefits

COG: center of gravity

COJ: *Classification of Jobs According to Worker Trait Factors*

COLA: cost of living adjustment

COLD: chronic obstructive lung disease

COM: center of mass or center of motion

CONTRA: contraindication

COPD: chronic pulmonary obstructive disease

CORF: comprehensive outpatient rehabilitation facility

CP: chest pain

CPE: certified professional ergonomist

CPE: continuing professional education

CPEF: Clinical Performance Evaluation Form (developed by the New England Consortium of Academic Coordinators of Clinical Education)

CPI: consumer price index

CPM: continuous passive motion

CPR: cardiopulmonary resuscitation

CPT: *Current Procedural Terminology*

CPU: central processing unit

CQI: continuous quality improvement

CRI: chronic renal insufficiency

CSF: cerebrospinal fluid

CSHN: Children with Special Health Needs

CSM: Combined Sections Meeting (APTA)

CT: computed tomography

CTS: carpal tunnel syndrome

cu: cubic

CV: cardiovascular

CVA: cerebrovascular accident

CVD: cardiovascular disease

CVP: central venous pressure

CXR: chest x-ray

D: distal

D&C: dilation and curettage

d/c: discharge

DD: developmental disabilities

Dep: dependent

Derm: dermatology

DFF: Directions for the Future

dia: diameter

DIP: distal interphalangeal

DJD: degenerative joint disease

DKA: diabetic ketoacidosis

dL: deciliter (=100 mL)

DM: diabetes mellitus

DME: durable medical equipment

DMEPOS: durable medical equipment protheses, orthotics, and supplies

DMERC: DME Regional Carrier (HCFA)

DMG: dimethylglycerine

DNA: deoxyribonucleic acid

DNR: "Do not resuscitate" orders

DOE: dyspnea on exertion

Doff: take off clothing

DOMS: delayed onset muscle soreness

Don: put on clothing

DOT: *Dictionary of Occupational Titles*

DRG: diagnosis related groups

DRS: disability rating scale

DSR: Dynamic Spatial Reconstructor

DT: delirium tremens

DTP: diphtheria-tetanus-pertussis (vaccine)

DTR: deep tendon reflex

DVT: deep vein thrombosis

Dx: diagnosis

DZ: disease

EAP: employee assistance program

ECF: extended care facility

E.C.F.: extracellular fluid

ECG: electrocardiogram

ECT: electroconvulsive therapy

ECU: environmental control unit

EDM: extensor digitorum minimi

EEG: electroencephalogram

EENT: eye, ear, nose, and throat

EKG: electrocardiogram

EMA: external moment arm

EMG: electromyelogram

EMI: educable mentally impaired

EMS: electrical muscle stimulation

EMS: emergency medical service

ENT: ear, nose, and throat

EOB: edge of bed

EOB: explanation of benefits

EOM: edge of mat

EPL: extensor pollicis longus

EPSDT: Early and Periodic Screening, Diagnostic, and Treatment

ER: emergency room

ER: external rotation

ERV: expiratory reserve volume

ESR: erythrocyte sedimentation rate

ESRD: end stage renal disease

ESTR: electrical stimulation for tissue repair

ETIOL: etiology

EVAL: evaluation, evaluate
Ex: example
EX: exercise
EXT: extension

F-: fair (40%)
F: Fahrenheit
F: fair (50%)
F: female
F+: fair (60%)
FAS: fetal alcohol syndrome
FCU: flexor carpi ulnaris
FEMS: functional electrical muscle stimulation
FES: functional electrical stimulation
FET: force expiratory technique
FEV1: forced expiratory volume
FH: family history
FIM: functional independence measure
FLEX: flexion
FOR: frame of reference
FRG: functional related groups
FSH: follicle-stimulating hormone
ft: foot, feet
FUNC: function
FUO: fever undetermined origin
FWB: full weightbearing
FWW: front-wheeled walker
FY: fiscal year
Fx: fracture

G-: good (70%)

G: good (80%)

G+: good (90%)

GABA: gamma-amionbutyric acid

GAS: general adaptation syndrome

GAU: geriatric assessment unit

GBS: Guillain-Barré syndrome

GCRC: General Clinical Research Center

GCS: Geriatric Certified Specialist

GEC: geriatric education center

GED: general educational development

GER: gerontology

GFR: glomerular filtration rate

GI: gastrointestinal

gm: gram(s)

GME: Graduate Medical Education

GNP: Gross National Product

GOE: *Guide for Occupational Exploration*

Gr: grain

GSR: galvanic skin response

GSW: gunshot wound

GU: genitourinary

GYN: gynecology

H2: histamine

H/A: headache

Hb: hemoglobin

HCFA: Health Care Finance Administration

HCO$_3$: bicarbonate

HCPCS: Health Care Financing Administration Common Procedure Coding System

HCS: Health Communication Services

Hct: hematocrit

HCVD: hypertensive cardiovascular disease

HDL: high density lipoprotein

HEA: Higher Education Act

Hemi: hemiplegia

HEP: home exercise program

HF: heart failure

Hg: mercury

Hgb: hemoglobin

HHA: home health agency

HHE: home health equipment

HI: head injury

HI: hearing impaired

HI: hospital insurance

HIV: human immunodeficiency virus

HL: human leukocyte

HMO: health maintenance organization

H&P: history and physical

HP: hot pack

HPI: history of present illness

HR: heart rate

Hr: hour

HS: high school

HS: hours of sleep

HSA: health systems agency

HSN: hospital satellite network

HTN: hypertension
HVPS: high-voltage pulsed stimulation
Hx: history
HYPO: hypodermic
Hz: hertz (cycles/second)

I: independent
IADL: instrumental activities of daily living
IAT: Inter-Agency Transfer
IC: inspiratory capacity
IC: integrated circuit
ICD: *International Classification of Diseases*
ICD-9: *International Classification of Diseases*, 9th Rev
ICF: intermediary care facility
I.C.F.: intracellular fluid
ICIDH: *International Classification of Impairments, Disabilities, and Handicaps*
ICIDH-2: *International Classification of Impairments, Disabilities, and Handicaps—2*
ICU: intensive care unit
IDDM: insulin-dependent diabetes mellitus
IDEA: Individuals with Disabilities Education Act
IDT: Inter-Departmental Transfer
IEP: individualized education plan
IFSP: individual family service plan
IgA, etc: immunoglobin A, etc
ILC: independent living center
IM: intramuscular
IME: Indirect Medical Education

IMP: impression (tentative diagnosis)

in: inch(es)

IND: indications

Indep: independent

inf: inferior

Inhal: inhalation

Inj: injection

IP: interphalangeal

IPA: independent practice association

IPPB: inspiratory positive pressure breathing

IR: internal rotation

IRV: inspiratory reserve volume

ITC: Information Technology and Communications

ITP: individual transition plan

IU: International Unit(s)

IV: intravenous

IVDU: intravenous drug user

IVP: intravenous pyelogram

JRA: juvenile rheumatoid arthritis

JROM: joint range of motion

K: potassium

KAFO: knee ankle foot orthosis

KB: kilobyte

kcal: kilocalorie (food calorie)

kg: kilogram(s)

KJ: knee jerk

KO: knee orthosis

KUB: kidney, ureter, bladder

(L): left
L: liter(s); lumbar
LAD: language acquisition device
Lat: lateral
lb: pound(s)
LBP: low back pain
LC: locus coeruleus
LCR: lifetime clinical record
LD: learning disabilities
LDH: lactic dehydrogenase
LDL: low-density lipoprotein
LDLR: Labor and Delivery, Recovery, Postpartum
LE: lower extremity
L.E.: lupus erythematosus
LH: lutenizing hormone
LLB: long leg brace
LLD: leg length discrepancy
LLE: left lower extremity
LLQ: left lower quadrant (of abdomen)
LMN: lower motor neuron
LMP: last menstrual period
LMT: Licensed Massage Therapist
LOA: leave of absence
LOC: loss of consciousness
LOS: length of stay
LP: lumbar puncture
LS: lumbosacral

LTC: long-term care
LTG: long-term goals
LUE: left upper extremity
L&W: living and well

M: male
m: meter(s)
m.: muscle
MA: mechanical advantage
ma: milliampere(s)
MAO: monoamine oxidase
MAS: mobile arm support
Max: maximum
MBD: minimal brain damage
MC: metacarpal
MCC: Medical Center Computing
MCE: medical care evaluation
mcg: microgram(s)
MCH: Maternal and Child Health
MCH: mean corpuscular hemoglobin
MCHC: mean corpusular hemoglobin concentration
MCO: managed care organization
MCP: metacarpalphalangeal
MCV: mean corpuscular volume
MD: muscular dystrophy
Mdn: median
MDS: minimum data set
med: medium, medial, median

MED: minimum effective dose

MEPS: motor evoked potentials

mEq: milliequivalent(s)

MFR: myofascial release

MFT: muscle function test

Mg: magnesium

mg: milligram(s)

MG: myasthenia gravis

MH: mental health

MHB: maximum hospital benefit

MHC: myosin heavy chain

MI: myocardial infarction

MIN: minimal

min: minute

MIS: Medical Information System

mL: milliliter(s)

mm: millimeter(s)

MMSE: Mini-Mental Status Exam

MMT: manual muscle testing

MNE: motor neuron excitability

mo: month

Mod: moderate

MP: metacarpophalangeal joint

mph: miles per hour

MPSMS: materials, products, subject matter, or services

MRI: magnetic resonance imaging

MRSA: methicillin-resistant staphylococcus aureus

MS: mitral stenosis

MS: multiple sclerosis

MSP: Medicare secondary payer

MSQ: mental status questionnaire

MT: massage therapist/massage therapy

MTEWA: machines, tools, equipment, and work aids used

MUP: motor unit potential

MVA: motor vehicle accident

MVC: maximum voluntary contraction

MVE: maximum voluntary effort

n.: nerve

N: normal; nitrogen

Na: sodium

N/A: not applicable or not available

NaC: normal saline

NCS: Neurology Certified Specialist

ND: new drugs

NDT: Neurodevelopmental Treatment

Neg: negative

ng: nanogram

NG-tube: nasogastric tube

NICU: neonatal intensive care unit

NIDDM: non-insulin-dependent diabetes mellitus

NKA: no known allergy

NKDA: no known drug allergy

NP: neuropsychiatry; nursing procedure

NPH: neutral protein Hagedorn (insulin)

NPN: non-protein nitrogen

NPO: nothing by mouth
NREM: non-rapid eye movement
NSAIDs: nonsteroidal anti-inflammatory drugs
NSG: nursing
NWB: non-weightbearing

O$_2$: oxygen
OA: osteoarthritis
OB: obstetrics
OBRA '87: Omnibus Budget Reconciliation Act of 1987
OBS: observation
OCS: Orthopedic Certified Specialist
OD: once daily
OD: right eye
OHT: orthotopic heart transplant
OLPR: Online Patient Record
OLT: orthotopic liver transplant
OOB: out of bed
OPD: outpatient department
OR: operating room
Orth: orthopedic
OS: left eye
OTC: over the counter
OU: both eyes
oz: ounce

P-: poor (10%)
P: phosphorus; pressure

P: poor (20%)

P+: poor (30%)

P$_{CO2}$: carbon dioxide pressure (or tension)

P$_{O2}$: oxygen pressure (or tension)

PA: posterior anterior

Pa$_{CO2}$: arterial carbon dioxide pressure

Pa$_{O2}$: arterial oxygen pressure

PA$_{O2}$: alveolar oxygen pressure

PAMs: physical agent modalities

PARA: paraplegia

PATH: pathology

PATRA: Professional and Technical Role Analysis

PCA: personal care attendant

PCS: Pediatric Certified Specialist

PCT: periarticular connective tissue

PD: physical disabilities

PDD: pervasive developmental disorder

PDR: *Physicians' Desk Reference*

PE: physical examination

Ped: pediatric

PES: Professional Examination Service

PET: Positron emission tomography

PFS: Patient Financial Services

PFT: pulmonary function test

PHYS: physical; physiology

Phys Dys: physical disabilities

PI: present illness

PI: proactive interface

PICU: pediatric intensive care unit

PID: pelvic inflammatory disease

PIP: proximal interphalangeal

PKU: phenylketoneuria

PMH: past medical history

PMR: physical medicine and rehabilitation

PMT: premotor time

PNF: proprioceptive neuromuscular facilitation

PNS: peripheral nervous system

PO: by mouth

PO: postoperative

POMR: problem-oriented medical record

Postop: postoperative

PPE: personal protective equipment

ppm: parts per million

PPO: preferred provider organization

PPS: prospective payment system (Medicare)

PRE: progressive resistive exercise

Preop: preoperative

PRN: whenever necessary

PRO: peer review organization

PROG: prognosis

PROM: passive range of motion

PROSTUD: Prospective Student Program Data Base

pt: pint(s)

PTA: prior to admission

PTB: patella tendon bearing

PTSD: posttraumatic stress disorder

PVD: peripheral vascular disease

PVE: prevocational evaluation

PWA: person with AIDS

PWB: partial weightbearing

Px: physical examination

q: every

q2h: every 2 hours

QA: quality assurance

qd: every day

qh: every hour

QI: quality improvement

qid: four times daily

qn: every night

qod: every other day

qt: quart

(R): right

R, r: roentgen(s)

RA: reasonable accommodation

RA: rheumatoid arthritis

RAM: random access memory

RAP: resident assessment protocol

RAS: reticular activating system

RBC: red blood count

RBRVS: Resource-Based Relative Value Scale (Medicare)

RC: rehabilitation counselor

RD: retinal detachment

Rehab: rehabilitation

REM: rapid eye movement
RET: rational emotive therapy
RF: renal failure
RF: rheumatoid factor; rheumatic fever
RHC: Rural Health Clinic
RHD: rheumatic heart disease
RLE: right lower extremity
RM: repetition maximum
RNA: ribonucleic acid
RPCH: Rural Primary Care Hospital
RO: rule out
ROH: Roster of Honor
ROM: range of motion
ROS: review of systems
RPE: rating of perceived exertion
RROM: resistive range of motion
RTI: routine task inventory
RUE: right upper extremity
RUG: resource utilization grouping
RV: residual volume
RVU: relative value unit
Rx: prescription

S: social history; sacral
SAD: seasonal affective disorder
Sa$_{O2}$: arterial oxygen saturation
SAQ: short arc quad
sat: saturated
SBE: subacute bacterial endocarditis

SBF: skin blood cell flux

s.c.: subcutaneous(ly)

SCI: spinal cord injury

SCS: Splint Classification System

SCS: Sports Certified Specialist

SE: side effects

sec: second(s)

SED: seriously emotionally disturbed

SEP: somatosensory evoked potential

SGOT: serum glutamic oxaloacetic transaminase

SGPT: serum glutamic pyruvic transaminase

SHUR: System for Hospital Uniform Reporting

SI: sensory integration

SICU: surgical intensive care unit

SIDS: sudden infant death syndrome

SLB: short leg brace

SLE: systemic lupus erythematosus

SLH: State and Local Hospitalization

SLR: straight leg raise

SMI: supplemental medical insurance

SMS: Shared Medical Systems

SNF: skilled nursing facility

SOAP: subjective, objective, assessment, plan

SOB: shortness of breath

soln: solution

SOP: standard operating procedure

SOS: if necessary

SP: speech

s/p: status post

SPEM: smooth pursuit eye movement

sp. gr.: specific gravity

S$_{PO2}$: pulse oxygen saturation

SPSS: *Statistical Package for Social Sciences*

SPT: student physical therapist

sq: square

SR: systematic review

SSI: supplemental security income

Stat: at once

STD: sexually transmitted disease

STG: short-term goals

STNR: symmetrical tonic neck reflex

SUDS: single use diagnostic system

sup: superior

Sup: supination

SVP: specific vocational preparation

Sx: symptom

SXI: severely multiply impaired

SYM: symptom

Sz: schizophrenia

Sz: seizure

T: trace (5%)

t$_{1/2}$: half-life

T&A: tonsils and adenoids

TAB: temporarily abled body

TAP: turning and positioning program

TB: tuberculosis

TBG: thyroxin-binding globulin

TBI: traumatic brain injury

TDD: telecommunication device for the deaf

TDWB: touch down weightbearing

TEFRA: Tax Equity and Fiscal Responsibility Act

TENS: transcutaneous electrical nerve stimulation

Th: thoracic

THR: total hip replacement

TIA: transient ischemic attack

tid: three times daily

TKR: total knee replacement

TLR: tonic labyrinthe reflex

TOWER: testing, orientation, and work evaluation in rehabilitation

TPR: temperature, pulse, respiration

TQM: total quality management

TSH: thyroid-stimulating hormone

TTWB: toe touch weightbearing

TTY: teletypewriter

TV: tidal volume

Tx: treatment

u: unit(s)

UAP: university-affiliated programs

UE: upper extremity

UMN: upper motor neuron

Un: unable

UR: utilization review

URI: upper respiratory infection

US: ultrasound

USA: unstable angina
UTI: urinary tract infection
UV: ultraviolet

VC: vital capacity
VER: visual evoked response
VI: volume index
VO: verbal order
V$_{O2}$: maximum oxygen consumption
VS: vestibular stimulation
VS: vital signs

WBAT: weightbearing as tolerated
WBC: white blood cell count
WBQC: wide base quad cane
W/C or WC: wheelchair
WD: well developed
WFL: within functional limits
WIC: Special Supplemental Nutrition Program for Women, Infants, and Children
Wk: week
WN: well nourished
WNL: within normal limits
WORK: *Work: A Journal of Prevention, Assessment & Rehabilitation*
wt: weight

x: times
y/n: yes/no

y/o: years old
yrs: years

Organization Acronyms

AA: Alcoholics Anonymous

AAA: Area Agencies on Aging

AAACE: American Association of Adult and Continuing Education

AAAS: American Association for the Advancement of Science

AACHP: American Association for Comprehensive Health Planning

AAFP: American Academy of Family Practitioners

AAHPERD: American Alliance for Health, Physical Education, Recreation, and Dance

AAMR: American Association on Mental Retardation

AAP: American Academy of Pediatrics

AAPC: American Association of Pastoral Counselors

AAPD: American Academy of Pediatric Dentists

AAPH: American Association of Partial Hospitalization

AARP: American Association for Retired Persons

AART: American Association for Respiratory Therapy

AART: Association for the Advancement of Rehabilitation Technology

ABMP: Associated Bodywork and Massage Professionals

ABPTS: American Board of Physical Therapy Specialists

ACA: American Counseling Association

ACALD: Association for Children and Adults with Learning Disabilities

ACCD: American Coalition of Citizens with Disabilities

ACCH: Association for the Care of Children's Health

ACCP: American College of Chest Physicians

ACDD: Accreditation Council on Services for People with Developmental Disabilities

ACF: Administration for Children and Families

ACHCA: American College of Health Care Administrators

ACIP: Advisory Committee on Immunization Practices

ACRE: American Council on Rural Education

ACRM: American Congress of Rehabilitation Medicine

ACSM: American College of Sports Medicine

ACYF: Administration on Children, Youth, and Families

ADA: American Dietetic Association

ADD: Administration on Developmental Disabilities

ADED: Association of Driver Educators for the Disabled

ADHA: American Dental Hygienists Association

ADRDA: Alzheimer's Disease and Related Disorders Association

AERA: American Educational Research Association

AF: Arthritis Foundation

AGA: American Geriatric Association

AGHE: Association for Gerontology in Higher Education

AHA: American Hospital Association

AHCA: American Health Care Association

AHCPR: Agency for Health Care Policy and Research

AHEA: American Home Economics Association

AHPA: Arthritis Health Professional Association

AICPR: American Institute of Certified Public Accountants

AMA: American Medical Association

AMDA: American Medical Directors Association

AMH: Accreditation Manual for Hospitals (JCAHO)

AMTA: American Massage Therapy Association

ANA: American Nurses Association

ANSI: American National Standards Institute

AOA: Administration on Aging (DHHS)

AOA: American Optometric Association

AOA: American Osteopathic Association

AOPA: American Orthotic and Prosthetic Association

AOTA: American Occupational Therapy Association

APA: American Psychiatric Association

APA: American Psychological Association

APHA: American Public Health Association

APTA: American Physical Therapy Association

ARC: Association for Retarded Citizens

ARCA: American Rehabilitation Counseling Association

ARF: Association of Rehabilitation Facilities

ASA: American Society on Aging

ASAE: American Society of Association Executives

ASAHP: American Society of Allied Health Professions

ASHA: American Speech-Language-Hearing Association

ASHT: American Society of Hand Therapists

ASI: Assessment Systems, Inc

ASPA: Association of Specialized and Professional Accreditors

BC/BC: Blue Cross/ Blue Shield Association

BCPE: Board for Certification in Professional Ergonomics

BHP: Bureau of Health Professions (DHHS)

BLS: Bureau of Labor Statistics (DOL)

BOC: Board of Commissioners (JCAHO)

BPD: Bureau of Policy Development (HCFA)

BPO: Bureau of Operations (HCFA)

CAAHEP: Commission on Accreditation of Allied Health Education Programs

CAHEA: Committee on Allied Health Education and Accreditation (AMA)

CAPTE: Commission on Accreditation in Physical Therapy Education

CARF: Commission on Accreditation of Rehabilitation Facilities

CBO: Congressional Budget Office

CCB: Child Care Bureau

CCD: Consortium for Citizens with Disabilities

CCR&R: Child Care Resource and Referral Agency

CCY: Coalition for Children and Youth

CDC: Centers for Disease Control and Prevention

CEC: Council for Exceptional Children

CHF: Coalition for Health Funding

CHHA/CHS: Council of Home Health Agencies and Community Health Services (NLN)

CLEAR: Clearinghouse on Licenser, Enforcement, and Regulation

CME: Council on Medical Education (AMA)

COMTA: Commission on Massage Therapy Accreditation

COPA: Council on Postsecondary Accreditation

CORE: Commission on Rehabilitation Education

CSG: Council of State Governments

CSN: Children's Safety Network

CSS: Children's Specialty Services

CWLA: Child Welfare League of America

DAHEA: Division of Allied Health Education and Accreditation (AMA)

DAHP: Division of Associated Health Professions (DHHS)

DHHS: Department of Health and Human Services

DOE: Department of Education

DOL: Department of Labor

ECELS: Early Childhood Education Linkage System

EFA: Epilepsy Foundation of America

EHA: Education of Handicapped Act

FAHD: Forum on Allied Health Data

FAO: United Nations Food and Agriculture Organization

FDA: Food and Drug Administration (DHHS)

FEC: Federal Election Commission

FEHBP: Federal Employees Health and Benefits Program

FM: Financial Management Department

FTC: Federal Trade Commission

FUSA: Families United for Senior Action

GAO: Government Accounting Office

GMENAC: Graduate Medical Education National Advisory Committee

GSA: Gerontological Society of America

GU: Generations United

GWSAE: Greater Washington Society of Association Executives

HBMN: Hospital Based Massage Network

HCFA: Health Care Financing Administration (DHHS)

HCPAC: Health Care Professionals Advisory Committee (AMA)

HCPDG: Health Care Professionals Discussion Group

HFMA: Healthcare Financial Management Association

HIAA: Health Insurance Association of America

HMHB: Healthy Mothers, Healthy Babies Coalition

HMO: Health Maintenance Organization

HRSA: Health Resources and Services Administration (DHHS)

HSF: Health Services Foundation

HSQB: Health Standards and Quality Bureau (HCFA)

HTCC: Hand Therapy Certification Commission

IAIM: International Association of Infant Massage
IHS: Indian Health Service
IMA: International Massage Association
IOM: Institute of Medicine
IRB: Institutional Review Board
IRS: Internal Revenue Service
IRSG: Insurance Rehabilitation Study Group

JCAHO: Joint Commission on Accreditation of
    Healthcare Organizations

LDA: Learning Disabilities Association

MCHB: Maternal and Child Health Bureau
    (DHHS)
MDAA: Muscular Dystrophy Association of
    America
MPI: Meeting Planners International
MRC: Medical Research Council

NAATRP: National Association of Activity
    Therapy and Rehabilitation Programs
NACCRRA: National Association of Child Care
    Resource and Referral Agencies
NACOSH: National Advisory Committee on
    Scouting for the Handicapped
NADT: National Association for Drama Therapy
NAEYC: National Association for Education of
    Young Children
NAHB/NRC: National Association of Home
    Builders/National Research Center
NAHC: National Association for Home Care

NAHHA: National Association of Home Health Agencies

NAMI: National Alliance for the Mentally Ill

NAMME: National Association of Medical Minority Educators

NAMT: National Association for Music Therapy

NANMT: National Association of Nurse Massage Therapists

NAPHS: National Association of Psychiatric Health Systems

NAPNAP: National Association of Pediatric Nurse Associates and Practitioners

NAPSO: National Alliance of Pupil Service Organizations

NARA: National Association of Rehabilitation Agencies

NARC: National Association for Retarded Citizens

NARF: National Association of Rehabilitation Facilities

NASA: National Aeronautics and Space Agency

NASDSE: National Association of State Directors of Special Education

NASL: National Association for Long-Term Care

NASMHPD: National Association of State Mental Health Program Directors

NASUA: National Association of State Units on Aging

NASW: National Association of Social Workers

NAVESP: National Association of Vocational Education Special Personnel

NCAHE: National Commission on Allied Health Education

NCBFE: National Center for a Barrier Free Environment

NCBTMB: National Certification Board for Therapeutic Massage and Bodywork

NCCNHR: National Citizens Coalition for Nursing Home Reform

NCD: National Council on Disability

NCDPEH: National Coalition for Disease Prevention and Environmental Health

NCEMCH: National Center for Education in Maternal and Child Health

NCES: National Center for Education Statistics (DHHS)

NCHC: National Council on Health Care Technologists

NCHCA: National Commission for Health Certifying Agencies

NCHHA: National Council of Homemakers and Home Health Aides

NCHP: National Council for Health Planning

NCHS: National Center for Health Statistics (DHHS)

NCIL: National Council on Independent Living

NCMRR: National Center for Medical Rehabilitation Research

NCOA: National Council on Aging

NCSL: National Conference of State Legislatives

NDTA: Neurodevelopmental Treatment Association

NHC: National Health Council

NHLA: National Health Lawyers Association

NHO: National Hospice Organization

NHTSA: National Highway Traffic Safety Administration

NIA: National Institute on Aging

NIAAA: National Institutes on Alcohol Abuse and Alcoholism (Public Health Service)

NICCYD: National Information Center for Children and Youth with Disabilities

NIDA: National Institute of Drug Abuse

NIDRR: National Institute on Disability and Rehabilitation Research

NIH: National Institutes of Health

NIHR: National Institute of Handicapped Research

NIMH: National Institute of Mental Health

NLN: National League for Nursing

NLRB: National Labor Relations Board

NMHA: National Mental Health Association

NMSS: National Multiple Sclerosis Society

NPSRC: National Professional Standards Review Council

NRA: National Rehabilitation Association

NRC: National Research Council

NRCA: National Rehabilitation Counseling Association

NRTI: National Rehabilitation Training Institutes

NUCEA: National University Continuing Education Association

NVOILA: National Voluntary Organizations for Independent Living for the Aging

OCR: Office of Civil Rights

OE: Office of Education

OH: Office of the Handicapped

OIG: Office of the Inspector General

OMB: Office of Management and Budget (Executive Office of the President)

OPM: Office of Personnel Management

OPRR: Office for Protection from Research Risks (DHHS)

OSEP: Office of Special Education Programs

OSERS: Office of Special Education and Rehabilitation Services (DOE)

OSG: Office of the Surgeon General

OSHA: Occupational Safety and Health Administration

OVR: Office of Vocational Rehabilitation

OWH: Office of Women's Health (DHHS)

PAC-APTA: Political Action Committee— American Physical Therapy Association

PATH: Partners Appropriate Technology for the Handicapped

PCMA: Professional Convention Management Association

PCPD: President's Committee on People with Disabilities

PPO: Preferred Provider Organization

PROPAC: Prospective Payment Assessment Commission

PRRB: Provider Reimbursement Review Board

PRSA: Public Relations Society of America

PSRO: Professional Standards Review Organization

PTAC: Professional and Technical Advisory Committee (JCAHO)

PVA: Paralyzed Veterans of America

RSA: Rehabilitation Services Administration (DOE)

SAMHSA: Substance Abuse and Mental Health Services Administration (DHHS)

SISSC: Special Interest Section Steering Committee

SNAP: Society of National Association Publications

SSA: Social Security Administration (DHHS)

TASH: The Association for Persons with Severe Handicaps

TRB: Transportation Research Board

UCPA: United Cerebral Palsy Association

USDA: United States Department of Agriculture

VA: Department of Veterans Affairs

VA DM&S: Veterans Administration Department of Medicine and Surgery

VEWAA: Vocational Evaluation and Work Adjustment Association (NRA)

WCPT: World Confederation of Physical Therapists

WFOT: World Federation of Occupational Therapists

WHCOA: White House Conference on Aging

WHIF: Washington Health Issues Forum

WHO: World Health Organization

WIC: Women in Communication

Selected National and International Massage Associations

AMERICAN MASSAGE THERAPY ASSOCIATION

500 Davis Street, Suite 900
Evanston, IL 60201-4695
Phone 847-864-0123
Fax 847-864-1178
www.amtamassage.org
info@amtamassage.org

AMERICAN POLARITY THERAPY ASSOCIATION

PO Box 19858
Boulder, CO 80308
Phone 303-545-2080
Fax 303-545-2161
www.polaritytherapy.org
HQ@polaritytherapy.org

ASSOCIATED BODYWORK & MASSAGE PROFESSIONALS

1271 Sugarbush Drive
Evergreen, CO 80439-9766
Phone 800-458-2267 or 303-674-8478
Fax 800-667-8260
www.abmp.com
expectmore@abmp.com

THE ASSOCIATION OF MASSAGE THERAPISTS AND WHOLISTIC PRACTITIONERS

#600, 10339 - 124 Street
Edmonton, AB, Canada
T5S 3W1
Phone 888-711-7701 or 780-484-2010
Fax 780-484-3605
www.amtwp.org
admin@amtwp.org

AMERICAN MEDICAL MASSAGE ASSOCIATION

1845 Lakeshore Drive, Suite 7
Muskegon, MI 49441
Phone 888-375-7245
Fax 231-755-2963
www.americanmedicalmassage.com

CANADIAN SPORT MASSAGE THERAPISTS ASSOCIATION

1849 Yonge Street, Suite 814
Toronto, ON M4S 1Y2
Phone 416-488-4414
Fax 416-488-3079
www.csmta.ca
natoffice@csmta.ca

INFORMATION FOR PEOPLE, INC

PO Box 1038
Olympia, WA 98507-1038
Phone 800-754-9790
Fax 360-705-3864
www.info4people.com
info@info4people.com

THE IMA GROUP

PO Box 421
25 South Fourth Street
Warrenton, VA 20188-0421
Phone 540-351-0800
Fax 540-351-0816
www.imagroup.com
info@imagroup.com

INTERNATIONAL ASSOCIATION OF ANIMAL MASSAGE
THERAPISTS

PO Box 56483
Virgina Beach, VA 23456
www.iaamt.com

INTERNATIONAL ASSOCIATION OF INFANT MASSAGE

1891 Goodyear Avenue, Suite 622
Ventura, CA 93003
Phone 805-644-8524
Fax 805-644-7699
www.iaim-us.com
iaim4us@aol.com

NATIONAL ASSOCIATION OF NURSE MASSAGE
THERAPISTS

PO Box 24004
Huber Hts, OH 45424
Phone 800-262-4017
www.nanmt.org
nanmtadmin@nanmt.org

Medical Roots: Etymology (Greek and Latin Derivations)

a-	negative prefix (n is added before words beginning with a vowel), eg, amtria
ab-	away from, eg, abducent
abdomin-	abdomen, eg, abdominis, abdominoscopy
ac-	*see* ad-, eg, accretion
acet-	acid, eg, acetum vinegar, acetometer
acid-	acid, eg, acidus sour, aciduric
acou-	hear, eg, acouesthesia (also spelled acu)
acr-	extremity, peak, eg, acromegaly
act-	drive, act, eg, reaction
actin-	ray, radius, eg, actinogenesis
acu-	hear, eg, osteoacusis
ad-	toward (d changes to c, f, g, p, s, or t before words beginning with those consonants), eg, adrenal
aden-	gland, eg, adenoma
adip-	fat, eg, adipocellular, adipose
-aemia	blood, eg, polycythaemia
aer-	air, eg, anaerobiosis
aesthe-	sensation, eg, aesthesioneurosis
af-	*see* ad-, eg, afferent
ag-	*see* ad-, eg, agglutinant
-agogue	leading, inducing, eg, galactagogue

-agra	catching, seizure, eg, podagra
alb-	white, eg, albocinereous
alg-	pain, eg, neuralgia, algesia
all-	other, different, eg, allergy
alve-	channel, cavity, eg, alveolar, alveous trough
amb-	both, on both sides, eg, ambulate
amph-	*see* amphi-, around, on both sides, eg, ampheclexis
amphi-	both, doubly (i is dropped before words beginning with a vowel), eg, amphicelous
amyl-	starch, eg, amylosynthesis
an-	*see* ana-, eg, anagogic
ana-	up, positive (final a is dropped before words beginning with a vowel), eg, anaphoresis
andr-	man, eg, gynandroid
angi-	vessel, eg, angiemphraxis
ankyl-	crooked, looped, eg, ankylodactylia (also spelled ancyl-)
ant-	*see* anti-, antophthalmic
ante-	before, eg, anteflexion
anti-	against, counter (i is dropped before words beginning with a vowel, or the word is hyphenated), eg, antipyogenic, anti-inflammatory (*see* also contra-)
antr-	cavern, eg, antrodynia
ap-	*see* ad-, eg, append
-aph-	touch, eg, dysaphia (*see* also hapt-)

apo-   away from, detached, opposed (o is dropped before words beginning with a vowel), eg, apophysis

arachn-   spider, eg, arachnodactyly

arch-   beginning, origin, eg, archenteron

arter(i)-   elevator, artery, eg, arteriosclerosis, periarteritis

arthr-   joint, eg, synarthrosis (*see* also articul)

articul-   articulus joint, eg, disarticulation (*see* also arthr-)

as-   *see* ad-, eg, assimilation

-ase   enzyme

at-   *see* ad-, eg, attrition

aur-   ear, eg, aurinasal (*see* also ot-)

aut-   self, eg, autechoscope

auto-   self, eg, autoimmune

aux-   increase, eg, enterauxe

ax-   axis, eg, axofugal

axon-   axis, eg, axonometer

ba-   go, walk, stand, eg, hypnobatia

bacill-   small staff, rod, eg, actinobacillosis (*see* also bacter-)

bacter-   small staff, rod, eg, bacteriophage (*see* also bacill-)

ball-   throw, eg, ballistics (*see* also bol-)

bar-   weight, eg, pedobarometer

bi-1   life, eg, aerobic

bi-2   two, twice, double, eg, bipedal

bil-   bile, eg, biliary

blast-   bud, child, a growing thing in its early stages, eg, blastoma, zygotoblast

blep-   look, see, eg, hemiablepsia

blephar-   eyelid, eg, blepharoncus

bol-   ball, eg, embolism

brachi-   arm, eg, brachiocephalic

brachy-   short, eg, brachycephalic

brady-   slow, eg, bradycardia

brom-   stench, eg, podobromidrosis

bronch-   windpipe, eg, bronchoscopy

bry-   be full of life, eg, embryonic

bucc-   cheek, eg, distobuccal

cac-   bad, evil, abnormal, eg, cacodontia, arthrocace (*see* also mal-, dys-)

calc-1   stone, limestone, lime, eg, calcipexy

calc-2   heel, eg, calcaneotibial

calor-   heat, eg, calorimeter (*see* also therm-)

cancr-   cancer, crab, eg, camcrology (*see* also carcin-)

capit-   head, eg, decapitate (*see* also cephal-)

caps-   container, eg, encapsulation

carbo-   coal, charcoal, eg, carbohydrate, carbonuria

carcin-   crab, cancer, eg, carcinoma (*see* also cancr-)

cardi-   heart, eg, lipocardiac

cat-   *see* cata-, eg, cathode

cata-   down, negative (final a is dropped before words beginning with a vowel), eg, catabatic

caud-   tail, eg, caudate

cav-	hollow, eg, concave
cec-	blind, eg, cecopexy
-cele	tumor, hernia, cyst, eg, gastrocele
cell-	room, eg, celliferous
cen-	common, eg, cenesthesia
cent-	one hundred, eg, centimeter, centipede
cente-	puncture, eg, enterocentesis, amniocentesis
centr-	central point, center, eg, neurocentral
cephal-	relating to the head, eg, encephalitis
cept-	take, receive, eg, receptor
cer-	wax, eg, ceroplasty, ceromel
cerebr-	relating to the cerebrum, eg, cerebrospinal
cervic-	neck, eg, cervicitis, cervical
chancr-	crab, cancer, eg, chancriform
chir-	hand, eg, chiromegaly
chlor-	green, eg, achloropsia
chol-	bile, eg, hepatocholangeitis
chondr-	cartilage, eg, chondromalcia
chord-	string, cord, eg, perichordal
chori-	protective fetal membrane, eg, endochorion
chrom-	color, eg, polychromatic
chron-	time, eg, synchronous
chy-	pour, eg, ecchymosis
-cid(e)	causing death, cut, kill, eg, infanticide, germicidal
cili-	eyelid, eg, superciliary (*see* also blephar-)

cine-   move, eg, autocinesis

-cipient   take, receive, eg, incipient

circum-   around, eg, circumferential (*see* also peri-)

-cis-   cut, kill, eg, excision

clas-   break, eg, osteoclast, cranioclast

clin-   bend, incline, make lie down, eg, clinometer

clus-   shut, eg, malocclusion

co-   *see* con-, eg, cohesion

cocc-   seed, pill, eg, gonococcus

coel-   hollow, eg, coelenteron(also spelled cel-)

col-1   pertaining to the lower intestine, eg, colic

col-2   *see* con-, eg, collapse

colon-   lower intestine, eg, colonic

colp-   hollow, vagina, eg, endocolpitis

com-   *see* con-, eg, commasculation

con-   with, together (becomes co- before vowels or h; col- before l; com- before b, m, or p; cor- before r), eg, contraction

contra-   against, counter, eg, contraindication (*see* also anti-)

copr-   dung, eg, coproma (*see* also sterco-)

cor-1   doll, little image, pupil, eg, isocoria

cor-2   *see* con-, eg, corrugator

corpor-   body, eg, intracorporal (*see* also somat-)

cortic-   bark, rind, eg, corticosterone

cost-   rib, eg, intercostal (*see* also pleur-)

crani-   skull, cranium, eg, pericranium

creat-	meat, flesh, eg, creatorrhea
-crescent	grow, eg, excrescent
cret-1	grow, eg, accretion
cret-2	distinguish, separate off, eg, discrete
crin-	distinguish, separate off, eg, endocrinology
crur-	shin, leg, eg, brachiocrural
cry-	cold, eg, cryesthesia
crypt-	hide, conceal, eg, cryptorchism
cult-	tend, cultivate, eg, culture
cune-	wedge, eg, sphencuneiform
cut-	skin, eg, subcutaneous [*see* also derm(at)-]
cyan-	blue, eg, anthocyanin
cycl-	circle, cycle, eg, cyclophoria
cyst-	bag, bladder, eg, nephrocystitis (*see* also vesic-)
cyt-	cell, eg, plasmocytoma (*see* also cell-)
dacry-	tear, eg, dacryocyst
dactyl-	finger, toe, digit, eg, hexadactylism
de-	down from, eg, decomposition
dec-1	ten, indicates multiple in metric system, eg, decagram
dec-2	ten, indicates fraction in metric system, eg, decimeter
deci-	tenth, eg, decibel
demi-	half, eg, demipenniform
dendr-	tree, eg, neurodendrite
dent-	tooth, eg, interdental (*see* also odont-)

derm-	skin, eg, endoderm, dermatitis (*see* also cut-)
desm-	band, ligament, eg, syndesmopexy
dextr-	handedness, eg, ambidextrous
di-1	two, eg, dimorphic (*see* also bi-2)
di-2	*see* dia-, eg, diuresis
di-3	*see* dis-, eg, divergent
dia-	through, apart, between, asunder (a is dropped before words beginning with a vowel), eg, diagnosis
didym-	twin, gemini, eg, epididymal
digit-	finger, toe, eg, digital (*see* also dactyl-)
diplo-	double, eg, diplomyelia
dis-	apart, away from, negative, absence of (s may be dropped before a word beginning with a consonant), eg, dislocation
disc-	disk, eg, discoplacenta
dors-	back, eg, ventrodorsal
drom-	course, eg, hemodromometer
-ducent	lead, conduct, eg, adducent
duct-	lead, conduct, eg, oviduct
dur-	hard, sclera, eg, induration
dynam(i)-	power, eg, dynamoneure, neurodynamic
-dynia	pain, eg, coxodynia
dys-	bad, improper, malfunction, difficult, eg, dystrophic
e-	out from, eg, emission
ec-	out of, on the outside, eg, eccentric

-ech-	have, hold, be, eg, synechotomy
ect-	outside, eg, ectoplasm (*see* also extra-)
-ectomy	a cutting out, eg, mastectomy
ede-	swell, eg, edematous
ef-	out of, eg, efflorescent
-elc-	sore, ulcer, eg, enterelcosis (*see* hel c-)
electr-	amber, eg, electrotherapy
em-	in, on, eg, embolism, empathy, emphlysis (*see* also en-)
-em-	blood, eg, anemia (*see* also hem[at]-)
-emesis	vomiting, eg, nemesis
-emia	blood, eg, bacteremia
en-	in, on, into (n changes to m before b, p, or ph), eg, encelitis
end-	inside, eg, end-angium (*see* also intra-)
endo-	within, eg, endocardium
enter-	intestine, eg, dysentery
epi-	upon, after, in addition (i is dropped before words beginning with a vowel), eg, epiglottis, epaxial
erg-	work, deed, eg, energy
erythr-	red, rubor, eg, erythrochromia
eso-	inside, eg, esophylactic (*see* also intra-, endo-)
esthe-	perceive, feel, sensation, eg, anesthesia
eu-	good, normal, well, eg, eupepsia, eugeric
ex-	out of, eg, excretion
exo-	outside, eg, exopathic (*see* also extra-)
extra-	outside of, beyond, eg, extracellular

faci-	face, eg, brachiofaciolingual
-facient	make, eg, calefacient
-fact-	make, eg, artefact
fasci-	band, eg, fascia
febr-	fever, eg, febrile, febricide
-fect-	make, eg, defective
-ferent	bear, carry, eg, efferent, afferent
ferr-	iron, eg, ferroprotein
fibr-	fibre, eg, chondofibroma
fil-	thread, eg, filament, filiform
fiss-	split, eg, fissure
flagell-	whip, eg, flagellation
flav-	yellow, eg, riboflavin
-flect-	bend, divert, eg, deflection
-flex-	bend, divert, eg, reflexometer, flexion
flu-	flow, eg, fluid
flux-	flow, eg, affluxion
for-	door, opening, eg, foramen, perforated
fore-	before, in front of, eg, forefront
-form	shape, form, eg, ossiform, cuniform
fract-	break, eg, fracture, refractive
front-	forehead, front, eg, nasofrontal
-fug(e)	to drive away, flee, avoid, eg, vermifuge, centrifugal
funct-	perform, serve, function, eg, function al, malfunction
fund-	pour, eg, infundibulum
fus-	pour, eg, diffusible
galact-	milk, eg, dysgalactia

gam-	marriage, reproductive union, eg, agamont
gangli-	swelling, plexus, eg, neurogangliitis
gastro-	stomach, belly, eg, gastrostomy
gelat-	freeze, congeal, eg, gelatin
gemin-	twin, double, eg, quadrigeminal
gen-	become, be produced, originate, formation, eg, genesis, cytogenic, gene
germ-	bud, a growing thing in its early stages, eg, germinal, ovigerm
gest-	bear, carry, eg, congestion
gland-	acorn, eg, intraglandular
-glia	glue, eg, neuroglia
gloss-	relating to the tongue, eg, lingutrichoglossia
glott-	tongue, language, eg, glottic
gluc-	sweet, eg, glucose
glutin-	glue, eg, agglutination
glyc(y)-	sweet, eg, glycemia, glycyrrhizin
gnath-	jaw, eg, orthognathous
gno-	know, discern, eg, diagnosis
gon-	produce, formulate, eg, gonad, amphigony
grad-	walk, take steps, eg, retrograde
-gram	scratch, write, record, eg, cardiogram
gran-	grain, particle, eg, lipogranuloma, granulation
graph-	scratch, write, record, eg, histography
grav-	heavy, eg, multigravida
gyn(ec)-	woman, wife, eg, androgyny, gynecologic

gyr-	ring, circle, eg, gyrospasm
haem(at)-	pertaining to blood, eg, haemorrhagia, haematoxylon
hapt-	touch, eg, haptometer
hect-	one hundred, indicates multiple in metric system, eg, hectometer
helc-	sore, ulcer, eg, helcosis
hem(at)-	blood, eg, hematocyturia, hemagioma
hemi	half, eg, hemiageusia (*see* also semi-)
hen-	one, eg, henogenesis
hepat-	liver, eg, gastrohepatic
hept(a)-	seven, eg, heptatomic, heptavalent
hered-	heir, eg, heredity
hetero-	other, indicating dissimilarity, eg, heterogeneous
hex-1	six, sex-, hexly-, eg, hexagram
hex-2	have, hold, be, eg, cachexy
hexa-	six, sex-, hexly-, eg, hexachromic
hidr-	sweat, eg, hyperhidrosis
hist-	web, tissue, eg, histodialysis
hod-	road, path, eg, hodoneuromere
holo-	all, eg, hologenesis
homo-	common, same, eg, homomorphic
horm-	impetus, impulse, eg, hormone
hydat-	water, eg, hydatism
hydr-	pertaining to water, eg, achlorhydria
hyp-	under, eg, hypaxial, hypodermic
hyper-	over, above, beyond, extreme, eg, hypertrophy

hypn-   sleep, eg, hypnotic

hypo-   under, below (o is dropped before words beginning with a vowel), eg, hypometabolism

hyster-   womb, eg, hysterectomy

-iasis   condition, pathological state, eg, hemiathriasis (*see* also -osis)

iatr-   specialty in medicine, eg, pediatrics

idio-   peculiar, separate, distinct, eg, idiosyncrasy

il-   negative prefix, eg, illegible; in, on, eg, illinition

ile-   pertaining to the ileum (ile- is commonly used to refer to the portion of the intestines known as the ileum), eg, ileostomy

ili-   lower abdomen, intestines, (ili- is commonly used to refer to the flaring part of the hip bone known as the ilium), eg, iliosacral

im-   in, on, eg, immersion; negative prefix, eg, imperfection

in-1   fiber, eg, inosteatoma

in-2   in, on (n changes to l, m, or r before words beginning with those consonants), eg, insertion

in-3   negative prefix, eg, invalid

infra-   beneath, eg, infraorbital

insul-   island, eg, insulin

inter-   among, between, eg, intercarpal

intra-   inside, eg, intravenous

ir-	in, on, eg, irradiation; negative prefix, eg, irreducible
irid-	rainbow, colored circle, eg, keratoiridocyclitis
is-	equal, eg, isotope
ischi-	hip, haunch, eg, ischiopubic
-ism	condition, theory, eg, hemiballism, agism
iso-	equal, eg, isotonic
-itis	inflammation, eg, neuritis
-ize	to treat by special method, eg, specialize
jact-	throw, eg, jactitation
ject-	throw, eg, injection
jejun-	hungry, not partaking of food, eg, gastrojejunostomy
jug-	yoke, eg, conjugation
junct-	yoke, join, eg, conjunctiva
juxta-	near, eg, juxtaposed
kary-	nut, kernel, nucleus, eg, megakarocyte
kerat-	horn, eg, keratolysis, keratin
kil-	one thousand, indicates multiple in metric system, eg, kilogram
kine-	move, eg, kinematics
-kinesis	movement, eg, orthokinesis
labi-	lip, eg, gingivolabial
lact-	milk, eg, glucolactone, lactose
lal-	talk, babble, eg, glossolalia
lapar-	flank, loin, abdomen, eg, laparotomy
laryng-	windpipe, eg, laryngendoscope

lat-   bear, carry, eg, translation

later-   side, eg, bentrolateral

lent-   lentil, eg, lenticonus

lep-   take, seize, eg, cataleptic, epileptic

lepto-   small, soft, eg, leptotene

leuk-   white, eg, leukocyte (also spelled leuc)

lien-   spleen, eg, lienocele

lig-   tie, bind, eg, ligate

lingu-   tongue, eg, sublingual

lip-   fat, eg, glycolipid

lith-   stone, eg, nephrolithotomy

loc-   place, eg, locomotion

log-   speak, give an account, eg, logorrhea, embryology

lumb-   loin, eg, dorsolumbar

lute-   yellow, eg, xanthluteoma

ly-   loose, dissolve, eg, keratolysis

-lysis   setting free, disintegration, eg, glycolysis

lymph-   water, eg, hydrlymphadenosis

macro-   long, large, eg, marcromyoblast

mal-   bad, abnormal, eg, malfunction

malac-   soft, eg, osteomalacia

mamm-   breast, eg, mammogram, mammary

man-   hand, eg, maniphalanx, manipulation

mani-   mental aberration, eg, kleptomania

mast-   breast, eg, mastectomy, hypermastia

medi-   middle, eg, medial, medifrontal

mega-   great, large, indicates multiple (1,000,000) in metric system, eg, megacolon, megadyne

megal-	great, large, eg, cardiomegaly, acromegaly
mel-	limb, member, eg, symmelia
melan-	black, eg, melanoma, melanin
men-	month, eg, menopause, dysmenorrhea
mening-	membrane, eg, encephalomeningitis
ment-	mind, eg, dementia
mer-	part, eg, polymeric
mes-	middle, eg, mesoderm
met-	after, beyond, accompanying, eg, met allergy
meta-	after, beyond, accompanying (a is dropped before words beginning with a vowel), eg, metacarpal, metatarsal
metr-1	measure, eg, stereometry
metr-2	womb, eg, endometritis
micr-	small, eg, photomicrograph
mill-	one thousand, indicates fraction in metric system, eg, milligram, millipede
mio-	smaller, less, eg, mionectic
miss-	send, eg, intromission
-mittent	send, eg, intermittent
mne-	remember, eg, pseudomnesia
mon-	only, sole, single, eg, monoplegia
morph-	form, shape, eg, morphonuclear
mot-	move, eg, vasomotor, locomotion
multi-	many, eg, multiple
my-	muscle, eg, myopathy
-myces	fungus, eg, myelomyces

myc(et)-	fungus, eg, ascomycetes, streptomycin
myel-	marrow, eg, poliomyelitis
myx-	mucus, eg, myxedema
narc-	numbness, eg, toponarcosis, narcolepsy
nas-	nose, eg, nasal
ne-	new, young, eg, neocyte, neonate
necr-	corpse, dead, eg, necrocytosis, necrosis
nephr-	kidney, eg, nephron, nephric
neur-	nerve, eg, neurology, estesioneure
nod-	knot, eg, nodosity
nom-	deal out, distribute, law, custom, eg, nominal, taxonomy
non-	nine, no, eg, nonacosane
nos-	disease, eg, nosology
nucle-	nut, kernel, eg, nucleus, nucleide
nutri-	nourish, eg, malnutrition
ob-	against, toward (b changes to c before words beginning with that consonant) eg, obtuse
oc-	*see* ob-, occlude
ocul-	eye, eg, oculomotor
-od-	road, path, eg, periodic
-ode1	road, path, eg, cathode
-ode2	form, eg, nematode
odont-	tooth, eg, orthodontia
-odyn-	pain, distress, eg, gastrodynia
-oid	form, eg, hyoid
-ol	oil, eg, cholesterol
-old	form, shape, resemblance, eg, scaffold

ole-	oil, eg, oleorsin
olig-	few, small, eg, oligospermia
-oma	tumor, eg, blastoma
omo-	shoulder, eg, omosternum
omphal-	navel, eg, periomphalic
onc-	bulk, mass, eg, oncology, hematoncometry
onych-	claw, nail, eg, anonychia
oo-	egg, ovum, eg, perioothecitis
oophor-	pertaining to the ovary, eg, oophorectomy
ophthalm-	eye, eg, ophthalmic
or-	mouth, eg, intraoral
orb-	circle, eg, suborbital
orchi-	testicle, eg, orchiopathy
organ-	implement, instrument, eg, organoleptic
orth-	straight, right, normal, eg, orthopedics
-osis	condition, disease, eg, osteoporosis
oss-	bone, eg, osseous, ossiphone
ost(e)-	bone, eg, enostosis, osteonecrosis
ot-	ear, eg, parotid (*see* also aur-)
-otomy	cutting, eg, osteotomy
ov-	egg, eg, synovia
oxy-	sharp, acid, eg, oxycephalic
pachy(n)-	thicken, eg, pachyderma, myopachynsis
pag-	fix, make fast, eg, thoracopagus
pan-	entire, all, eg, pancytosis, pandemic
par-1	bear, give birth to, eg, primiparous
par-2	*see* para-, eg, parepigastric

para-	beside, beyond, along side of (final a is dropped before words beginning with a vowel), eg, paramastoid
part-	bear, give birth to, eg, parturition
path-	that which one undergoes, sickness, disease, eg, pathology, psychopathic
pec-	fix, make fast, eg, sympectothiene (*see* also pex-)
ped-	child, eg, pediatric, orthopedic
pell-	skin, hide, eg, pellagra
-pellent	drive, eg, repellent
pen-	need, lack, eg, erythrocytopenia
pend-	hang down, eg, appendix
pent(a)-	five, eg, pentose, pentaploid
peps-	digest, eg, bradypepsia
pept-	digest, eg, dyspeptic
per-	through, excessive, eg, pernasal
peri-	around, eg, periphery
pet-	seek, tend toward, eg, centripetal
pex-	fix, make fast, eg, hepatopexy
pha-	say, speak, eg, dysphasia
phac-	lentil, lens, eg, phacosclerosis (also spelled phak-)
phag-	eat, eg, lipphagic
phak-	lentil, lens, eg, phakitis
phan-	show, be seen, eg, diaphanoscopy
pharmac-	drug, eg, pharmacology
pharyng-	throat, eg, glossopharyngeal
phen-	show, be seen, eg, phosphene

pher-	bear, support, eg, periphery
phil-	like, have affinity for, eg, eosinophilia, philosophy
phleb-	vein, eg, periphlebitis, phlebotomy
phleg-	burn, inflame, eg, adenophlegmon
phlog-	burn, inflame, eg, antiphlogistic
phob-	fear, dread, eg, claustrophobia
phon-	sound, eg, echophony
phor-	bear, support, eg, exophoria
phos-	light, eg, phosphorus
phot-	light, eg, photerythrous
phrag-	fence, wall off, stop up, eg, diaphragm
phrax-	fence, wall off, stop up, eg, emphraxis
phren-	mind, midriff, eg, metaphrenia, metaphrenon
phthi-	decay, waste away, eg, opthalmophthisis
phy-	beget, bring forth, produce, be by nature, eg, nosophyte, physical
phyl-	tribe, kind, eg, phylogeny
phylac-	guard, eg, prophylactic
-phylaxis	protection, eg, prophylaxis
-phyll	leaf, eg, xanthophyll
phys(a)-	blow, inflate, eg, physocele, physalis
physe-	blow, inflate, eg, emphysema
pil-	hair, eg, epilation
pituit-	phlegm, eg, pituitous
placent-	cake, eg, extraplacental
plas-	mold, shape, eg, cineplasty, plastazode
platy-	broad, flat, eg, platyrrhine
pleg-	strike, eg, diplegia, paraplegia

plet-   fill, eg, depletion

pleur-   rib, side, eg, peripleural

plex-   strike, eg, apoplexy

plic-   fold, eg, complication

plur-   more, eg, plural

pne-   breathing, eg, traumatopnea

pneum(at)-breath, air, eg, pneumodynamics, pneumatothorax

pneumo(n)-lung, eg, pneumocentesis, pneumontomy

pod-   foot, eg, podiatry

poie-   make, produce, eg, sarcopoietic

pol-   axis of a sphere, eg, peripolar

poly-   much, many, eg, polyspermia

pont-   bridge, eg, pontocerebellar

por-1   passage, eg, myelopore

por-2   callus, eg, porocele

posit-   put, place, eg, deposit, repositor

post-   after, behind in time or place, eg, postnatal, postural

pre-   before in time or place, eg, prenatal, prevesical

press-   press, eg, pressure, pressoreceptive

pro-   before in time or place, eg, progamous, prolapse

proct-   anus, eg, ecteroproctia

prosop-   face, eg, prosopus

proto-   first, eg, prototype

pseud-   false, eg, pseudoparaplegia

psych-   soul, mind, eg, psychosomatic

pto-	fall, eg, nephroptosis
pub-	adult, eg, puberty, ischiopubic
puber-	adult, eg, puberty
pulmo(n)-	lung, eg, cardiopulmonary, pulmolith
puls-	drive, eg, propulsion
punct-	prick, pierce, eg, puncture, punctiform
pur-	pus, eg, puration
py-	pus, eg, nephropyosis
pyel-	trough, basin, pelvis, eg, nephropyelitis
pyl-	door, orifice, eg, pylephlebitis
pyr-	fire, eg, galactopyra
quadr-	four, eg, quadraplegic, quadrigeminal
quinque-	five, eg, quinquecuspid
rachi-	spine, eg, alorachidian
radi-	ray, eg, irradiation
re-	back, again, eg, retraction
ren-	kidneys, eg, adrenal
ret-	net, eg, retothelium
retro-	backwards, eg, retrodeviation, retrograde
rhag-	break, burst, eg, hemorrhagic
rhaph-	suture, stitching, eg, gastrorrhaphy
rhe-	flow, discharge, eg, disrrheal
rhex-	break, burst, eg, metrorrhexis
rhin-	nose, eg, basirhinal
rot-	wheel, eg, rotator
rub(r)-	red, eg, bilirubin, rubrospinal
racchar-	sugar, eg, saccharin
sacro-	pertaining to the sacrum, eg, sacroiliac

salping-	tube, trumpet, eg, salpingitis
sanguin-	blood, eg, sanguineous
sarc-	flesh, eg, sarcoma
schis-	split, eg, schistorachis, rachischisis
scler-	hard, eg, sclerosis, scleraderma
scop-	look at, observe, eg, endoscope
sect-	cut, eg, sectile, resection
semi-	half, eg, semiflexion
sens-	perceive, feel, eg, sensory
sep-	rot, decay, eg, sepsis
sept-1	fence, wall off, stop up, eg, septal
sept-2	seven, eg, septan
ser-	whey, watery substance, eg, serum, serosynovitis
sex-	six, eg, sexdigitate
sial-	saliva, eg, polysialia
sin-	hollow, fold, eg, sinobronchitis
sit-	food, eg, parasitic
solut-	loose, dissolve, set free, eg, dissolution
-solvent	loose, dissolve, eg, dissolvent
somat-	body, eg, somatic, psychosomatic
-some	body, eg, dictyosome
spas-	draw, pull, eg, spasm, spastic
spectr-	appearance, what is seen, eg, spectrum, microspectroscope
sperm(at)-	seed, eg, spermacrasia, spermatozoon
spers-	scatter, eg, dispersion
sphen-	wedge, eg, sphenoid
spher-	ball, eg, hemisphere

sphygm- pulsation, eg, sphygmomanometer

spin- spine, eg, cerebrospinal

spirat- breathe, eg, inspiratory

splanchn- entrails, vicera, eg, neurosplanchnic

splen- spleen, eg, splenomegaly

spor- seed, eg, sporophyte, sygospore

squam- scale, eg, squamus, despuamation

sta- make stand, stop, eg, genesistasis

stal- send, eg, peristalsis (*see* also stol-)

staphyl- bunch of grapes, uvula, eg, staphylococcus, staphylectomy

stear- fat, eg, stearodermia

steat- fat, eg, steatopygous

sten- narrow, compressed, eg, stenocardia

ster- solid, eg, cholesterol

sterc- dung, eg, stercoporphyrin

sthen- strength, eg, asthenia

stol- send, eg, diastole

stom(at)- mouth, orifice, eg, anastomosis, stom atogastric

strep(h)- twist, eg, strephosymbolia, streptomycin (*see* also stroph-)

strict- draw tight, compress, cause pain, eg, constriction

-stringent draw tight, compress, cause pain , eg, astringent

stroph- twist, eg, astrophic [*see* also strep(h)-]

struct- pile up (against), eg, obstruction

sub- under, below (b changes to f or p before words beginning with those consonants), eg, sublumbar

suf-	*see* sub-, eg, suffusion
sup-	*see* sub-, eg, suppository
super-	above, beyond, extreme, eg, supermobility
sy-	*see* syn-, eg, sytole
syl-	*see* syn-, eg, syllepsiology
sym-	*see* syn-, eg, symbiosis, symmetry, sympathetic, symphysis
syn-	with, together (n disappears before s, changes to l before l, and changes to m before b, m, p, and ph), eg, myosynizesis
ta-	stretch, put under pressure, eg, ectasis
tac-	order, arrange, eg, atactic
tact-	touch, eg, contact
tax-	order, arrange, eg, ataxia, taxotomy
tect-	cover, eg, protective
teg-	cover, eg, integument
tel-	end, eg, telosynapsis
tele-	at a distance, eg, teleceptor, telescope
tempor-	time, timely or fatal spot, temple, eg, temporomalar
ten(ont)-	tight stretched band, eg, tenodynia, tenonitis, tenontagra
tens-	stretch, eg, extensor
test-	pertaining to the testicle, eg, testitis
tetra-	four, eg, tetragenous
the-	put, place, eg, synthesis
thec-	repository, case, eg, thecostegnosis
thel-	teat, nipple, eg, thelerethism
therap-	treatment, eg, hydrotherapy

therm-	heat, eg, diathermy
thi-	sulfur, eg, thiogenic
thorac-	chest, eg, thoracoplasty
thromb-	lump, clot, eg, thrombophlebitits, thrombopenia
thym-	spirit, eg, dysthymia
thyr-	shield, shaped like a door, eg, thyroid
tme-	cut, eg, axonotmesis
toc-	childbirth, eg, dystocia
tom-	cut, eg, appendenctomy
ton-	stretch, put under pressure, eg, tonus, peritoneum
top-	place, eg, topesthesia
tors-	twist, eg, extorsion
tox-	arrow poison, poison, eg, toxemia
trache-	windpipe, eg, tracheotomy
trachel-	neck, eg, tracheloplexy
tract-	draw, drag, eg, protraction
trans-	across, eg, transport
traumat-	wound, eg, traumatic
tri-	three, eg, trigonad
trich-	hair, eg, trichoid
trip-	rub, eg, entripsis
trop-	turn, react, eg, sitotropism
troph-	nurture, relating to nourishment, eg, atrophy
tuber-	swelling, node, eg, tubercle, tuberculosis
typ-	type, eg, atypical
typh-	for, stupor, eg, adenotyphus

typhl-	blind, eg, typhlectasis
uni-	one, eg, unioval
ur-	urine, eg, polyuria
vacc-	cow, eg, vaccine
vagin-	sheath, eg, invaginated
vas-	vessel, eg, vascular
ventro-	abdomen, in front of, eg, ventrolateral, ventrose
vers-	turn, eg, inversion
vert-	turn, eg, diverticulum
vesic-	bladder, eg, vesicovaginal
vit-	life, eg, devitalize
vuls-	pull, twitch, eg, convulsion
xanth-	yellow, blond, eg, xanthophyll
-yl-	substance, eg, cacodyl
zo-	life, animal, eg, microzoaria
zyg-	yoke, union, eg, zygote, zygodactyly
zym-	ferment, eg, enzyme

Massage Techniques and Modalities Contact Information

ACUPRESSURE

- www.acupressure.com
- www.crystalinks.com/acupressure.html
- www.dishant.com/acupressure/whatis.html

ACU-YOGA

- www.acuyogatherapy.com/
- www.polisa.co.uk/AcuYoga/yogaIntro.html
- www.4integrativetherapy.com/htm/acuyoga.htm

ADAMANTINE SYSTEM

- www.adamantinesystem.com/site
- www.awakening-healing.com/AHS/AdamantineParticles.htm
- www.naturaw.com

ALEXANDER TECHNIQUE

* Alexander Technique International, Inc
  1692 Massachusetts Avenue, 3rd Floor
  Cambridge, MA 02138
  Tel: 617-497-2242 or 888-668-8996
  Fax: 617-497-2615
  E-mail: alexandertechnique@compuserve.
  com
  Web site: www.ati-net.com
* www.alexandertechnique.com/at.htm
* www.life.uiuc.edu/jeff/at_descrip tion.html
* www.alexandercenter.com/#1Anchor

AMMA/ANMA

* www.aobta.org/Style%20Long%20Definitio
  ns/Amma.htm
* www.tcmpractitioners.com/amma.php
* www.bubishi.com/nwwiobt/whatisamma.
  html

ANIMAL MASSAGE

* www.amtil.com/
* members.aol.com/petassage/main.html
* www.drschoen.com/articles_L2_2_.html

APPLIED KINESIOLOGY

- www.icak.com/about/whatis.shtml
- www.naturalhealers.com/qa/kinesiology.shtml

APPLIED PHYSIOLOGY

- www.eis2win.co.uk/tex/wha_sposci_whatis_physio.aspx
- www.appliedphysiology.com/class_info.html
- www.iask.org/appliedphysiology.html

ASHIATSU ORIENTAL BAR THERAPY

- www.deepfeet.com/howitworks.html
- www.vineyardmassage.com/ashiat su.htm
- www.massagemedicine.com/ashiat su.html

ASTON-PATTERNING

- www.astonenterprises.com
- www.ziasite.com/apmed.html
- www.spine-inc.com/glossary/a/aston.htm

ATTUNEMENT

- International Association of Attunement
  Practitioners
  1600 Genessee Street, Suite #500
  PO Box 014064
  Kansas City, MO 64102
  E-mail: attunement@attunement.com
  Web site: www.attunementpractitioners.org
- www.csaprocess.com/page2.html
- www.geocities.com/wayneak/#L3

AYURVEDIC MASSAGE

- www.sanatansociety.org/ayurvedic _mas
  sage/ayurvedic_massage_techniques.htm
- www.tantra-ifc-the-art-of-conscious-
  love.com/ayurvedic_massage1.html
- www.hindubooks.org/david_frawley/river
  heaven/natures_medicine_ayurve da/treat-
  ment.pg3.htm

BALINESE MASSAGE

- www.ibahbali.com/spa.html
- www.experiencebali.com/spa/wellbeing
  spa/
- www.hotelviking.com/viking_spa.pdf

BIOFEEDBACK

- Association For Applied Psychophysiology and Biofeedback
  10200 W. 44th Avenue, Suite 304
  Wheat Ridge, CO 80033-2840
  Tel: 303-422-8436
  E-mail: aapb@resourcenter.com
  Web site: www.aapb.org
- webideas.com/biofeedback/whatis
- www.holistic-online. com/Biofeedback.htm

BIO-SYNC

- www.biosync.com
- www.biosync.com/articles.htm
- ahha.org/wellnessarticles.htm

BODY ALIGNMENT TECHNIQUE

- www.gkindia.com/therapies/bodyalignment.htm
- www.silentpond.com/bodyalignment.htm
- www.bodyalignment.org

BODY LOGIC

- www.bodylogic.com
- www.yamunabodyrolling.com

BODY ORIENTED PSYCHOTHERAPY

- www.sfhakomi.org/about.html
- www.usabp.org/displaycommon. cfm?an=8

BODY ROLLING

- www.bodylogic.com
- www.yamunabodyrolling.com
- membrane.com/philanet/fitness/body_ rolling.html

BODY-MIND CENTERING

- Body-Mind Centering Association, Inc.
  16 Center Street, Suite 530
  Northampton, MA 01060
  Tel: 413/594-1273
  E-mail: admin@bmcassoc.org
  Web site: www.bmcassoc.org/
- www.bodymindcentering.com/About
- www.yogameditationcentercalgary.ca/ body_mind_centering.htm
- www.schulmanmd.com/html/ dr__schulman__body_mind_center.html

BODYTALK

- International BodyTalk Association
  2750 Stickney Point Road, Suite 203
  Sarasota, FL 3423
  Tel: 877-519-9119
  Fax: 941-924-3779
  Web site: www.bodytalksystem.com
- www.innatewisdom.net/bodytalk.shtml
- www.goldenspirit.com/althealth/
  bodytalk/chucknannettewkshop.htm

BONNIE PRUDDEN MYOTHERAPY

- www.bomi.info/bodywork/mo.htm
  #Trigger%20Point%20Myotherapy
- www.myotherapy.to/north_bay_myothera-
  py001.htm
- www.myotherapyseminars.com

BOWEN TECHNIQUE

  Bowtech
  337 North Rush St.
  Prescott, AZ 86301
  Tel: 866-862-6936
  E-mail: usbr@bowtech.com
  Web site: www.bowtech.com
- www.bowtech.com/public/about/
  overview.do
- www.bowentherapytechnique.com/
  BowenPat/Bowen-Technique.html

Brain Gym

- Brain Gym International
  1575 Spinnaker Drive, Suite 204B
  Ventura, CA 93001
  Tel: 800-356-2109
  E-mail: edukfd@earthlink.net
  Web site: www.braingym.org
- esl.about.com/library/lessons/
  blbraingym.htm
- www.brainwise.co.uk
- members.aol.com/braingym/bg.html

Breath Therapy

- breathmastery.com/principles.htm
- www.breaththerapy.net/page0003 .htm
- www.bcreativ.com.au/breath.html

Breema Bodywork

- homepage.eircom.net/~bomi/bodywork/
  b.htm
- www.breemahealth.com
- www.kinajoy.com/breema.html

Budzek Medical Massage Therapy

- www.massagetherapy.com/glossary/
  index.php#B
- home.earthlink.net/~massage911

CHAIR MASSAGE

- www.naturalhealers.com/qa/chairmass age.shtml
- www.holisticonline.com/massage/ mas_workplace.htm
- www.aurorahealthcare.org/services/ compmedicine/chairmassage.asp

CHAMPISSAGE

- www.indianchampissage.com/indian champissag.html
- www.stressresponse.com/head.htm
- www.indianheadmassages.co.uk/right.html

CHI GONG

- acupuncture.com/QiKung/Intent.htm
- acupuncture.com/QiKung/QikunInd.htm
- www.nqa.org

CHI NEI TSANG

- www.chineitsang.com
- www.chionline.com/cnt
- www.bomi.info/bodywork/c.htm#Chi% 20Nei%20Tsang

CONNECTIVE TISSUE MASSAGE

- www.activemassage.com/ctm.htm
- www.ultimatewatermassage.com/massage-types-connective-tiss.htm
- www.johnlatz.com/articles.html

CORE ENERGETICS

- www.stephenshostek.com
- www.core-energetics-south.com/Developing%20Capacity.htm
- www.coreenergeticinstitute.com

CORE STRUCTURAL INTEGRATIVE THERAPY

- www.massagetoday.com/archives/2001/03/07.html
- www.healtouch.com/health&harmony/massage.html
- www.thebodyworker.com/modalitiesR.htm

CRANIOSACRAL THERAPY

- www.upledger.com
- www.craniosacral.co.uk
- www.craniosacraltherapy.org/Whatis.htm
- www.craniosacral.com

CRYOTHERAPY

- www.massagetherapy.com/glossary/ index.php#C
- www.jointhealing.com/pages/product-pages/cryotherapy.html
- www.uni-patch.com/PDF/Cryotherapy.pdf

DEEP TISSUE MASSAGE

- www.mamashealth.com/massage/ dtissue.asp
- www.thebodyworker.com/deeptissue.htm
- membrane.com/philanet/massage/styles. html

DEGRIEFING

- www.massagetherapy.com/glossary/ index.php#D
- massagetherapy.com/articles/index.php? article_id=28
- www.degriefing.net

DO-IN (DAOYIN, DAO-IN, TAO-IN)

- www.chisuk.org.uk/bodymind/whatis/ do_in.php
- www.be-you.com/Display.php?ID=332
- www.holistic-online.com /shiatsu/hol_ shiatsu_related.htm

Dr. Vodder Manual Lymph Drainage

- www.chisuk.org.uk/bodymind/whatis/manlydra.php
- www.massagemag.com/2001/issue93/lymph.htm
- www.ipekcaldemir.com/eng/mld-eng.htm

EMF Balancing Technique

- www.emfbalancingtechnique.com
- www.magnificentvoyage.com/emf/about_emf.htm
- www.the-reflectory.com/emf.html

Equine Massage

- American Association of Equine Practitioners
  4075 Iron Works Parkway
  Lexington, KY 40511-8462
  Tel: 859-233-0147
  Fax 859-233-1968
  E-mail: aaepoffice@aaep.org
  Web site: www.aaep.org
- www.equinesportsmassage.com
- www.equissage.com/therapy.htm
- home.earthlink.net/~equihands/new_page_2.htm

ESALEN MASSAGE

- Esalen Institute and Bodywork Association
  55000 Highway 1
  Big Sur, CA 93920-9616
  Tel: 831-667-3018
  Fax: 831-667-3008
  E-mail: info@esalen.org
  Web Site: www.esalenmassage.org
- www.esalen.org/info/massage.shtml
- www.unitone.org/luciarose/esalemsg.asp
  www.zeusfitness.com/swedish.htm

ESOTERIC HEALING

- www.ineh.org/Healing/WhatisEH.htm
- www.samirarao.net/esoteric.shtml

EUCAPNIC BREATH RETRAINING:

- www.massagetherapy.com/glossary/
  index.php#E
- www.alivewell.com/resources/resource
  _articles.html
- www.breathresource.com/heathlybreath-
  ing.html

Exerssage

- www.massagetherapy.com/glossary/ index.php#E
- www.starface.com/VideoMenu.htm

Feldenkrais

- www.feldenkrais.com/method/standards/ index.html#what
- www.feldenkrais-resources. com/back groundinfo.htm
- www.feldenkrais-method.org

Five Element Shiatsu

- www.ofspirit.com/sucousineau1.htm
- membrane.com/philanet/dvwn/director/ chinese.html

Foot Zone Therapy

- www.bow-mac.com/034Foot.html
- www.energybalancing.com/therapy/zone. html

Four Hand Massage

- www.handinhandmassage.com/ services/four_hands_massage.html
- www.mayaubud.com/spa/spa_programs. htm

GERIATRIC MASSAGE

- daybreak-massage.com
- www.healthfulhands.net/massage/archives/2003_10.php
- www.heavenshands.com/geriatric.htm

GRINBERG METHOD

- www.yvelia.com/yvettenahmia/grinberg.htm
- www.grinbergmethod.com
- www.selfgrowth.com/articles/Ron2.html

GUA SHA

- www.guasha.com
- www.redwingbooks.com/products/books/GuaShaNie.cfm
- discoveringwellness.hdmenterprises.com/gua_sha.htm

HAKOMI INTEGRATIVE SOMATICS

- www.hakomiinstitute.com
- www.sfhakomi.org
- www.nas.com/~richf/hakomi.htm

HANNA SOMATIC EDUCATION

- The Association for Hanna Somatic
  Education
  925 Golden Gate Drive
  Napa, CA 94558-9601
  Tel: 877-766-2473
  E-mail: info@hannasomatics.com
  Web site: www.hannasomatics.com

HEALING TOUCH

- Healing Touch International, Inc,
  445 Union Boulevard, Suite 105
  Lakewood, CO 80228
  Tel: 303-989-7982
  Fax: 303-980-8683
  E-Mail: Htiheal@aol.com
  Web Site: www.healingtouch.net
- www.healingtouch.net/hti.shtml
- stevehtouch.bizland.com/Info/
  Information.htm
- healingtouchforanimals.com/whatisit.htm

HELLERWORK

- Jack Schultz
  Hellerwork International
  3435 M Street
  Eureka, CA 95503
  Tel: 800/392-3900 or 707/441-4949
  E-Mail: Hellerwork@hellerwork.com
  Web Site: www.hellerwork.com
- www.hellerwork.com/intro.html
- www.bodytherapy.co.nz
- www.naturalhealers.com/qa/hellerwork. shtml

HEMME APPROACH

- www.affordablemassage.com/some.htm#21
- www.holistic.com/holistic/learning.nsf/ Title/Hemme+Approach
- www.hemmeapproach.com/page-1.html

HOSHINO THERAPY

- homepage.tinet.ie/~bomi/bodywork/h. htm#Hoshino%20Therapy
- www.biotherapeutics.net
- www.karinya.com/bodywk1.htm

Huna Kane

- www.holisticpractitionersnetwork.com/MONIQUE/what_is.htm
- www.tapintoheaven.com/2huna/huna home.shtml
- www.trance-action.com/articles/hk.htm

Hydrotherapy

- www.holistic-online.com/hydrotherapy.htm
- health.yahoo.com/health/alternative _medicine/alternative_therapies/Hydrotherapy
- www.naturalhealers.com/qa/hydrotherpy.shtm

Infant Massage

- International Association of Infant Massage — US
  1891 Goodyear Avenue Suite 622
  Ventura, CA 93003
  Tel: 805-644-8524
  Fax: 805-644-7699
  E-mail: IAIM4US@aol.com
  Web site: www.iaim-us.com
- www.infantmassage.com
- www.childbirth.org/articles/baby/infant massage.htm

INGHAM METHOD

- www.thenaturalhealer.ca/reflexology/ingham.php
- www.reflexologyny.com/images/how.pdf

INTEGRATIVE MANUAL THERAPY

- www.centerimt.com
- www.centerimt.com/WhatisCenteri mt.asp
- members.bellatlantic.net/~billgpt/IMT.htm
- www.massagetherapy101.com/massage-techniques/integrative-manual-therapy.aspx

INSIGHT BODYWORK

- www.bodhiwork.org/#INSIGHT.html
- www.bomi.info/bodywork/i-j-l.htm#Insight_Bodywork

INTEGRATED KABBALISTIC HEALING

- www.janemoody.ca/ikh/home.html
- www.asoulconnection.com/ikh.htm
- www.kabbalah.org

JAMU MASSAGE

- www.jamuspa.com/jamu_massage.html
- www.evalu8.org/staticpage?page=review&siteid=498
- www.capjuluca.com/sparituals.asp

Japanese Restoration Therapy

- www.kodenkan.com/restoration.html# kodenkan
- www.pckilohana.com/PCA/massage.htm
- jayacarl.abmp.com

Jin Shin Do

- www.bctravel.com/strollers1.html
- members.aol.com/NJTouch/index28.html

Jin Shin Jyutsu

- www.jinshinjyutsu.com/Artof/artof.htm

Korean Martial Therapy

- www.urban4est.com/202.htm
- www.bomi.info/bodywork/j-k-l.htm

Kripalu Bodywork

- www.rejuvenationroom.ca/massage.html
- www.nykripalu.org/YogaCommunity.htm
- www.canoe.ca/AltmedDictionary/k.html

Kriya Massage

- hahafarm.com/massage/km.htm
- www.dovestar.edu/questions.htm
- www.moondancemassage.com/kriya.shtml

LaStone Therapy

- www.ipekcaldemir.com/eng/hotrocktherapy.htm
- thepath-tulsa.com/lastone.html
- www.lastonetherapy.com/_Final/Index.asp

Lenair Technique

- www.massageandbodywork.com/Articles/DecJan2003/LenairTechnique.htm
- www.addictionrecoveryguide.org/holistic/bioelectric.html
- www.lenair.com

Lomi Lomi

- Hawaiian Lomilomi Association
  15-156 Puni Kahakaai Loop
  Pahoa, HI 96778
  Tel: 808/965-8917
  E-mail: Hla@haleola.com
  Web site: www.lomilomi.org
- www.bby-biz.com/somatichealing
- www.somatherapy.com/lomilomi.html
- www.coffeetimes.com/apr98.htm

Lymph Drainage Therapy

- www.susanmonkrmt.com/lymph.html
- www.upledger.com/therapies/ldt.htm
- www.awayofwellness.com/lymph.html

LYPPOSAGE

- www.susanmonkrmt.com/lypossage.html
- www.lypossageofloveland.com/facs.html
- www.wrightcenter.com/NewPage.html

MACROBIOTIC SHIATSU

- www.enjoy-life.com/macro.html
- www.imss.macrobiotic.net
- junior.apk.net/~rncjr

MANUAL LYMPH DRAINAGE

- North American Vodder Association of
  Lymphatic Therapy
  8324 Loma del Norte NE
  Albuquerque, NM 87109
  Tel: 888-462-8258
  Web site: www.navalt.org
- www.acols.com/introduction.htm
- www.chisuk.org.uk/bodymind/whatis/
  manlydra.php

MECHANICAL LINK

- www.iahe.com/html/therapies/ml.jsp
- www.upledger.com/therapies/ml.htm
- www.aquabilities.com/massage.asp

MIDDENDORF BREATHWORK

- www.breathexperiencenyc.com
- www.breathexperience.com/breathwork2.
  htm

MOVEMENT THERAPY

- Association for Dance Movement Therapy
  C/O Quaker Meeting House
  Wedmore Vale, Bristol, UK BS3 5HX
  E-mail: queries@admt.org.uk
  Web site: www.admt.org.uk
- www.nccata.org/dance.html

MUSCLE ENERGY TECHNIQUE

- www.massagetherapy101.com/
  massage_techniques/muscle-energy-tech
  nique.aspx
- www.harmonycentre.org/met.html
- www.boisestate.edu/recreation/services/
  massage.asp#clinical

MUSCLE RELEASE TECHNIQUE

- www.mrtherapy.com/muscle_release.html
- www.yin-yang-colonics.com/mrt.htm
- alpine-valley.com/FancherMassage/repeti
  tive_use_injuries.htm

MYOFASCIAL RELEASE

- members.aol.com/NJTouch/index33.html
- www.wholehealthmd.com/refshelf/sub
  stances_view/1,1525,10156,00.html
- www.yoga.com/ydc/enlighten/enlighten
  _category.asp?section=5&cat=70

Myofascial Trigger Point Therapy

- www.frontiernet.net/~painrel/ NewFiles/AboutMTPT.html
- www.myofascialtherapy.org/home.htm
- members.aol.com/fibroworld/mps.htm

Myomassology

- reachoutmag.com/jan02/sandee.html

Myopractic Muscle Therapy

- www.myopractic.com/Default.htm
- www.myopractic.com.au/myopractic _explained.htm
- www.health-and-beauty-directory.com/ massage/deep-tissue-massage.htm

Nambudripad's Allergy Elimination Technique

- www.healthplusweb.com/alt_directory/ naet.html
- remedyfind.com/rm-128-Nambudripads.asp

NAPRAPATHY

- American Naprapathic Association
  164 Division Street, Suite 202
  Elgin, IL 60120
  Tel: 847-214-8642
  Fax: 847-214-8645
  E-mail: anafordns@aol.com
  Web site: www.naprapathy.org
- www.painreliefprofessionals.com/naprap athy.htm
- personal.inet.fi/palvelu/ergo/frmain01. htm
- www.naprapathy.org/naprapathy.asp

NEUROMUSCULAR REPROGRAMMING

- www.medicalmassage.org/NeuroMuscular %20Reprogramming.htm
- www.ahpweb.org/articles/healthcare.html
- www.pilatesenergy.com/50-Foundations Modalities.html

NEUROMUSCULAR THERAPY

- www.spine-health.com/topics/co-serv/ massage/massage2.html
- www.positivehealth.com/permit/Articles/ Bodywork/lane47.htm
- www.iahe.com/controller/Iahe CurriculumDisplay?curriculum Code=NMT

Nikon Restorative Massage/ Okazaki Restorative Massage

- www.iwu.edu/~wellness/mas_folder/ okazaki.htm
- www.realpagessites.com/satori/page4.html
- www.palmettomassage.com/TypesOf Massage.htm#Okazaki

Nuat Thai

- www.thaibodywork.com/aboutthaimass age.html
- homepage.tinet.ie/~bomi/bodywork/ thaimassage.htm
- www.thaimassage.com/itta/curriculum. html

Ohashiatsu

- www.ohashiatsu.org
- www.healingshiatsu.com/content/ ohashiatsu.htm
- www.ohashi.com

On-site Massage

See Chair Massage

ONSEN TECHNIQUE

- Onsen International
  Linda Leeson, Head Onsen Instructor
  #10-2070 Harvey Avenue
  Kelowna, BC, Canada VIY 8P8
  Tel: 877-717-1210
  Web site: onsentherapy.com
- onsentherapy.com/what_is_onsen.htm
- www.backinbalancemassage.com/technique.html#onsen

ORTHO-BIONOMY

- Society of Ortho-Bionomy International
  5335 North Tacoma Street, Suite 21G
  Indianapolis, IN 46220
  Tel: 800-809-3747
  Fax: 317-356-0065
  E-mail: office@ortho-bionomy.org
  Web Site: www.ortho-bionomy.org
- www.ortho-bionomy.org/develop ment.htm
- ortho-bionomy.ws.futuresite.register.com/
  _wsn/page3.html
- www.handson-boise.com

ORTHOPEDIC MASSAGE

- www.omeri.com/orthopedic.htm
- www.massagetoday.com/archives/2004/02/
  03.html

- www.spring-training.com/html/ortho_
  mass.html

OSTEOPATHIC MEDICINE

- www.aacom.org/om.html
- history.aoa-net.org
- www.studentdoctor.net/do/index.asp

PFRIMMER DEEP MUSCLE THERAPY

- Therese C. Pfrimmer International
  Association of Deep Muscle Therapists
  103 Carriage Court
  Arthur, IL 61911
  Tel: 217-484-7774 or 217-484-3404
  Fax: 937-845-3909
  Web site: www.pfrimmer.com
- members.aol.com/NJTouch/index26.html
- www.devinemuscletherapy.com/pfrimmer.
  htm

PHOENIX RISING YOGA THERAPY

- www.pryt.com/about/yoga.html
- www.marylandyogatherapy.com/session.
  htm
- www.varunayoga.com/pryt.html

PHYTOTHERAPY

- www.collegeofphytotherapy.com/phyto.htm
- www.herbs.org/current/phytbenzo.html

PILATES METHOD

- www.pilatesmethodalliance.org/whatis.html
- www.pilates-method-exercise.com
- www.pilates-studio.com/docs/method/methwhat.htm

POLARITY THERAPY

- The American Polarity Therapy Association
  PO Box 19858
  Bolder, CO 80308
  Tel: 303-545-2080
  Fax: 303-545-2161
  E-mail: hq@polaritytherapy.org
  Web site: www.polaritytherapy.org
- www.polaritytherapy.org/polarity/index.html
- www.masterworksinternational.com/polarity/WhatisPol.htm
- www.personal.u-net.com/~ct/polarity.htm

POSTURAL INTEGRATION
AND ENERGETIC INTEGRATION

- www.bodymindintegration.com/english.html
- www.opencentre.com/ocsz.html
- www.energeticintegration.info/english.html

PRANIC HEALING

- pranichealingusa.com
- www.pranichealing.com
- www.pranichealingontario.ca/aboutpranic.htm

PRENATAL/PREGNANCY MASSAGE

- National Association of Pregnancy Massage Therapy
  1007 Mopac Circle #202
  Austin, TX 78746
  Tel: 888-451-4945 or 512-323-5925
  Fax: 512-306-8190
- www.bodywisdomschool.com/prenatal_massage.htm
- www.massagetherapy101.com/massage-techniques/prenatal-massage.aspx
- www.yogainthepearl.com/therapies.asp

QI GONG

See Chi Gong

Qi Gong Meridian Therapy

- www.meridianqigong.com/whatis.htm

Quantum Energetics

- www.perfectbalance101.com/services.htm
- www.healthythoughts.com/ht14/energetics.htm
- www.compwellness.org/eGuide/quantum.htm

Quantum Touch

- www.quantumtouch.com/QTOverviewReport.php
- www.awakening-healing.com/Quantum_Touch.htm
- www.sevadeva.com/healing/quantumtouch.htm

Radiance Technique

- www.authenticreiki.org/ • www.geocities.com/fascin8or/reiki_Radiance_Technique.html
- www.aegis.com/pubs/books/1997/BK970723.html

RADIX

- homepage.tinet.ie/~bomi/bodywork/ r.htm#Radix
- www.tarrin.net/radix.htm
- www.melodybrooke.com/pages/3

RAINDROP TECHNIQUE

- www.webdeb.com/oils/raindrop.htm
- rainbowhealingarts.com/docs/rain droptechnique.html
- www.healingenergies.com/raindrop.html

RAYID METHOD

- www.rayid.com/main/whatis.htm
- www.geocities.com/masteringwellness/ rayid.html

REBALANCING

- homepage.tinet.ie/~bomi/bodywork/ r.htm#Osho%20Rebalancing
- www.bomi.info/bodywork/r.htm#Osho% 20Rebalancing
- www.oshorebalancing.com/rebalancing_ eng.htm

Reflexognosy

- www.naturalapproach.com.au
- www.nctm.com.au/courses/diplomas/
  reflexognosy
   massagetherapy.com/articles/index.
  php?article_id=391

Reflexology

- Reflexology Association of America
  Administration Office
  79 Hudson Road
  Bolton, MA 01740
  Tel: 978-779-0255
  Fax: 978-779-0855
  E-mail: infoRAA@relexology-usa.org
  Web site: www.reflexology-usa.org
- www.reflexology.org
- www.reflexology-usa.org/refexolo.htm
- www.reflexology-usa.net/facts.htm

Reiki

- The International Center for Reiki Training
  21421 Hilltop Street, Unit #28
  Southfield, MI 48034
  Tel: 800-332-8112 or 248-948-8112
  Fax: 248-948-9534
  E-mail: center@reiki.org
  Web site: www.reiki.org
- reiki.7gen.com/index.html#Intro duction
- reiki.forplanetearth.com
- www.reiki.com/reiki.html

REPOSTURING DYNAMICS

- www.reposturingdynamics.com/whatis.htm
- www.aaronparnell.com/vitality7.com/Posture/index.html
- coastclick.com/pressreleases/index.cfm?ID=200009031048

RESONANT KINESIOLOGY

- vtmassageguild.org/services2 .htm#17
- www.aquathought.com/idatra/symposium/96/atwater.html
- www.nekn.org/ART.htm

RO-HUN TRANSFORMATIONAL THERAPY

- www.localaccess.com/HealingHands/RoHun.htm
- www.spiritleap.com/whatwedo/rohun.html
- www.delphi-center.com/programs/what is rohun.htm

RESTORATION THERAPY

- www.kodenkan.com
- www.pckilohana.com/PCA/massage.htm
- www.danzanryu.com/ort.html

ROLFING STRUCTURAL INTEGRATION

- www.rolf.org/about/index.html
- www.rolfguild.org/aboutsi.html

ROSEN METHOD BODYWORK

- www.rosenmethod.com/
- www.naturalhealers.com/qa/rosen.shtml
- members.cruzio.com/~bsamsel

RUBENFELD SYNERGY METHOD

- National Association of Rubenfeld
  Synergists
  7 Kendall Road
  Kendall Park, NJ 08824
  Tel: 877-RSM-2468
  E-mail: NARS@rubenfeldsynergy.com
  Web site: www.rubenfeldsynergy.com
- www.naturalhealers.com/qa/rubenfeld.
  shtml
- www.rubenfeldsynergy.com/synergy.htm
- www.health-alliance.com/learnabout/
  learn_rubenfeld.htm

RUSSIAN MASSAGE

- www.findarticles.com/cf_dls/g2603/0006/
  2603000638/p1/article.jhtml
- www.buyphilly.com/Shop/Product.Asp?
  ProdID=1967
- shell.ihug.co.nz/~nzig/Bioenergy.htm

SEATED MASSAGE

- TouchPro Association of Chair Massage
  584 Castro Street #555
  San Francisco, CA 94119
  Tel: 800-999-5026
  Fax: 415-612-1260
  E-mail: info@touchpro.com
  Web site: www.touchpro.org
- mysite.freeserve.com/mass_reflex/page1.html
- www.estt.com.au/about/corp.html#workplacestress

SHEN THERAPY

- www.naturalhealers.com/qa/shen.shtml

SHIATSU

- The Shiatsu Society
  Eastlands Court
  St Peters Road
  Rugby, UK CV21 3QP
  Tel: 0845 130 4560
  Fax: 01788 555052
  E-mail: admin@shiatsu.org
  Web site: www.shiatsu.org
- www.rianvisser.nl/shiatsu/e_watis .htm
- homepage.ntlworld.com/mikeflanagan/shiatsu

Soft Tissue Release

- www.massagecourses.gbr.fm/reasons.asp

Soma

- my.name-services.com/26818/page99.htm
- www.somabodywork.org
- www.gupbodyworks.com/intro.html

Soma Neuromuscular Integration

- www.bomi.info/bodywork/s.htm
- www.soma-institute.org
- www.massagetherapy.com/careers/
  enhanced_detail.php?state=WA&school
  =soma

Somatic Education

- www.somatics.com
- www.edmaupin.com/somatic
- www.susankramer.com/somatic. html

Somatic Experiencing

- www.traumahealing.com
- www.bomi.info/bodywork/s.htm# Somatic_
  Experiencing

Somatic Psychology

- www.sbgi.edu/html/som1.html
- www.centerforbody-mindintegration.com/
  somatic.php

SOMATOEMOTIONAL RELEASE

- www.craniosacralthpy.com/Somato Emotional.html
- www.upledger.co.uk/webser.htm

SOUND THERAPY

- www.biowaves.com/Info/WhatIsSound .cfm
- health.yahoo.com/health/alternative_medi cine/alternative_therapies/Sound_Therapy
- www.heartlandhealing.com/pages/archive/ sound_therapy

SPORTS MASSAGE

- Canadian Sport Massage Therapists Association
  1849 Yonge Street Suite 814
  Toronto, On, Canada M4s 1Y2
  Tel: 416/488-4414
  Fax: 416/488-3079
  E-mail: natoffice@csmat.ca
  Web site: www.csmta.ca
- www.thebodyworker.com/sportsmassage strokes.html
- csmta.ca/massage.htm
- www.bris.ac.uk/sport/sportsmedicine/mas sage.html

STRAIN/COUNTERSTRAIN

- www.hendrickhealth.org/rehab/strain.htm
- www.mission-hills-pt.com/strain.html
- www.chiroweb.com/archives/21/12/08. html

STRUCTURAL ENERGETIC THERAPY

- www.structuralenergetictherapy.com
- www.gregspindler.com/massage

STRUCTURAL INTEGRATION

See Rolfing.

SWEDISH MASSAGE

- www.mamashealth.com/massage/sweed. asp

SYNTROPY INSIGHT BODYWORK

- www.syntropy.net/What%20is.html

TAI CHI CHIH

- www.taichichih.org
- www.enhancing.com/taichichih.html
- www.wellspan.org/HealthServices/mind body_taichichih.htm

TAI CHI CHUAN

- www.chebucto.ns.ca/Philosophy/Taichi/chen.html
- ronperfetti.com/overview.html
- www.taichichuan.org/

TAIKYO SHIATSU

- www.gayatrihealing.com/massage.html
- www.massageandbodywork.com/Articles/AprilMay2003/TaikyoShiatsu.html

TARA APPROACH

- The TARA Approach
  2910 Country Road 67
  Boulder, CO 80303
  Tel: 303-499-9990
  Fax: 303-499-4454
  Web site: www.tara-approach.org
- www.tara-approach.org/#whatis
- www.ancient-holistic-healing-arts.com/taraapproach.htm#history
- www.boulderhealers.com/Calendar/tara.htm

TERA-MAI SEICHEM

- www.geocities.com/HotSprings/Resort/1239/1Seichem.html
- www.healingrays.com/Seichem
- www.lifepositive.com/Body/energy-healing/reiki/seichem.asp

THAI MASSAGE

- International Thai Therapists Association, Inc.
  PO Box 1048
  Palm Springs, CA 92263
  Tel: 760-641-0756
  E-mail: itta@cove.com
  Web site: www.thaimassage.com
- www.ancientmassage.com
- www.thai-massage.org/history.html

THALASSOTHERAPY

- www.spahealthspecialists.com/thalasso.htm
- www.alternativegreece.gr/WebForms/CategoryDisplay.aspx?ID=17

Therapeutic Touch

- Nurse Healer-Professional Associates
  International
  Alamo Plaza, Suite 111R
  4550 W. Oakey Boulevard
  Las Vegas, NV 89102
  Tel: 702-870-5507
  Fax: 702-870-5508
  E-mail: NH-PAI@therapeutic-touch.org
  Web site: www.therapeutic-touch.org
- www.therapeutic-touch.org/content/
  ttouch.asp
- www.phact.org/e/tt
- www.quackwatch.org/01Quackery
  RelatedTopics/tt.html

Touch For Health

- TFHIAA
  PO Box 5088
  Frankston South Vic. 3199
  Australia
  Tel/Fax: 0500 888 199
  E-mail: email@touch4health.org.au
  Web site: www.touch4health.org.au
- www.bomi.info/bodywork/t.htm#
  Touch%20For%20Health

TRAGER

- Trager International
  24800 Chagrin Boulevard, Suite 205
  Beachwood, OH 44122
  Tel: 250-337-5556
  E-mail: trager@trager.com
  Web site: www.trager.com
- www.trager.com/history.html
- www.naturalhealers.com/qa/trager.shtml
- health.yahoo.com/health/alternative_med icine/alternative_therapies/Trager _Integration/

TRAUMA TOUCH THERAPY

- www.csha.net/program_frames/ttt/ttt_ frameset.html
- www.birthjoy.com/articles/article_2002_ 08_8_1011.html

TRIGGER POINT MYOTHERAPY

See Bonnie Prudden Myotherapy
- www.bomi.info/bodywork/mo.htm
- www.painschool.com/trigger.html

Tui Na

- tcm.health-info.org/tuina/tcm-tuina-mass age.htm
- www.acupuncture.com/TuiNa/Tuina Ind.htm
- www.calmspirit.com/tuina.htm

Vibrational Healing Massage Therapy

- www.shareguide.com/vibrational.html
- www.upayacenter.org/practitioners/ crystal.htm

Visceral Manipulation

- www.upledger.com/therapies/vm.htm
- www.iahe.com/controller/IaheCurriculum Display?curriculumCode=VM
- www.craniosacralacupuncture.com/visceral manipulation.htm

Vortex Healing Energetic Therapy

- www.sweetmotherloves.com/pages/ener getic.html
- www.vortexhealing.com
- britishregister.tripod.com/healing/id14.html

Watsu

- Worldwide Aquatic Bodywork Association
  PO Box 889
  Middletown, CA 95461
  Tel: 707-987-3801
  Fax: 707-987-9638
  E-mail: info@waba.edu
  Web site: www.waba.edu
- www.waba.edu/#WATSU
- www.dolphinheart.com/watsu.html
- www.watsunorthwest.com

Yoga

- www.yogasite.com/yogastyles.html
- www.yogajournal.com/newtoyoga/
  160_1.cfm
- www.yogaworld.org

Yogassage

- www.growinghealthier.com/mystical
  massage.html
- www.infinitejoy.com/yoga

Zen Shiatsu

- www.zshiatsu.com/new_page_3.htm
- www.bcmt.org/training/zen-shiatsu .htm

ZERO BALANCING

- The Zero Balancing Health Association
  801 West Main Street Suite 202
  Charlottesville, VA 22903
  Tel: 434-244-2458
  Fax: 434-244-2645
  E-mail: zbaoffice@zerobalancing.com
  Web site: www.zerobalancing.com
- homepage.eircom.net/~bomi/bodywork/
  zero_balancing/introduction.htm
- www.naturalhealers.com/qa/zerobalancing.
  shtml

Range of Motion

Upper Extremity ROM

Cervical Spine

Flexion	0-45°
Extension	0-45°
Lateral flexion	0-45°
Rotation	0-60°

Shoulder

Flexion	0-170°
Extension	0-60°
Abduction	0-170°
Adduction	0°
Horizontal abduction	0-40°
Horizontal adduction	0-130°
Internal rotation	0-(60-70)°
External rotation	0-90°

Elbow & Forearm

Extension-flexion	0-150°
Supination	0-(80-90)°
Pronation	0-(80-90)°

Thumb (1st digit)

MP flexion	0-(50-90)°
MP hyperextension	0-(15-45)°
IP flexion	0-(80-90)°
Abduction	0-50°
Opposition	0 (cm.)

Fingers

MP flexion	0-90°
PIP flexion	0-(100-110)°
DIP flexion	0-80°
Abduction	0-25°

Lower Extremity ROM

Hip

Flexion	0-120°
Extension	0-30°
Abduction	0-40°
Adduction	0-35°
Internal rotation	0-45°
External rotation	0-45°

Knee

Extension-flexion	0-135°

Ankle-Foot

Dorsiflexion	0-15°
Plantarflexion	0-50°
Inversion	0-35°
Eversion	0-20°

Wrist

Flexion	0-(80-90)°
Extension	0-70°
Ulnar deviation	0-(30-35)°
Radial deviation	0-20°

Adapted from Trombly CA. Evaluation of biomechanical and physiological aspects of motor performance. In Trombly CA, ed. *Occupational therapy for physical dysfunction*, 4th edition. Baltimore, Md: Williams & Wilkins; 1995 and from Duesterhaus Minor MA and Duesterhaus Minor S. *Patient evaluation methods for the health professional*. Reston, Va: Reston Publishing Co, Inc; 1985.

Bones of the Body

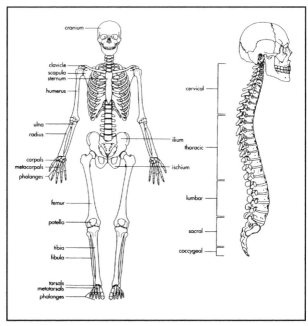

Figure 13-1. Reprinted from Sladyk K. *OT Student Primer: A Guide to College Success*. Thorofare, NJ: SLACK Incorporated; 1997.

MUSCLES OF THE BODY

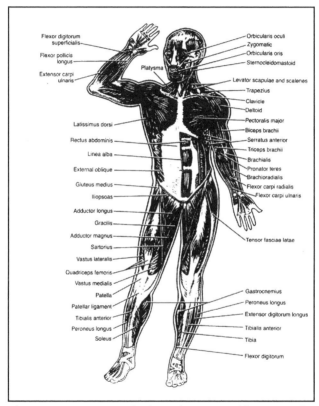

Figure 14-1. Anterior superficial muscles. Reprinted from Leonard P. Quick and Easy Terminology, 2nd ed; 1995 with permission from Elsevier Science.

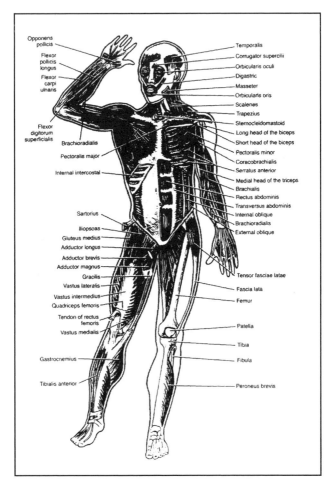

Figure 14-2. Anterior deep muscles. Reprinted from Leonard P. *Quick and Easy Terminology,* 2nd ed; 1995 with permission from Elsevier Science.

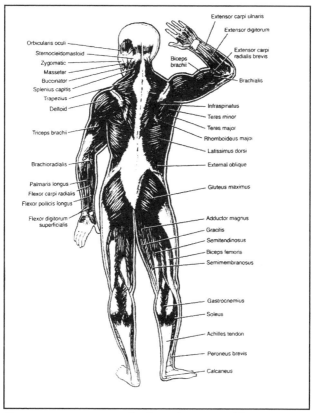

Figure 14-3. Posterior superficial muscles.Reprinted from Leonard P. *Quick and Easy Terminology*, 2nd ed; 1995 with permission from Elsevier Science.

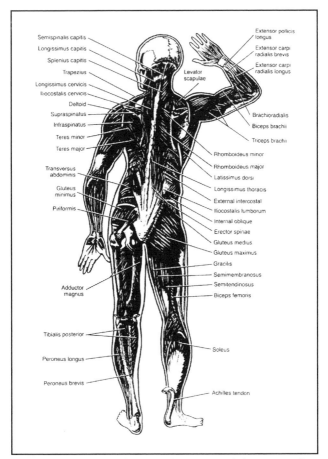

Figure 14-4. Posterior deep muscles. Reprinted from Leonard P. *Quick and Easy Terminology*, 2nd ed; 1995 with permission from Elsevier Science.

Muscles: Origin/Insertion/Action—Innervation—Blood Supply

Muscle	Origin	Insertion	Action	Nerve	Artery
Neck					
Sternocleido-mastoid (SCM)	Med or sternal head cranial part of ventral surface of manubrium; lat or clavicular head—sup border & ant surface of med 1/3 clavicle	Lat surface mastoid process & lat 1/2 sup nuchal line of occipital bone	↻ opp side lat ✓same side ✓ forward	Spinal accessory n. C2 & C3 ant rami	Subclavian a.
Platysma	Fascia covering sup part of pectoralis major & deltoid	Some fibers into bone below oblique line, others into skin	Draws lip inf & post	Cervical branch of facial n.	Subclavian a. (branch)
Suprahyoid group					
Digastricus	Post belly: mastoid notch of temporal bone; Ant belly: a depression on inner side of inf border of mandible	Post belly: hyoid bone by fibrous loop; Ant belly: same as post belly	▲ hyoid bone Post: draws backwards Ant: draws forward	Post: facial n. Ant: mylohyoid n.	Lingual a.
Stylohyoideus	Post & lat surface of styloid process	Body of hyoid bone	Draws hyoid sup & post	Facial n. (branch)	Lingual a.

*See Appendix 7 for helpful abbreviations.

Muscle	Origin	Insertion	Action	Nerve	Artery
Mylohyoideus	Whole length of mylohyoid line of mandible	Body of hyoid bone	▲ hyoid & tongue	Mylohyoid n.	Lingual a.
Geniohyoideus	Inf mental spine on inner surface of symphysis menti	Ant surface of hyoid	Draws hyoid & tongue ant	1st cervical n. (through hypoglossal n.)	Lingual a.
Infrahyoid Group					
Sternohyoideus	Post surface of med end of clavicle, post sterno-clav lig & sup & post part of manubrium sterni	Inf border of hyoid bone	Draws hyoid inferiorly	Branch of ansa cervicalis (1st three cervical nerves)	Lingual a. Subclavian a.
Sternothyroideus	Dorsal surface of manubrium sterni (caudal of origin of sternohyoideus)	Oblique line on lamina of thyroid cartilage	Draws thyroid caudally	Branch of ansa cervicalis (1st three cervical nerves)	Lingual a. Subclavian a.
Thyrohyoideus	Oblique line on lamina of thyroid cartilage	Inf border of greater cornu of hyoid bone	Draws hyoid inferiorly Draws thyroid cartilage sup	1st & 2nd cervical n.	Lingual a. Subclavian a.
Omohyoideus	Cranial border of scapula (near or crossing scapular notch)	Caudal border of hyoid bone	Draws hyoid caudally	Branch of ansa cervicalis (1st three cervical nerves)	Subclavian a.

Muscle	Origin	Insertion	Action	Nerve	Artery
Longus Colli	Vertical: ant surface of C5, C6, C7, T1, T2, & T3; Sup: ant tubercles of transverse processes C3, C4, C5; Inf: ant surface of T2 & T3	Vertical: ant surface of C2, C3, C4; Sup: narrow tendon into tubercle on ant arch of atlas; Inf: ant tubercles of transverse processes C5 & C6	✓ of neck ↻ neck (min)	Branches of 2nd to 7th cervical nerves	Subclavian a. (thyrocervical)
Longus Capitus	Four tendinous slips from ant tubercles of transverse processes C3, C4, C5, & C6	Inf surface of the basilar part of occipital bone	Head ✓	Branches from 1st, 2nd, & 3rd cervical nerves	Subclavian a.
Rectus Capitus Anterior	Ant surface of lat mass of the atlas & from root of its transverse process	Inf surface of basilar part of occipital bone	Head ✓	Branch of 1st & 2nd cervical nerves	Subclavian a.
Rectus Capitus Lateralis	Sup surface of transverse process of atlas	Inf surface of jugular process of occipital bone	Lat ✓ head	Branch of 1st & 2nd cervical nerves	Subclavian a.
Scalenus Anterior	Ant tubercles of transverse processes of C3, C4, C5, & C6	Scalene tubercle on inner border of 1st rib & ridge on cranial surface of rib	▲ 1st rib ✓ head ↻ head	Branches of lower cervical nerves	Subclavian a. (thyrocervical)

Muscle	Origin	Insertion	Action	Nerve	Artery
Scalenus Medius	Post tubercles of transverse processes of C2, C3, C4, C5, C6, & C7	Cranial surface of 1st rib between tubercle & subclavian groove	▲ 1st rib / head ↻ head	Branches from cervical nerves	Subclavian a. (thyrocervical)
Scalenus Posterior	Post tubercles of transverse processes of C5, C6, & C7	Outer surface of 2nd rib (deep to serratus anterior)	▲ 2nd rib / head ↻ head	Ventral primary branches C5, C6 & C7	Subclavian a.
Back/Neck					
Serratus Posterior Superior	Caudal part of ligamentum nuchae, spinous processes C7, T1, T2, & T3; supraspinal ligament	Four digitations—cranial borders of ribs 2, 3, 4, & 5	Respiratory ▲ ribs	Ventral rami T1 to T4	Subclavian a.
Serratus Posterior Inferior	Spinous processes T11, T12, L1, L2, & L3; supraspinal ligament	Four digitations into inf borders last 4 ribs (a little beyond their angles)	Respiratory Draws ribs ◄► & ▼	Ventral rami T9 to T12	Subclavian a.
Splenius Capitis Cervicis	Caudal ½ ligamentum nuchae & spinous processes C7, T1, T2, T3, & sometimes T4	Occipital bone just inf to lat 1/3 of sup nuchal line; into mastoid process of temporal bone	/ head & neck lat ✓ same side ↻ same side	Lat branches dorsal primary cervical nerves	Subclavian a. (branches)

Muscle	Origin	Insertion	Action / spine	Nerve Branch dorsal primary spinal nerves	Artery Branch dorsal Thoracic aorta (branch)
Spinalis Capitis	Usually inseparable from semispinalis capitis				
Semispinalis Capitis	Tips of transverse processes C7, T1, T2, T3, T4, T5, T6, and sometimes T7	Between sup & inf nuchal lines of occipital bone	/ head & neck ↻ opp side	Dorsal rami	Subclavian a. (branches)
Longissimus Capitis	Transverse processes T4 and T5 and cervicis and articular processes C4, C5, C6, and C7	Post margin of mastoid process (deep to splenius capitis and SCM)	/ head ↺ same side ✓ same side	Dorsal primary mid and lower cervical n(s).	Subclavian a. (branches)
Obliquus Capitis Inferior	Arises from apex of spinous process of axis	Inf & dorsal transverse process of atlas	↻ same side	Branch dorsal primary division suboccipital n.	Subclavian a. (branch)
Obliquus Capitis Superior	Tendinous fibers from sup surface transverse process of atlas	Occipital bone between sup & inf nuchal lines (lat to semispinalis capitis)	/ head	Branch dorsal primary division suboccipital n.	Subclavian a. (branch)
Rectus Capitis Posterior Major	Spinous process of the axis	Lat part of inf nuchal line of occipital bone and surface immediately inf	/ head ↺ same side	Branch dorsal primary division suboccipital n.	Subclavian a. (branch)

Muscle	Origin	Insertion	Action	Nerve	Artery
Rectus Capitis Posterior Minor	Tendon from tubercle on post arch of atlas	Med part of the inf nuchal line of occipital bone & surface between it and foramen magnum	/ head	Branch dorsal primary division suboccipital n.	Subclavian a. (branch)
Longissimus Cervicis	Long thin tendons from apex transverse processes upper 4 or 5 thoracic vertebrae	Post tubercles of transverse processes of C2 to C6	/ spine lat ✓ ▼ ribs	Dorsal primary branch spinal nerves	Thoracic aorta (branches)
Iliocostalis Cervicis	Angles of the 3rd, 4th, 5th & 6th ribs	Post tubercles of transverse processes of C4, C5, & C6	/ spine lat ✓ ▼ ribs	Dorsal primary branch spinal nerves	Thoracic aorta (branches)
Spinalis Cervicis	Caudal part of ligamentum nuchae, spinous process C7; sometimes T1 and T2	Spinous processes of axis; sometimes spinous process C1 & C2	/ spine	Dorsal primary branch spinal nerves	Thoracic aorta (branch)
Semispinalis Cervicis	Transverse processes of 1st five or six thoracic vertebrae	Cervical spinous processes from axis to C5	/ spine ↻ opp side	Dorsal primary branch spinal nerves	Thoracic aorta (branch)

Muscle Back	Origin	Insertion	Action	Nerve	Artery
Longissimus Thoracis	Arising from erector spinae and post surfaces transverse and accessory processes of lumbar vertebrae and ant layer lumbocostal aponeurosis	Transverse processes of all thoracic vertebrae and lower 9 or 10 ribs between tubercles and angles	/ spine lat ✓ ▼ ribs	Dorsal primary branch spinal nerves	Thoracic aorta (branch)
Iliocostalis Thoracis	Flattened tendons from upper borders of angles of lower 6 ribs (med to iliocostalis lumborum)	Cranial borders of angles of 1st 6 ribs and into dorsum of transverse process C7	/ spine lat ✓ ▼ ribs	Dorsal primary branch spinal nerves	Thoracic aorta (branch)
Spinalis Thoracis	Med continuation of sacrospinalis. Arises from spinous processes of T11, T12, L1, & L2	Spinous processes of upper thoracic vertebrae	/ spine	Dorsal primary branch spinal nerves	Thoracic aorta (branch)
Semispinalis Thoracis	Transverse processes of T6 to T10	Spinous processes of C6, C7, T1, T2, T3, & T4	/ spine ↻ opp side	Dorsal primary branch spinal nerves	Thoracic aorta (branch)
Iliocostalis Lumborum	Flattened tendons from upper portion of erector spinae	Inf borders of angles of last 6 or 7 ribs	/ spine lat ✓ ▼ ribs	Dorsal primary branch spinal nerves	Thoracic aorta (branch)

Muscle	Origin	Insertion	Action	Nerve	Artery
Sacrospinalis (Erector Spinae)	Arises from broad tendon attached to mid crest of sacrum; spinous processes T11 to T12 and lumbar vertebrae; supraspinal ligament to lip of iliac crests and lat crest of sacrum	Splits into longissimus, iliocostalis, spinalis, and semispinalis muscles (see respective muscles)	/ spine ↻ spine ▶ ribs lat ✓	Spinal nerves	Thoracic aorta
Multifidus	Spinous processes of each vertebra from sacrum to axis. Arises from back of sacrum from aponeurosis of sacrospinalis, from med surface of post sup iliac spine and post sacroiliac ligaments	Each ascends obliquely crossing over 2 to 4 vertebrae and inserted into spinous process of vertebra from last lumbar to axis	/ spine ↻ opp side	Branches of dorsal primary spinal nerves	Thoracic aorta
Rotatores	Transverse process of one vertebra and insert at base of spinous process of vertebra above from the sacrum to the axis	*Rotatores longi* cross one vertebra in their oblique course. *Rotatores breves* insert in next succeeding vertebra and run horizontal	/ spine ↻ opp side	Branches of dorsal primary spinal nerves	Thoracic aorta

Muscle	Origin	Insertion	Action	Nerve	Artery
Quadratus Lumborum	Sup borders of the transverse processes L2 to L5	Inf border of last rib and transverse process L1 to L4	▼ last rib lat ✓	12th thoracic n. 1st lumbar n.	Iliac circumflex
Shoulder Girdle					
Trapezius	Ext occipital protuberance; med 1/3 sup nuchal line; spinous process C7, T1 to T12	Post border of lat 3rd clavicle; med margin acromion; spine of the scapula	▲ &/shoulder Abd same side ⟲ opp side Retraction ▲ ⟲ glen fossa ▲ glenoid fossa	Spinal accessory n. C3 & C4 spinal nerves	Suprascapular
Levator Scapulae	Transverse processes C1 to C4	Med border scapula between sup angle and spine	Elevation Protraction / cervical spine Abd same side ⟲ same side	Dorsal scapular n. C3 & C4 spinal nerves	Superficial cervical a. Transverse cervical a.
Romboideus Minor	Spinous process of C7 and T1	Med border scapula at level of the spine	Elevation Retraction ▼ ⟲ glen fossa	Dorsal scapular n.	Descending scapular a.
Romboideus Major	Spinous process of T2 to T5	Med border scapula between spine and inf angle	Elevation Retraction ▼ ⟲ glen fossa	Dorsal scapular n.	Descending scapular a.

Muscle	Origin	Insertion	Action / shoulder	Nerve	Artery
Latissimus Dorsi	Lumbar aponeurosis; spinous processes of T6 to T12, L1 to L5, & sacral vertebrae	Distal part of intertubercular groove of humerus	Abd shoulder Med ↻ Elevation Retraction	Thoracodorsal n. C6 to C8 spinal nerves	Subscapular a.
Pectoralis Major	Ant surface sternal 1/2 clavicle; ventral surface sternum; aponeurosis of externus abdominis	Crest of greater tubercle of humerus	✓ shoulder Add shoulder Med ↻ Protract; ▲▼	Med and lat pectoral n. C5 to C8 spinal nerves 1st thoracic n.	Thoraco-acromial a. obliquus
Pectoralis Minor	Ext surfaces of ribs 3, 4, and 5 near their cartilages	Caracoid process of scapula	Protraction Depression ▼ ↻ glen fossa	Med pectoral n.	Thoraco-acromial a.
Subclavius	1st rib and its cartilage near their junction	Inf aspect of clavicle in the mid 3rd	Protraction Depression	Branch from brachial plexus (sup trunk)	Thoraco-acromial a.
Serratus Anterior	Ext surfaces of ribs 1 to 9	Ant aspect of med border of scapula from sup to inf angle	Protraction Depression ▲ ↻ glen fossa	Long thoracic n.	Lat thoracic a.
Subscapularis	Mid 2/3 subscapular fossa; inf 2/3 groove on axillary	Lesser tubercle of humerus	Med ↻ ✓ & / Abd & add	Subscapular n.	Circumflex scapular a.

Muscle	Origin	Insertion	Action	Nerve	Artery
Supraspinatus	Mid 2/3 supraspinatous fossa	Sub impression of greater tubercle of humerus	Abd Lat ↻ (weak) ✓ (weak)	Suprascapular n.	Supra-scapular
Infraspinatus	Med 2/3 infraspinatus fossa	Mid impression of greater tubercle of humerus	Lat ↻ Abd and add	Suprascapular n.	Supra-scapular
Teres Minor	Dorsal surface of axillary border of scapula	Inf impression of greater tubercle of humerus distal to inf impression	Lat ↻ Add	Branch of axillary n.	Post humeral circumflex a.
Teres Major	Oval area on dorsal surface of inf angle of scapula	Crest of lesser tubercle of humerus	Add / shoulder Med ↻	Lower subscapular n.	Circumflex scapular a.
Deltoideus	Ant border and sup surface of lat 3rd of clavicle; lat margin & sup surface of acromion; inf lip post border scapular spine	Deltoid prominence on mid of lat body of humerus	Abd shoulder ✓ shoulder / shoulder Med & lat ↻	Axillary n. from brachial plexus	Post humeral circumflex a.
Shoulder/Elbow					
Triceps Brachii	Long head: infraglenoid tuberosity of scapula;	Post proximal surface of olecranon	/ elbow / shoulder	Branches radial n. collateral a.	Profunda brachii a.

Muscle	Origin	Insertion	Action	Nerve	Artery
					Inf ulnar
Brachialis	Lat head: post surface of humerus; Med head: post surface of humerus distal to radial groove. Distal 1/2 of ant aspect of humerus	Tuberosity of ulna; rough depression on ant surface of coronoid process	Add shoulder ✓ elbow	Musculocutaneous n. Radial & med n.	Brachial a.
Biceps Brachii	Short head: apex of coracoid process; Long head: supraglenoid tuberosity at sup margin of glenoid	Rough post portion tuberosity of radius	✓ shoulder ✓ elbow Supination	Musculocutaneous n.	Brachial a.
Coracobrachialis	Apex of coracoid process	Impression at med surface & border of humerus	✓ shoulder Add shoulder	Musculocutaneous n.	Brachial a.
Forearm/Wrist					
Pronator Teres	Humeral head: proximal to med epicondyle of humerus; Ulnar head: med side of coronoid process of ulna	Rough impression at mid of lat surface of radius	Pronation	Median n.	Inf ulnar collateral a.

Muscle	Origin	Insertion	Action	Nerve	Artery
Flexor Carpi Radialis	Med epicondyle of humerus	Base of 2nd metacarpal bone	✓ wrist Radial ✓	Median n.	Radial a.
Palmaris Longus	Med epicondyle of humerus	Palmar aponeurosis	✓ wrist	Median n.	Volar interosseous a.
Flexor Carpi Ulnaris	Humeral head: med epicondyle of humerus; Ulnar head: med margin olecranon; proximal 2/3 dorsal border of ulna	Pisiform bone	✓ wrist Add wrist	Ulnar n.	Ulnar a.
Flexor Digitorum Superficialis	Humeral head: med epicondyle of humerus; Ulnar head: med side of coronoid process; Radial head: oblique line of radius	Divides into 4 tendons which are inserted into the sides of the 2nd phalanx	✓ PIPs ✓ MCPs ✓ wrist	Median n.	Ulnar a.
Flexor Digitorum Profundus	Proximal 3/4 of volar & med surfaces of body of ulna	Bases of last phalanges	✓ DIPs ✓ PIPs ✓ MCPs ✓ wrist	Palmar interosseous n. from median n. Branch of ulnar n.	Ulnar a. Volar interosseous a.
Flexor Pollicis Longus	Grooved volar surface of body of the radius	Base of distal phalanx of the thumb	✓ IP digit 1 ✓ MCP digit 1 ✓ & add wrist	Palmar interosseous n. from median n.	Radial a.

Muscle	Origin	Insertion	Action	Nerve	Artery
Pronator Quadratus	Pronator ridge on distal part of palmar surface of body of ulna; med part of palmar surface of distal 1/4 of ulna	Distal 1/4 of lat border and palmar surface of body of the radius	Pronation	Palmar interosseous from median n.	Ulnar and radial
Brachioradialis	Proximal 2/3 of lat supracondylar ridge of humerus	Lat side of base of styloid process of radius	✓ elbow	Branch of radial n.	Radial a.
Extensor Carpi Radialis Longus	Distal 1/3 lat supracondylar ridge of humerus	Dorsal surface of base of 2nd metacarpal bone—radial side	/ extension Abd wrist	Radial n.	Radial a.
Extensor Carpi Radialis Brevis	Lat epicondyle of humerus	Dorsal surface of base of 3rd metacarpal bone—radial side	/ wrist Abd wrist	Radial n.	Radial a.
Extensor Carpi Ulnaris	Lat epicondyle of humerus	Prominent tubercle on ulnar side of base of metacarpal V	/ wrist Add wrist	Deep radial n.	Ulnar a.
Extensor Digitorum	Lat epicondyle of humerus	2nd & 3rd phalanges of fingers; dorsal surface of distal phalanx	/ PIPs and DIPs / MCPs	Deep radial n.	Ulnar a.
Extensor Digiti Minimi	Common extensor tendon	Expansion of ext digitorum tendon on dorsum of 1st phalanx of little finger	/ wrist / PIPs, DIPs, and MCP digit V	Deep radial n.	Ulnar a.

Muscle	Origin	Insertion	Action	Nerve	Artery
Anconeus	Separate tendon from dorsal part of lat epicondyle of humerus	Side of olecranon; proximal 1/4 of dorsal surface of body of ulna	/ elbow	Radial n.	Ulnar a.
Abductor Pollicis Longus	Lat part of dorsal surface of body of ulna	Radial side of base of 1st metacarpal bone	Abd IP, MCP of digit I Abd wrist	Deep radial n.	Radial a.
Extensor Pollicis Brevis	Dorsal surface of body of radius distal to that muscle and interosseous membrane	Base of 1st phalanx of thumb	/ IP, MCP of digit I / wrist	Deep radial n.	Radial a.
Extensor Pollicis Longus	Lat part of mid 1/3 of dorsal surface of body of ulna distal to origin of abductor pollicis longus	Base of last phalanx of thumb	/ IP, MCP of digit I / wrist	Deep radial n.	Radial a.
Extensor Indicis	Dorsal surface of body of ulna below origin of extensor pollicis longus	Joins ulnar side of tendon of extensor digitorum	/ and add of IP, MCP digit II	Deep radial n.	Radial a.
Supinator	Lat epicondyle of humerus from ridge of ulna	Lat edge of radial tuberosity and oblique line of radius and med surface of radius posteriorly	Supination	Deep radial n.	Radial a.

Muscle Hand	Origin	Insertion	Action	Nerve	Artery
Abductor Pollicis Brevis	Transverse carpal ligament, tuberosity of scaphoid, ridge of trapezium	Radial side of base of 1st phalanx thumb	Abd thumb	Median n.	Radial a.
Opponens Pollicis	Ridge of trapezium	Length of metacarpal bone of thumb on radial side	Abd thumb ✓ thumb Med ↷	Median n.	Radial a.
Flexor Pollicis Brevis	Distal ridge of trapezium; ulnar side of 1st metacarpal	Radial side of base of proximal phalanx of thumb; ulnar side of base of 1st phalanx	✓ thumb Add thumb	Median & ulnar n.	Radial a.
Adductor Pollicis	Capitale bone, bases of 2nd & 3rd metacarpals	Ulnar side of base of proximal phalanx of thumb	Add thumb	Deep palmar branch of ulnar	Ulnar n.
Palmaris Brevis	Tendinous fasciculi from palmar aponeurosis	Skin on ulnar border of palm of hand	Draws skin midpalm	Ulnar n.	Superficial ulnar a.
Abductor Digiti Minimi	Pisiform bone	Ulnar side of base of 1st phalanx of digit V	Abd digit V ✓ proximal phalanx	Ulnar n.	Ulnar a.
Flexor Digiti Minimi Brevis	Convex surface of hamulus of hamate bone	Ulnar side of base of 1st phalanx of digit V	✓ digit V	Ulnar n.	Ulnar a.

Muscle	Origin	Insertion	Action	Nerve	Artery
Opponens Digiti Minimi	Convexity of hamulus of hamate bone	Length of metacarpal bone of digit V along ulnar margin	Abd digit V ✓ digit V Med ↻ V	Ulnar n.	Ulnar a.
Lumbricals	Originate from the profundus tendons. 1 and 2: radials sides and palmar surfaces of tendons of digits II and III; 3: contiguous sides of mid and ring fingers; 4: contiguous sides of tendons of ring & little finger	Tendinous expansion of extensor digitorum	✓ MCPs / PIPs and DIPs	1 and 2: median n. 3 and 4: ulnar n.	Median a. Ulnar a.
Interosseous Dorsales	Two heads from adjacent sides of metacarpal bone	Bases of 1st phalanx	Abd—midline (digit III)	Deep palmar branch n.	Ulnar a.
Interossei	All from entire length of metacarpal bones	Side of base of 1st phalanx	Add—midline (digit III) ✓ MCPs / PIPs and DIPs	Deep palmar branch n.	Ulnar a.

Muscle Hip	Origin	Insertion	Action	Nerve	Artery
Psoas Major (Iliopsoas)	Ventral surface of bases and caudal borders of transverse process of lumbar spine; sides and corresponding intervertebral disks of last thoracic and all lumbar vertebrae	Lesser trochanter of femur	✓ of hip ✓ of spine in lumbar region	2nd and 3rd lumbar n.	Lumbar of iliolumbar a.
Psoas Minor (Iliopsoas)	Vertebral margins of T12 and L1 & corresponding disks	Pectineal line; iliopectineal eminence	✓ of spine in lumbar region	1st & 2nd lumbar n.	Lumbar branch of iliolumbar a.
Iliacus (Iliopsoas)	Upper 2/3 of iliac fossa; iliac crest	Lesser trochanter of femur	✓ at hip	Femoral n. (muscular branches)	Lumbar branch of iliolumbar a.
Tensor Fasciae Latae (TFL)	Ant part of outer lip of iliac crest; ant border of ilium	Lat part of fascia lata at junction of proximal and mid thirds of thigh (proximal end of iliotibial band)	Tenses TFL 3 at hip Abd at hip Int ↻ at hip	Sup gluteal n.	Sup gluteal a.

Muscle	Origin	Insertion	Action	Nerve	Artery
Gluteus Maximus	Post gluteal line; dorsal surface of sacrum and coccyx	Gluteal tuberosity; lat part of TFL at junction of proximal and mid thirds of thigh (proximal end of iliotibial band)	/ at hip Add at hip Ext ↻ at hip / lower spine	Inf gluteal n.	Inf gluteal a.
Gluteus Medius	Outer surface of ilium from iliac crest and post gluteal line above to ant gluteal line below	Lat surface of greater trochanter	Abd at hip Int ↻ at hip	Sup gluteal n.	Sup gluteal a.
Piriformis	Pelvic surface of sacrum between ant sacral foramina and margin of greater sciatic foramen	Upper border of greater trochanter of femur	Ext ↻ at hip Abd at hip	1st and 2nd sacral n.	Sup gluteal a.
Obturator Internus	Margins of obturator foramen; pelvic surface of hip bone; post and sup obturator foramen	Med surface of greater trochanter	Ext ↻ at hip Abd at hip	Obturator n. to obturator internus and gemellus sup	Obturator a. Sup gluteal a.
Gemellus Superior	Outer surface of ischial spine	Med surface of greater trochanter	Ext ↻ at hip	Obturator n. to obturator internus and gemellus sup	Obturator a. Sup gluteal a.

Muscle	Origin	Insertion	Action	Nerve	Artery
Gemellus Inferior	Upper part of ischial tuberosity	Med surface of greater trochanter	Ext ↻ at hip	Obturator n. to quadratus femoris & gemellus inf	Sup gluteal a.
Quadratus Femoris	Lat margin of ischial tuberosity	Quadrate tubercle of femur; linea quadrata	Add at hip Ext ↻ at hip	Obturator n. to quadratus femoris & gemellus inf	Sup gluteal a.
Obturator Externus	Outer margin of obturator foramen	Trochanteric fossa of femur	Add at hip Ext ↻ at hip	Post branch of obturator n.	Obturator a.
Hip/Thigh					
Sartorius	Ant-sup iliac spine; upper half of iliac notch	Upper part of med surface of tibia	✓ at hip Ext ↻ at hip ✓ at knee Abd hip (weak)	Muscular branches of femoral n.	Femoral a.
Quadriceps Femoris					
Rectus Femoris	Ant-inf iliac spine	Patella by the patellar ligament to the tibial tuberosity	/ at knee ✓ at hip	Muscular branches of femoral n.	Femoral a.
Vastus Lateralis	Lat aspect of the shaft of the femur	Patella by the patellar ligament to the tibial tuberosity	/ at knee	Muscular branches of femoral n.	Femoral a.
Vastus Medialis	Med aspect of the shaft of the femur	Patella by the patellar ligament to the tibial tuberosity	/ at knee draws patella medially	Muscular branches of femoral n.	Femoral a.

Muscle	Origin	Insertion	Action	Nerve	Artery
Vastus Intermedius	Ant aspect of the shaft of the femur	Patella by the patellar ligament to the tibial tuberosity	/ at knee	Muscular branches of femoral n.	Femoral a.
Gracilis	Lower 1/2 of pubic symphysis; upper 1/2 of pubic arch	Proximal part of med surface of tibia	✓ at knee; Int ↻ at knee; Add at hip	Ant branch of obturator n.	Med femoral circumflex a. (ascending)
Pectineus	Pubic pectineal line and an area of bone ant to it	Line leading from the lesser trochanter to the linea aspera	✓ at hip; Int ↻ hip; Add at hip	Muscular branches of femoral & obturator n.	Med femoral circumflex a.
Adductor Longus	Ant portion of pubis in angle between crest and symphysis	Mid part of linea aspera	Add at hip; ✓ at hip	Ant branch of obturator n.	Profunda femoris a.
Adductor Brevis	Ext surface of inf ramus of pubis	Proximal part of linea aspera	Add at hip; ✓ at hip	Ant branch of obturator n.	Mid femoral circumflex a.
Adductor Magnus	Pubic arch & ischial tuberosity	Oblique line along entire shaft of the femur	Add at hip; ✓ hip (upper); / hip (lower)	Post branch of obturator & sciatic n.	Profunda femoris & med femoris circumflex a.
Biceps Femoris	Long head: from ischial tuberosity; Short head: lat lip of linea aspera, lat supracondylar line of femur	Head of fibula, lat condyle of tibia, deep fascia on lat side of leg	✓ at knee; / at hip; Ext ↻ knee (semiflexed)	Sciatic n. tibial branch to long head; peroneal branch to short head	Profunda femoris a.

Muscle	Origin	Insertion	Action	Nerve	Artery
Semitendinous	Upper & mid impression of ischial tuberosity (with tendon of the biceps femoris)	Proximal part of ant border & med surface of the tibia	✓ at knee / at hip; Int ⤸ knee (semiflexed)	Sciatic n.	Perforating branch profunda femoris a.
Semimembranous	Proximal & lat facet of ischial tuberosity	Med-post surface of med condyle of tibia	✓ at knee / at hip; Int ⤸ knee (semiflexed)	Sciatic n.	Perforating branch profunda femoris a.
Leg					
Tibialis Anterior	Lat surface of shaft of tibia; med aspect of fibula; ant interosseus membrane	Med & plantar surface of med cuniform bone; base of 1st metatarsal bone	Dorsiflexion inversion	Deep peroneal n.	Ant tibial a.
Popliteus	Lat condyle of femur	Triangular area on post surface of tibia above ideal line	✓ at knee; Int ⤸ at knee	Tibial n. (med & int popliteal)	Post tibial a.
Leg/Foot					
Extensor Hallucis Longus	Lat surface of shaft of tibia; med aspect of fibula; ant interosseous membrane	Base of distal phalanx of great toe	/ MTP & IP Dorsiflexion	Deep peroneal n. (ant tibial)	Ant tibial a.

Muscle	Origin	Insertion	Action	Nerve	Artery
Extensor Digitorum Longus (EDL)	Lat surface of shaft of tibia; med aspect of fibula; ant interosseous membrane	Dorsal surface of mid and distal phalanges of lat 4 digits	/ IPs digits II to V Dorsiflexion	Deep peroneal n. (ant tibial)	Ant tibial a.
Extensor Digitorum Brevis (EDB)	Proximal and lat surface of calcaneus; lat talocalcaneal ligament	1st tendon dorsal surface of base of proximal phalanx of hallux; other 3 tendons lat sides of tendons of EDL	/ IPs	Deep peroneal n.	Ant tibial a.
Flexor Digitorum Longus	Post surface of shaft of tibia; post aspect of fibula; post interosseous membrane	Plantar surface of base of distal phalanx of lat 4 digits	✓ digits II to V Plantarflexion	Tibial n. (med & int popliteal)	Post tibial a.
Flexor Hallucis Longus	Post surface of shaft of tibia; post aspect of fibula; post interosseous membrane	Base of distal phalanx of hallux	✓ digit I Plantarflexion	Tibial n. (med & int popliteal)	Post tibial a.

Muscle	Origin	Insertion	Action	Nerve	Artery
Tibialis Posterior	Post surface of shaft of tibia; post aspect of fibula; post interosseous membrane	Tuberosity of navicular; plantar surface of cuniform bones; plantar surface of base of 2nd, 3rd and 4th metatarsals, cuboid, sustentaculum tali	Plantarflexion Inversion	Tibial n. (med & int popliteal)	Post tibial a.
Peroneus Tertius	Lat surface of shaft of tibia; med aspect of fibula; ant interosseous membrane	Dorsal surface of base of 5th metatarsal bone	Dorsiflexion Eversion	Deep peroneal n. (ant tibial)	Ant tibial a.
Peroneus Longus	Lat condyle of tibia; head and upper 2/3 of lat surface of fibula	Lat side of med cuniform bone, base of 1st metatarsal bone	Plantarflexion Eversion	Superficial peroneal n. (musculocu-taneous)	Peroneal a.
Peroneus Brevis	Lower 2/3 of lat surface of fibula	Lat side of base of 5th metatarsal bone	Plantarflexion Eversion	Superficial peroneal n. (musculocu-taneous)	Peroneal a.

Muscle	Origin	Insertion	Action	Nerve	Artery
Gastrocnemius	Med head: med condyle & adjacent part of femur; capsule of knee; Long head: lat condyle and adjacent part of femur; capsule of knee	Calcaneus by the calcaneal tendon	Plantarflexion ✓ at knee	Tibial n. (med popliteal)	Popliteal a.
Soleus	Post surface of head & proximal 1/3 of shaft of fibula; mid 1/3 of med border of tibia	Calcaneus by the calcaneal tendon	Plantarflexion	Tibial n. (med popliteal)	Post tibial a.
Plantaris	Lat supracondylar line of femur	Med side of post part of calcaneus	Plantarflexion	Tibial n. (med popliteal)	Post tibial a.
Foot					
Quadratus Plantae	Med head: med surface of calcaneus and med border of long plantar ligament; Lat head: lat border of plantar surface of calcaneus and lat border of long plantar ligament	Attached to tendons of flexor digitorum longus	✓ last IP digits II to V	Lat plantar n.	Lat plantar a.

Muscle	Origin	Insertion	Action	Nerve	Artery
Lumbricals (4)	Tendons of flexor digitorum longus	Tendons of EDL & interossei into bases of last phalanges of digits II to V	✓ MP joints / IP joints	Med plantar n. Deep lat plantar n.	Med plantar a.

Key

✓ flexion
/ extension
↻ rotation
▼ depression, downward, caudal
▲ elevation, upward, cephalic
◆▶ outward, expand
n. = nerve
a. = artery
Lat = lateral
Med = medial
Ext = external
Sup = superior
Ant = anterior

Min = minimal
MTP = metatarsalphalangeal
MCP = metacarpalphalangeal
IP = interphalangeal
PIP = proximal interphalangeal
DIP = distal interphalangeal
Opp = opposite
Abd = abduction
Add = adduction
Mid = middle
Int = internal
Inf = inferior
Post = posterior

Metric System

Linear Measure
10 millimeters = 1 centimeter
10 centimeters = 1 decimeter
10 decimeters = 1 meter
10 meters = 1 dekameter
10 dekameters = 1 hectometer
10 hectometers = 1 kilometer

Liquid Measure
10 milliliters = 1 centiliter
10 centiliters = 1 deciliter
10 deciliters = 1 liter
10 liters = 1 dekaliter
10 dekaliters = 1 hectoliter
10 hectoliters = 1 kiloliter

Square Measure
100 square millimeters = 1 square centimeter
100 square centimeters = 1 square decimeter
100 square decimeters = 1 square meter
100 square meters = 1 square dekameter
100 square dekameters = 1 square hectometer
100 square hectometers = 1 square kilometer

Weights
10 milligrams = 1 centigram
10 centigrams = 1 decigram
10 decigrams = 1 gram
10 grams = 1 dekagram
10 dekagrams = 1 hectogram
10 hectograms = 1 kilogram
100 kilograms = 1 quintal
10 quintals = 1 ton

Cubic Measure

1,000 cubic millimeters = 1 cubic centimeter
1,000 cubic centimeters = 1 cubic decimeter
1,000 cubic decimeters = 1 cubic meter

Weight and Measure Conversions

ENGLISH SYSTEM

Linear Measure
12 inches = 1 foot
3 feet = 1 yard (0.9144 meter)
5.5 yards = 1 rod
40 rods = 1 furlong/220 yards
8 furlongs = 1 statute mile/1760 yards
5280 feet = 1 statute or land mile
3 miles = 1 league
6,076.11549 feet = 1 international nautical mile
(1852 meters)

Dry Measure
2 pints = 1 quart
8 quarts = 1 peck
4 pecks = 1 bushel/2150.42 cubic inches

Angular and Circular Measure
60 seconds = 1 minute
60 minutes = 1 degree
90 degrees = 1 right angle
180 degrees = 1 straight angle
360 degrees = 1 circle

Square Measure
144 square inches = 1 square foot
9 square feet = 1 square yard
30.25 square yards = 1 square rod
160 square rods = 1 acre
640 acres = 1 square mile

Troy Weight
24 grains = 1 pennyweight
20 pennyweights = 1 ounce
12 ounces = 1 pound, Troy

Cubic Measure
1728 cubic inches = 1 cubic foot
27 cubic feet = 1 cubic yard

Liquid Measure
4 gills = 1 pint
2 pints = 1 quart
4 quarts = 1 gallon/231 cubic inches

Avoirdupois Weight
27.34375 grains = 1 dram
16 drams = 1 ounce
16 ounces = 1 pound/0.45359237 kilogram
100 pounds = 1 short hundredweight
20 short hundredweights = 1 short ton

The Metric System

Linear Measure
10 millimeters = 1 centimeter
10 centimeters = 1 decimeter
10 decimeters = 1 meter
10 meters = 1 dekameter
10 dekameters = 1 hectometer
10 hectometers = 1 kilometer

Liquid Measure
10 milliliters = 1 centiliter
10 centiliters = 1 deciliter
10 deciliters = 1 liter
10 liters = 1 dekaliter
10 dekaliters = 1 hectoliter
10 hectoliters = 1 kiloliter

Square Measure
100 square millimeters = 1 square centimeter
100 square centimeters = 1 square decimeter
100 square decimeters = 1 square meter
100 square meters = 1 square dekameter
100 square dekameters = 1 square hectometer
100 square hectometers = 1 square kilometer

Weights
10 milligrams = 1 centigram
10 centigrams = 1 decigram
10 decigrams = 1 gram
10 grams = 1 dekagram
10 dekagrams = 1 hectogram
10 hectograms = 1 kilogram
100 kilograms = 1 quintal
10 quintals = 1 ton

Cubic Measure
1000 cubic millimeters = 1 cubic centimeter
1000 cubic centimeters = 1 cubic decimeter
1000 cubic decimeters = 1 cubic meter

ENGLISH AND METRIC CONVERSION

Linear Measure
1 centimeter = 0.3937 inch
1 inch = 2.54 centimeters
1 foot = 0.3048 meter
1 meter = 39.37 inches/1.0936 yards
1 yard = 0.9144 meter
1 kilometer = 0.621 mile
1 mile = 1.609 kilometers

Square Measure
1 square centimeter = 0.1550 square inch
1 square inch = 6.452 square centimeters
1 square foot = 0.0929 square meter
1 square meter = 1.196 square yards
1 square yard = 0.8361 square meter
1 hectare = 2.47 acres
1 acre = 0.4047 hectare
1 square kilometer = 0.386 square mile
1 square mile = 2.59 square kilometers

Weight Measure
1 gram = 0.03527 ounce
1 ounce = 28.35 grams
1 kilogram = 2.2046 pounds
1 pound = 0.4536 kilogram
1 metric ton = 0.98421 English ton
1 English ton = 1.016 metric tons

Volume Measure
1 cubic centimeter = 0.061 cubic inch
1 cubic inch = 16.39 cubic centimeters
1 cubic foot = 0.0283 cubic meter
1 cubic meter = 1.308 cubic yards
1 cubic yard = 0.7646 cubic meter
1 liter = 1.0567 quarts
1 quart dry = 1.101 liters
1 quart liquid = 0.9463 liter
1 gallon = 3.78541 liters
1 peck = 8.810 liters
1 hecroliter = 2.8375 bushels

Reprinted with permission from Bottomley J. *Quick Reference Dictionary for Physical Therapy.* Thorofare, NJ: SLACK Incorporated; 2000.

Peripheral Nerve Innervations: Upper Extremity

Peripheral Nerve	Sensory Area	Manual Muscle Test (see Figures 1 and 2 for complete list)
Axillary (C5-6)	Upper deltoid area	Deltoid, teres minor
Musculocutaneous (C5-7)	Interior and lateral upper arm	Biceps brachii
Radial (C5-T1)	Posterior arm, dorsum of hand	Triceps, wrist extensors
Ulnar (C7-T1)	Anterior/medial forearm, 4th and 5th fingers	Ulnar flexion, flexor digitorum profundus for last two digits
Median (C6-T1)	Anterior/lateral forearm, palmer thumb, 1st, 2nd finger, half of 3rd finger	Thenar eminence, pronators

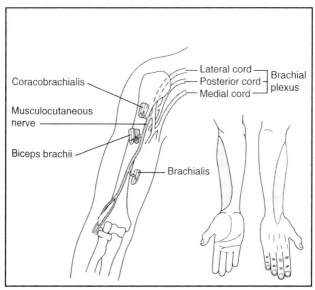

Figure 17-1. Motor and sensory distribution of musculocutaneous nerves. Reprinted with permission from Magee D. *Orthopedic Physical Assessment*. 3rd ed. Philadelphia, Pa: WB Saunders; 1997.

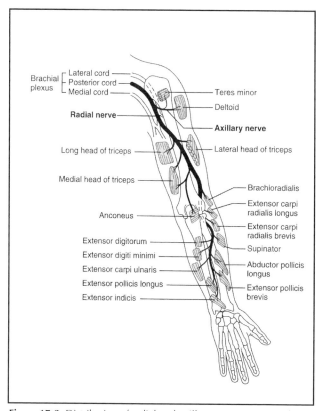

Figure 17-2. Distribution of radial and axillary nerves. Reprinted with permission from Magee D. *Orthopedic Physical Assessment.* 3rd ed. Philadelphia, Pa: WB Saunders; 1997.

Peripheral Nerve Innervations: Lower Extremity

Peripheral Nerve	Sensory Area	Manual Muscle Test (See Figures 1 through 5 for complete list)
Femoral	Medial thigh and leg	Quadriceps
Sciatic	Posterior thigh and leg	Hamstrings
Obturator	Mid anterior thigh	Adductors
Common peroneal	See deep and superficial peroneal	See deep and superficial peroneal
Deep peroneal	Web space between 1st and 2nd toes	Dorsiflexors
Superficial peroneal	Medial dorsal surface of foot	Evertors
Tibial	Posterior leg	Plantar flexors

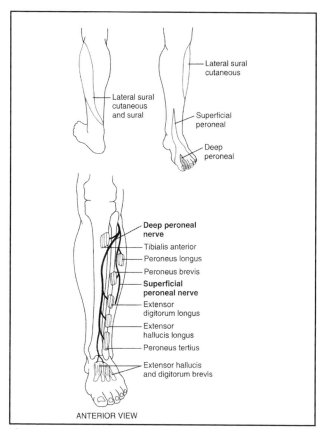

Figure 18-1. Common peroneal nerve. Reprinted with permission from Magee D. *Orthopedic Physical Assessment.* 3rd ed. Philadelphia, Pa: WB Saunders; 1997.

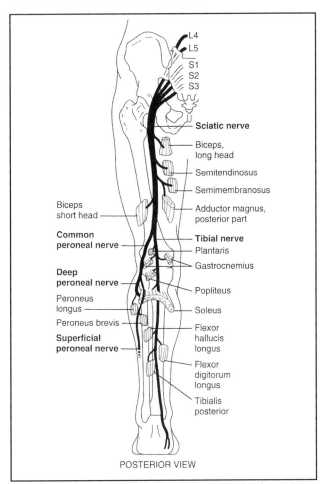

Figure 18-2. Sciatic nerve and its branches. Reprinted with permission from Magee D. *Orthopedic Physical Assessment.* 3rd ed. Philadelphia, Pa: WB Saunders; 1997.

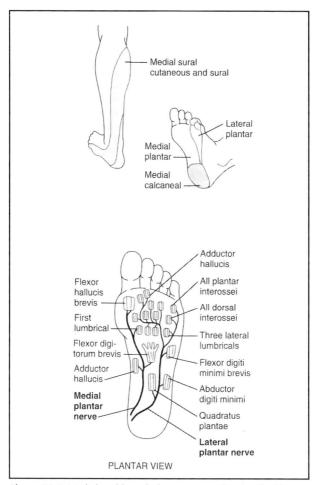

Figure 18-3. Medial and lateral plantar nerves. Reprinted with permission from Magee D. *Orthopedic Physical Assessment.* 3rd ed. Philadelphia, Pa: WB Saunders; 1997.

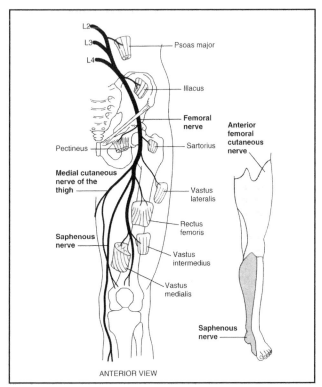

L2
L3
L4

Psoas major

Illacus

Femoral nerve

Pectineus

Sartorius

Medial cutaneous nerve of the thigh

Vastus lateralis

Rectus femoris

Saphenous nerve

Vastus intermedius

Vastus medialis

Anterior femoral cutaneous nerve

Saphenous nerve

ANTERIOR VIEW

Figure 18-4. Femoral nerve. Reprinted with permission from Magee D. *Orthopedic Physical Assessment.* 3rd ed. Philadelphia, Pa: WB Saunders; 1997.

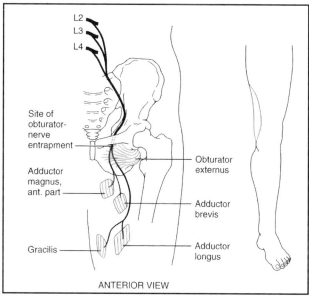

Figure 18-5. Obturator nerve. Reprinted with permission from Magee D. *Orthopedic Physical Assessment.* 3rd ed. Philadelphia, Pa: WB Saunders; 1997.

Diseases, Pathologies, and Syndromes Defined

achlorhydria: A condition resulting in the absence of hydrochloric acid in the gastric juice.

acquired immunodeficiency syndrome (AIDS): AIDS is characterized by progressive destruction of cell-mediated (T cell) immunity (as well as humoral immunity), resulting in susceptibility to opportunistic diseases. It is a syndrome caused by the human immunodeficiency virus that renders immune cells ineffective, permitting opportunistic infections, malignancies, and neurologic diseases to develop; it is transmitted sexually or through exposure to contaminated blood.

acromegaly: A disease that develops after closure of the epiphyses of the long bones affecting the bones of the face, jaw, hands, and feet. Acromegaly (ie, hyperpituitarism) occurs as a result of excessive secretion of growth hormone after normal completion of body growth. It results in increased bone thickness and hypertrophy of the soft tissues due to growth hormone-secreting adenomas of the anterior pituitary gland.

Adams-Stokes syndrome: A condition characterized by sudden attacks of unconsciousness, with or without convulsions. It frequently accompanies heart block.

Addison's disease: A disease characterized by a bronze-like pigmentation of the skin, severe prostration, progressive anemia, low blood pressure, diarrhea, and digestive disturbance. It is due to disease (hypofunction) of the adrenal glands and is usually fatal.

adhesive capsulitis: Also known as *periarthritis* or *frozen joints*, it is characterized by diffuse joint pain and loss of motion in all directions, often with a positive painful arc test and limited joint accessory motions.

adult respiratory distress syndrome (ARDS): ARDS is a group of symptoms that accompany acute respiratory failure following a systemic or pulmonary insult. It is also called *shock lung, wet lung, stiff lung, adult hyaline membrane disease, posttraumatic lung,* or *diffuse alveolar damage (DAD).*

allergy: *See* hypersensitivity disorder.

Alzheimer's disease (AD): Alzheimer's disease is a progressive dementia characterized by a slow decline in memory, language, visuospatial skills, personality, cognition, and motor skills. It is a disabling neurological disorder that may be characterized by memory loss; disorientation; paranoia; hallucinations; violent changes of mood; loss of the ability to read, write, eat, or walk; and, finally, dementia. It usually affects people over the age of 65 and has no known cause or cure.

amyotrophic lateral sclerosis (ALS): ALS is a progressive motor neuron disease in which degeneration and scarring of the motor neurons in the lateral aspect of the spinal cord, brainstem, and cerebral cortex result in progressive weakness and profound limitation of movement. ALS attacks the upper motor neurons of the medulla oblongata and the lower neurons of the spinal cord. It is also called *Lou Gehrig disease.*

anemia: Anemia is a reduction in the oxygen-carrying capacity of the blood owing to an abnormality in the quantity or quality of erythrocytes (RBC). Hemoglobin is < 14 g/dL for men and < 12 g/dL for women. Hematocrit is < 41% for men and < 37% for women.

anencephaly: The most severe form of neural tube defect in which there is no development above the brainstem; absence of the brain.

aneurysm: A condition in which there is an abnormal stretching (dilation) in the wall of an artery, a vein, or the heart. The dilation can weaken to the point of rupture.

ankylosing spondylitis: Ankylosing spondylitis is an inflammatory arthropathy of the axial skeleton, including the sacroiliac joints, apophyseal joints, costovertebral joints, and the intervertebral disk articulations. It results in the dissolution of a vertebrae.

anorexia nervosa: Anorexia nervosa is an eating disorder in which the individual refuses to eat. It is characterized by severe weight loss in the absence of physical cause and attributed to emotions such as anxiety, irritation, anger, and fear. It is characterized by distortion of body image and the fear of becoming fat. The individual does not eat enough to maintain appropriate weight (maintenance of weight 15% below normal for age, height, and body type is indicative of anorexia). It most often occurs in adolescent girls and young women.

anterior cerebral artery syndrome: Infarction in the territory of the anterior cerebral artery is uncommon, but when it occurs, it results in profound abulia, or a delay in verbal and motor response with paraplegia.

anterior cord syndrome: Damage to the anterior and anterolateral aspect of the cord results in bilateral loss of motor function, pain, and temperature sensation due to interruption of the anterior and lateral spinothalamic tracts and corticospinal tract. It is frequently associated with flexion injuries.

anterior inferior cerebellar artery syndrome: A stroke-related syndrome in which the principle symptoms include ipsilateral deafness, facial weakness, vertigo, nausea and vomiting, nystagmus (or rhythmic oscillations of the eye), and ataxia. Horner's syndrome ptosis, miosis (ie, constriction of the pupil), and loss of sweating over the ipsilateral side of the face may also occur. A paresis of lateral gaze may be seen. Pain and temperature sensation are lost on the contralateral side of the body.

anterograde amnesia: A disorder of recent memory in which there is failure of new learning.

anxiety disorder: A generalized emotional state of fear and apprehension that is usually associated with a heightened state of physiologic arousal, such as elevation in heart rate and sweat gland activity.

aortic stenosis: Progressive valvular calcification of the bicuspid valve.

appendicitis: Inflammation of the vermiform appendix that often results in necrosis and perforation with subsequent localized or generalized peritonitis.

Arnold-Hilgartner hemophilic arthropathy: A condition in hemophilic individuals beginning with soft tissue swelling of the joints, osteoporosis, and overgrowth of epiphysis with no erosion or narrowing of cartilage space; leading to subchondral bone cysts, squaring of the patella, significant cartilage space narrowing; and ending in fibrous joint contracture, loss of joint cartilage space, marked enlargement of the epiphyses, and substantial disorganization of the joints.

arrhythmia: Disturbance of heart rate or rhythm caused by an abnormal rate of electrical impulse generation by the sinoatrial (SA) node or the abnormal conduction of impulses. Sinus arrhythmia is an irregularity in rhythm that may be a normal variation or may be caused by an alteration in vagal stimulation. Atrial fibrillation, or involuntary, irregular muscular contractions of the atrial myocardium, is the most common chronic arrhythmia; it occurs in rheumatic heart disease, dilated cardiomyopathy, atrial septal defect, hypertension, mitral valve prolapse, and hypertrophic cardiomyopathy. Ventricular fibrillation, or involuntary contractions of the ventricular muscle, is a frequent cause of cardiac arrest. Heart block is a disorder of the heartbeat caused by an interruption in the passages of impulses through the heart's electrical system. Causes include CAD, hypertension, myocarditis, overdose of cardiac medications (such as digitalis), and aging.

arteriosclerosis (obliterans): Atherosclerosis in which proliferation of the intima has caused complete obliteration of the lumen of the artery. Arteriosclerosis represents a group of diseases characterized by thickening and loss of elasticity of the arterial walls, often referred to as *hardening of the arteries*.

arteritis: A vasculitis primarily involving multiple sites of the temporal and cranial arteries.

arthrogryposis multiplex congenita (AMC): A nonprogressive neuromuscular syndrome in which multiple congenital contractures, either in flexion or extension, are present at birth. There are 3 types of AMC: contracture syndromes, amyoplasia (ie, lack of muscle formation), and distal arthrogryposis, primarily affecting the hands and feet. The child is born with stiff joints and weak muscles.

ascites: An abnormal accumulation of serous (edematous) fluid within the peritoneal cavity, the potential space between the lining of the liver, and the lining of the abdominal cavity. It is most often caused by cirrhosis, but other diseases associated with ascites include heart failure, constrictive pericarditis, abdominal malignancies, nephrotic syndrome, and malnutrition.

asthma: An inflammatory condition of the lungs with secondary bronchospasm marked by recurrent attacks of dyspnea, with wheezing due to the spasmodic constriction of the bronchi.

atelectasis: The collapse of normally expanded and aerated lung tissue at any structural level (eg, lung parenchyma, alveoli, pleura, chest wall, bronchi) involving all or part of the lung.

atherosclerosis: This condition represents a group of diseases characterized by thickening and loss of elasticity of the arterial walls, often referred to as *hardening of the arteries*.

athetoid cerebral palsy (Vogt's syndrome): A type of cerebral palsy characterized by continuous, slow, twisting motions of the upper and lower extremities and facial and trunk musculature.

attention deficit disorder (ADD): Characterized by an inability to focus attention and impulsiveness; often diagnosed in children.

attention deficit hyperactivity disorder (ADHD): Characterized by an inability to focus attention, impulsiveness, and hyperactivity; often diagnosed in children.

autism: Developmental disorder characterized by a severely reduced ability to communicate and emotionally relate to other people; self-absorption.

autoimmune disease: Autoimmune diseases fall into a category of conditions in which the cause involves immune mechanisms directed against self-antigens. The body fails to distinguish self from nonself, causing the immune system to direct immune responses against normal (ie, self) tissue and become self-destructive.

avascular necrosis (AVN): Death of bone and/or cartilaginous tissue as a result of having a poor or absent blood supply (*see also* osteonecrosis).

bacterial infection(s): An infection process in which a bacterial organism establishes a parasitic relationship with its host.

Barlow's syndrome: Mitral valve prolapse. A slight variation in the shape or structure of the mitral valve causes prolapse. This syndrome is also referred to as *floppy valve syndrome* or *click-murmur syndrome*.

basal cell carcinoma: A slow-growing surface epithelial skin tumor originating from undifferentiated basal cells contained in the epidermis. This type of carcinoma rarely metastasizes beyond the skin and does not invade blood or lymph vessels but can cause significant local damage.

basilar artery syndrome: Atheromatous lesions along the basilar trunk resulting in ischemia as a result of occlusion affect the brainstem, including the corticospinal tracts, corticobulbar tracts, medial and superior cerebellar peduncles, spinothalamic tracts, and cranial nerve nuclei. If the basilar artery is occluded, the brainstem symptoms are bilateral. When a branch of the basilar artery is occluded, the symptoms are unilateral, involving sensory and motor aspects of the cranial nerves.

Bell's palsy: Facial paralysis due to a functional disorder of the seventh cranial nerve. A condition in which the facial nerve is unilaterally affected. Etiology is uncertain, although it is suggested that it occurs as an inflammatory response in the auditory canal. Any agent that causes inflammation and swelling creates a compression that initially causes demyelination.

benign prostatic hyperplasia (BPH): An age-related, nonmalignant enlargement of the prostate gland.

biliary cirrhosis: Primary biliary cirrhosis is one type of cirrhosis characterized by chronic, progressive, inflammatory liver disease. Secondary biliary cirrhosis can occur with prolonged, partial, or complete obstruction of the common bile duct or its branches.

boil: A painful nodule, formed in the skin by inflammation of the dermis and subcutaneous tissue, enclosing a central slough or "core;" also called *furuncle*.

botulism: Classified as a bacterial infection, botulism is a rare paralytic disease that has a predilection for the cranial nerves and then progresses caudally and symmetrically to the trunk and extremities. It is often caused by the ingestion of neurotoxins in food that resist gastric digestion and proteolytic enzymes and are readily absorbed into the blood from the proximal small intestine.

brain abscess: Brain abscesses occur when microorganisms reach the brain and cause a local infection.

brainstem syndrome: This syndrome reflects lesions of cranial nerves III through XII at the root, nuclear, or bulbar level. Common symptoms are gaze palsies, a loss of active control of eye movement; nystagmus, involving rhythmic tremor of the eye; and dysarthria, abnormal speech resulting from poor control of the muscles of speech. It is commonly associated with multiple sclerosis.

breast cancer: Breast cancer is the most common malignancy of females in the United States. Most breast carcinomas are adenocarcinomas derived from the glandular epithelium of the terminal duct lobular unit.

bronchiectasis: This is a form of obstructive lung disease that is actually an extreme form of bronchitis. There is chronic dilation of the bronchi and bronchioles that develops when the supporting structures (ie, bronchial walls) are weakened by chronic inflammatory changes associated with secondary infection.

bronchiolitis: Bronchiolitis is a commonly occurring acute, diffuse, and often severe inflammation of the lower airways (bronchioles) caused by a viral infection.

Brown-Séquard's syndrome: A set of symptoms, caused by a primary intraspinal tumor, in which there is nerve root pain followed by motor weakness and wasting of muscle supplied by the nerve. This syndrome involves motor changes of extramedullary lesions beginning with segmental weakness at the lesion site and progressing to damage of half of the spinal cord. There is paralysis of motion on one side of the body and loss of sensation on the other side, depending on the site of the lesion involving one side of the spinal cord.

Buerger's disease: Also called *thromboangiitis obliterans*, this condition is a vasculitis that causes inflammatory lesions of the peripheral blood vessels accompanied by thrombus formation and vasospasm occluding blood vessels. The pathogenesis of Buerger's disease is unknown; however, it is generally considered an inflammatory process.

bulimarexia: An eating disorder in which anorexia nervosa and bulimia nervosa coexist. This is characterized by a period of starving to lose weight, alternating with periods of bingeing and purging.

bulimia nervosa: Bulimia nervosa is a compulsive eating disorder characterized by episodic binge eating (ie, consuming large amounts of food at one time) followed by purging behavior, such as self-induced vomiting, fasting, laxative and diuretic abuse, and excessive exercising.

burns: Injuries that result from direct contact or exposure to any thermal, chemical, electrical, or radiation source. The depth of injury is a function of temperature or source of energy and duration of exposure.

cachexia: A state of ill health, malnutrition, and wasting. It may occur in many chronic diseases, such as Alzheimer's disease; certain malignancies; and advanced pulmonary tuberculosis.

cancer: *Cancer* is a term that refers to a large group of diseases characterized by uncontrolled growth and spread of abnormal cells. Other terms used interchangeably for cancer are *malignant neoplasm, tumor, malignancy,* and *carcinoma.* Cancer in its various forms is a genetic disease characterized by deviations of the normal genetic mechanisms that regulate cell growth.

Caplan's syndrome: A condition associated with pneumoconiosis (*see* pneumoconiosis) and characterized by the presence of rheumatoid nodules in the periphery of the lung.

carbuncle: A circumscribed inflammation of the skin and deeper tissues that terminates in a slough and suppuration or boil. It results in a painful node that is covered by tight, reddened skin and contains pus.

carcinoma: A new growth or malignant tumor enclosing epithelial cells in connective tissue and tending to infiltrate and give rise to metastases. It may affect almost any organ or part of the body and spread by direct extension or through lymphatics or the blood stream.

cardiomyopathy (CM): A group of conditions affecting the heart muscle so that contraction and relaxation of myocardial muscle fibers are impaired.

carpal tunnel syndrome (CTS): Entrapment and compression of the median nerve within the carpal tunnel of the wrist. It is characterized by pain, tingling, numbness, and paresthesia, progressing to muscular weakness in the distribution of the median nerve.

celiac disease: This describes the condition that is a symptom complex including steatorrhea (ie, fat in feces), general malnutrition, abdominal distention, and secondary vitamin deficiencies. The disease is defined by an inability to digest gluten, one of the proteins found in wheat, barley, rye, and oats.

central cord syndrome: A result of damage to the central aspect of the spinal cord, often caused by hyperextension injuries in the cervical region. Characteristically, there is more severe neurologic involvement in the upper extremities than in the lower extremities. Function is typically retained in the thoracic, lumbar, and sacral regions, including the bowel, bladder, and genitals as peripherally located fibers are not affected.

cerebellar syndrome: Cerebellar syndrome deficits are usually symmetrical with all 4 limbs involved. Manifestations of cerebellar lesions are ataxia hypotonia and truncal weakness causing postural and movement disorders. Dysarthria of cerebellar origin (scanning speech, producing a prolonged, monotone sound) is common.

cerebral palsy (CP): A nonhereditary and nonprogressive lesion of the cerebral cortex resulting in a group of neuromuscular disorders of posture and voluntary movement, including lack of voluntary control; spasticity; impaired speech, vision, hearing, and perceptual functions; seizure disorder; hydrocephalus; microcephaly; or mental retardation. Damage to the motor area of the brain occurs during fetal life, birth, or infancy.

cerebral syndrome: Characterized by optic neuritis, the manifestation of demyelination of the optic nerve seen in multiple sclerosis and associated with visual field defects, decreased color vision, and reduced clarity of vision.

cerebrovascular accident (CVA): *See* stroke.

cerebrovascular disease: Intrinsic damage to the vessels of the brain caused by atherosclerosis, lipohyalinosis, inflammation, amyloid deposition, arterial dissection, developmental malformation, aneurysm, or venous thrombosis resulting in a stroke.

Charcot-Marie-Tooth disease: This is a peroneal muscular atrophy that is an inherited autosomal dominant disorder affecting motor and sensory nerves. Initially, the disorder involves the peroneal nerve and affects muscles in the foot and lower leg. It later progresses to the hands and forearms.

childhood disintegrative disorder: Marked regression in multiple areas of functioning following a period of at least 2 years of apparently normal development. The onset of the disorder takes place before the age of 10. Loss of previously acquired skills in at least two of the following areas: expressive or receptive language, social skills or adaptive behavior, bowel or bladder control, play, or motor skills.

cholangitis: Sclerosing cholangitis is an inflammatory disease of the bile ducts that has been linked to altered immunity, toxins, and infectious agents and is thought to be of genetic etiology.

cholecystitis: Inflammation of the gallbladder as a result of impaction of gallstones in the cystic duct causing painful distention of the gall bladder.

choledocholithiasis: Calculi in the common bile duct in persons with gallstones.

cholelithiasis (gallstones): Cholelithiasis is the formation or presence of gallstones that remain in the lumen of the gallbladder or are ejected with bile into the cystic duct.

chondrosarcoma: Chondrosarcoma is a tumor in which the neoplastic cells produce cartilage rather than the osteoid seen with the osteosarcoma.

chronic fatigue syndrome (CFS): CFS is a combination of symptoms hypothesized to be an autoimmune system response to stress. It is associated with severe and prolonged fatigue, low-grade fever, sore throat, painful lymph nodes, muscle weakness, discomfort or myalgia, sleep disturbances, headaches, migratory arthralgias without joint swelling or redness, photophobia, forgetfulness, irritability, confusion, depression, transient visual scotomata, difficulty in thinking, and inability to concentrate.

chronic obstructive bronchitis: This condition is clinically defined as a condition of productive cough lasting for at least 3 months per year for 2 consecutive years. The primary distinction between chronic obstructive bronchitis and chronic obstructive pulmonary disease is the chronic cough.

chronic obstructive pulmonary disease (COPD): Also called *chronic obstructive lung disease*, this condition refers to a number of disorders that affect movement of air in and out of the lungs, particularly within the small airways. There is blockage of air and abnormalities of the lungs, causing an effect on expiratory flow. The most important of these disorders are obstructive bronchitis, emphysema, and asthma.

chronic pain disorder (syndrome): Chronic pain has been recognized as pain that persists part of the normal healing time. Chronic pain is often associated with depressive disorders, whereas acute pain appears to be associated with anxiety disorders.

chronic renal failure (CRF): The loss of nephrons results in progressive deterioration of glomerular filtration, tubular reabsorption, and endocrine functions of the kidneys. This ultimately leads to failure of the kidneys and affects all other body systems.

cirrhosis: Cirrhosis of the liver is a group of chronic end-stage diseases of the liver resulting from a variety of chronic inflammatory, toxic, metabolic, or congestive damage most commonly associated with alcohol abuse.

click-murmur syndrome: *See* Barlow's syndrome or mitral valve prolapse.

cluster headache: Cluster headaches are severe unilateral headaches of relatively short duration. The episodic cluster headache is defined as the period of susceptibility to headache, called *cluster periods*, alternating with periods of remission. *Chronic cluster headache* is a term used when remissions have not occurred for at least 12 months.

coal workers' pneumoconiosis: Lung disease resulting from inhalation of coal dust.

colitis: An irritable bowel syndrome in which there is a suppression of normal gastrointestinal flora, the bacteria normally residing in the lumen of the intestines, allowing yeasts and molds to flourish.

collagen vascular disease: Also called *connective tissue disease*, this condition is associated with pulmonary manifestations, including exudative pleural effusion, pulmonary nodules, rheumatoid nodules, interstitial fibrosis, and pulmonary vasculitis.

congenital heart disease: An anatomic defect in the heart that develops in utero during the first trimester and is present at birth. There are 2 categories: cyanotic defects resulting from obstruction of blood flow to the lungs or mixing of desaturated blue venous blood with fully saturated red arterial blood within the chambers of the heart; and acyanotic defects primarily involving left-to-right shunting of blood through an abnormal opening.

congenital hip dysplasia: Developmental dysplasia of the hip that is unilateral or bilateral and occurs in 3 forms: unstable hip dysplasia in which the hip is positioned normally but can be dislocated by manipulation, subluxation or complete dislocation in which the femoral head remains intact with the acetabulum but the head of the femur is partially displaced or uncovered, and complete dislocation in which the femoral head is totally outside the acetabulum.

congestive heart failure (CHF): A heart condition in which the heart is unable to pump sufficient blood to supply the body's needs. Congestive heart disease represents a group of clinical manifestations caused by inadequate pump performance from either the cardiac valves or the myocardium.

There is excessive or abnormal accumulation of blood (congestion) in the heart. It causes mechanical or functional inadequacy to fully empty the blood from the heart, due to hypertrophic cardiac muscle changes.

connective tissue disease: A rheumatoid disease, such as systemic lupus erythematosus (SLE), scleroderma, or polymyositis (*see* systemic lupus erythematosus (SLE), scleroderma, and polymyositis).

Conn's syndrome: Conn's syndrome, or primary aldosteronism, is a metabolic disorder that occurs when an adrenal lesion results in hypersecretion of aldosterone, the most powerful of the mineralocorticoids (aldosterone's primary role is to conserve sodium, and it also promotes potassium excretion). There is an excess of sodium in the blood (ie, hypernatremia), indicating water loss exceeding sodium loss, and fluid volume excess (ie, hypervolemia), leading to an increase in the volume of circulating fluid or plasma in the body; low blood levels of potassium (ie, hypokalemia), and metabolic alkalosis. All of these factors lead to blood pressure increases.

constipation: A condition in which fecal matter is too hard to pass easily or in which bowel movements are so infrequent that discomfort and other symptoms interfere with activities of daily living.

contact dermatitis: An acute or chronic skin inflammation caused by exposure to a chemical, mechanical, physical, or biological agent.

conversion disorder: A psychodynamic phenomenon rather than a behavioral response to illness or injury defined as a transformation of an emotion into a physical manifestation.

coronary heart (or artery) disease (CAD): Blockage of the coronary arteries of the heart leading to myocardial infarction, arrhythmias, or failure.

cor pulmonale: Also called *pulmonary heart disease* in which there is an enlargement of the right ventricle secondary to pulmonary hypertension that occurs in diseases of the thorax, lung, and pulmonary circulation. It is a term that describes the pathologic effects of lung dysfunction as it affects the right side of the heart. There is hypertrophy or failure of the right ventricle. Heart disease is secondary to disease of the lungs or of the lungs' blood vessels.

corticospinal syndrome: This syndrome involves the corticospinal tract and dorsal column and results in stiffness, slowness, and weakness of the limbs.

Creutzfeldt-Jakob disease: Presenile dementia that is chronic in nature. It is a rapidly dementing disease thought to be activated by a slow virus of genetic predisposition. It results in memory deficits and electroencephalographic changes, and myoclonus is prevalent. Involves the frontal lobe with symptoms of apathy, lack of personal care, and the display of psychomotor retardation. Motor symptoms include incontinence and seizures.

Crohn's disease: Crohn's disease is a chronic lifelong inflammatory disorder of the bowel that can affect any segment of the intestinal tract and even tissues in other organs. It is characterized by exacerbations and periods of remission.

Cushing's syndrome: A metabolic disorder, also referred to as *hypercortisolism* (ie, hyperfunction of the adrenal gland), in which there is increased secretion of cortisol by the adrenal cortex, resulting in liberation of amino acids from muscle tissue with resultant weakening of protein structures.

The end results include a protuberant abdomen with striae ("stretch marks"), poor wound healing, generalized muscle weakness, and marked osteoporosis.

cystic fibrosis (CF): An inherited disease of the exocrine glands affecting the hepatic, digestive, male reproductive (the vas deferens is functionally disrupted in nearly all cases), and respiratory systems. The majority of morbidity and mortality is caused by lung disease and almost all persons develop obstructive lung disease associated with chronic infection that leads to progressive loss of pulmonary function. Cystic fibrosis is a chronic, progressive disorder characterized by abnormal mucous secretion in the glands of the pancreas and lungs. It is usually diagnosed early in life due to frequent respiratory infections or failure to thrive.

cystitis: Lower urinary tract infection.

cystocele: A herniation of the urinary bladder into the vagina.

cytomegalovirus (CMV): A commonly occurring DNA herpes virus infection occurring congenitally, peri- or postnatally, or disseminated in immunocompromised persons. This infection increases in frequency with age.

dactylitis: Painful swelling of the hands or feet that occurs as a result of clot formation. Occurs most often in those individuals affected by sickle cell disease.

degenerative intervertebral disk disease: A degenerative joint process that applies to any synovial joint, including the facet joints, or any intervertebral disk articulation of the spinal column. Events leading to disk degeneration include impaired cellular nutrition, reduced cellular viability, cellular senescence, accumulation of degraded matrix macromolecules, or fatigue failure of the matrix.

dehydration: Removal or loss of water from the body or a tissue; water deficit; severe dehydration may lead to acidosis, accumulation of waste products in the body (ie, uremia), and fatal shock.

dementia: Irrecoverable deteriorative mental state, the common end result of many entities.

depression: A morbid sadness, dejection, or a sense of melancholy, distinguished from grief, which is a normal response to a personal loss.

dermatitis: Infection of the skin. *Eczema* and *dermatitis* are terms that are used interchangeably. A superficial inflammation of the skin due to irritant exposure, allergic sensitization (delayed hypersensitivity), or genetically determined idiopathic factors (eg, eczema, atopic dermatitis, seborrheic dermatitis, etc).

dermatomyositis: Diffuse, inflammatory myopathies that produce symmetrical weakness of striated muscle, primarily the proximal muscles of the shoulder and pelvic girdles, neck, and pharynx. This inflammatory disorder is related to the family of rheumatic diseases and has periods of exacerbations and remissions.

dermatophytoses: Fungal infections, such as ringworm, that are caused by a group of fungi that invade the stratum corneum, hair, and nails. These are superficial infections that live on, not in, the skin and are confined to the dead keratin layers, unable to survive in the deeper layers.

diabetes insipidus: Diabetes insipidus, a rare disorder, involves a physiologic imbalance of water secondary to antidiuretic hormone (ADH) deficiency. Injury or loss of function of the hypothalamus, the neurohypophysial tract, or the posterior pituitary gland can result in diabetes insipidus.

diabetes mellitus (DM): A metabolic disorder in which the pancreas is unable to produce insulin, a substance the body needs to metabolize glucose as an energy source. A chronic, systemic disorder characterized by hyperglycemia (ie, excess glucose in the blood) and disruption of the metabolism of carbohydrates, fats, and proteins. Insufficient insulin is produced in the pancreas, resulting in high blood glucose levels. Over time, DM results in small- and large-vessel vascular complications and neuropathies.

diarrhea: Frequent, watery stools; results in poor absorption of water, nutritive elements, and electrolytes; fluid volume deficit; and acidosis as a result of potassium depletion. Other systemic effects of prolonged diarrhea are dehydration, electrolyte imbalance, and weight loss.

diplopia: Damage to the third cranial nerve, causing double vision.

discitis: A spinal infection affecting the disk, discitis can range from a self-limiting inflammatory process to a pyogenic infection. It may involve the intervertebral disk, vertebral end plates, or both.

discoid lupus erythematosus: A condition marked by chronic skin eruptions that, if left untreated, can lead to scarring and permanent disfigurement. Evidence suggests that this is an autoimmune defect.

disseminated intravascular coagulation (DIC):
Sometimes referred to as *consumption coagulopathy*, it is a thrombotic disease caused by overactivation of the coagulation cascade. It is an acquired disorder of platelet function, with diffuse or widespread coagulation occurring within arterioles and capillaries all over the body.

diverticular disease: *Diverticular disease* is the term used to describe diverticulosis (uncomplicated disease) and diverticulitis (disease complicated by inflammation). *Diverticulosis* refers to the presence of outpouchings (diverticula) in the wall of the colon or small intestine, a condition in which the mucosa and submucosa herniate through the muscular layers of the colon to form outpouchings containing feces.

Down syndrome: A genetic disorder attributed to a chromosomal aberration referred to as *trisomy 21*. Down syndrome is characterized by muscle hypotonia, cognitive delay, abnormal facial features, and other distinctive physical abnormalities. Distinct physical characteristics include a large tongue, poor muscle tone, a flat face, and heart problems.

Duchenne's muscular dystrophy: Progressive fatal disorder of the skeletal muscles beginning in early childhood caused by a hereditary sex-linked gene on the X chromosome.

Dupuytren's contracture: A finger deformity characterized by the formation of a flexion contracture and thickening band of palmar fascia, usually involving the third and fourth digits accompanied by pain and decreased extension. Characterized by progressive fibrosis (increase in fibrous tissue) of the palmar aponeurosis, resulting in the shortening and thickening of the fibrous bands that extend from the aponeurosis to the bases of the phalanges. These fibrous bands pull the digits into such marked flexion at the metacarpophalangeal joints that they cannot be straightened.

dysphagia: Difficulty swallowing. It may be caused by neurologic conditions, local trauma and muscle damage, or mechanical obstruction.

dysplasia: A general diagnostic category that indicates a disorganization of cells in which an adult cell varies from its normal size, shape, or organization.

dystonia: A neurologic syndrome dominated by sustained muscle contractions frequently causing twisting and repetitive movements or abnormal postures often exacerbated by active voluntary movements. Dystonia is both a symptom and the name for a collection of neurologic disorders characterized by these movements and postures.

ectopic pregnancy: A pregnancy marked by the implantation of a fertilized ovum outside the uterine cavity.

eczema: *See* dermatitis.

edema: Excessive accumulation of interstitial fluid (fluid that bathes the cells) that may be localized or generalized.

emphysema: Emphysema is defined as a pathologic accumulation of air in tissues, particularly in the lungs. Distention of tissues is caused by gas or air in the interstices. In chronic pulmonary disease, there is a characteristic increase beyond the normal in the size of air spaces distal to the terminal bronchiole with destructive changes in the alveolar sac walls.

encephalitis: An acute inflammatory disease of the brain caused by direct viral invasion or hypersensitivity initiated by a virus.

encephalocele: Hernia protrusion of brain substance and meninges through a congenital or traumatic opening in the skull.

encephalocystocele: Hernia protrusion of the brain distended by fluid.

enchondroma: A common, benign tumor that arises from residual cartilage in the metaphysis of bone. The hand, femur, and humerus are common sites.

endocarditis: Infective, or bacterial, endocarditis is an infection of the endocardium, the lining inside the heart, including the heart valves.

endometriosis: A condition marked by functioning endometrial tissue found outside the uterus, resulting in ectopic pregnancy.

entrapment syndromes: Entrapment or compression of peripheral nerves resulting from their proximity to bony, muscular, and vascular structures (*see* specific disorders: carpal tunnel syndrome, sciatica, Bell's palsy, tardy ulnar palsy, thoracic outlet syndrome, Saturday night palsy).

ependymoma: A neoplasm derived from the ependymal cell lining of the ventricular system and the central canal of the spinal cord. It is usually reddish, lobulated, and well circumscribed, resembling a cauliflower in shape.

epilepsy: Defined as a chronic disorder of various causes characterized by recurrent seizures due to excessive discharge of cerebral neurons.

Epstein-Barr virus (EBV): Also known as *infectious mononucleosis*, it is an acute infectious disease caused by EBV, a member of the herpes virus group.

Erb's palsy: A paralysis of the upper limb resulting from a traction injury to the brachial plexus at birth. Erb-Duchenne palsy affects the C5 to C6 nerve roots, whole-arm palsy affects C5 to T1, and Klumpke's palsy affects the C8 and T1 (lower plexus) nerve roots.

Ewing's sarcoma: A malignant primary bone tumor. The pelvis and lower extremity are the most common sites. This malignant bone tumor often attacks the shaft of the long bones.

facioscapulohumeral dystrophy: A mild form of muscular dystrophy beginning with weakness and atrophy of the facial muscles and shoulder girdle. The inability to close the eyes may be the earliest sign; the face is expressionless when laughing or crying, forward shoulders and scapular winging develop, and the person has difficulty raising the arms overhead.

factitious disorder: A psychophysiologic disorder characterized by somatic symptom production that is intentional or self-induced for the purpose of gaining attention by deceiving health care personnel or for personal gain.

fecal incontinence: Inability to control bowel movements. Psychological factors include anxiety, confusion, disorientation, and depression. Physiologic causes include neurologic sensory and motor impairment, anal distortion secondary to traumatic childbirth, sexual assault, hemorrhoids, and hemorrhoidal surgery; altered levels of consciousness; and severe diarrhea.

fibromyalgia: Fibromyalgia or fibromyalgia syndrome, often mislabeled or misdiagnosed as fibrocytis, fibromyositis, nonarticular arthritis, myofascial pain, chronic fatigue syndrome, or systemic lupus erythematosus, is a chronic muscle pain syndrome with no known cause and no known cure. Fibromyalgia has been defined as pain that is widespread with multiple tender points.

fibrositis: A term that means inflammation of the fibrous connective tissue, although muscle biopsy studies have failed to demonstrate an inflammatory process.

floppy valve syndrome: *See* mitral valve prolapse.

Friedreich's ataxia: A disease involving neurologic degeneration due to cell loss in the dorsal root ganglia and secondary degeneration in the ascending and descending posterior columns and spinocerebellar tracts. It is primarily a disorder of movement with ataxic gait the most common presenting symptom.

frontal lobe syndrome: Lesions affecting the frontal lobe result in change from the premorbid personality in terms of a person's character and temperament, slowness in processing information, lack of judgment based on known consequences, withdrawal, and irritability. Disinhibition and apathy are common clinical dysfunctions of the frontal lobe. The person may lack insight into the deficits; therefore, behavior can be difficult to control.

fulminant hepatitis: A rare form of hepatitis (occurs in less than 1% of persons with acute viral hepatitis) is defined as hepatic failure with stage III or IV encephalopathy (confusion, stupor, and coma) as a result of massive hepatic necrosis.

furuncle: *See* boil.

furunculosis: Persistent sequential occurrence of boils (furnucles) over a period of weeks of months.

gallstone(s): Gallstones, also called *cholelithiasis*, is the formation or presence of gallstones that remain in the lumen of the gallbladder or are ejected with bile into the cystic duct. Gallstones are stone-like masses called *calculi* (singular: calculus) that form in the gallbladder as a result of changes in the normal components of bile.

gangrene: Death of body tissue usually associated with loss of vascular (nutritive, arterial circulation) supply, and followed by bacterial invasion and putrefaction. The 3 major types of gangrene are dry, moist, and gas. Dry and moist gangrene result from loss of blood circulation due to various causes; gas gangrene occurs in wounds infected by anaerobic bacteria, leading to gas production and tissue breakdown.

gastric adenocarcinoma: A malignant neoplasm arising from the gastric mucosa, it constitutes more than 90% of the malignant tumors of the stomach.

gastritis: Inflammation of the lining of the stomach (gastric mucosa). It is not a single disease but represents a group of the most common stomach disorders.

gastroesophageal reflux disease (GERD): Also called *esophagitis*, it may be defined as an inflammation of the esophagus, which may be the result of reflux (backward flow) of gastric juices, infections, chemical irritants, involvement by systemic diseases, or physical agents, such as radiation and nasogastric intubation.

gigantism: An overgrowth of the long bones resulting from growth hormone-secreting adenomas of the anterior pituitary gland. Gigantism develops in children before the age when epiphyses of the bones close and results in generalized "largeness," with heights often reaching 8 to 9 feet.

gliomas: Primary tumors of the brain, gliomas are the most prevalent and are tumors of the glial cells, the group of cells that support, insulate, and metabolically assist the neurons.

goiter: An enlargement of the thyroid gland that may be the result of lack of iodine, inflammation, or tumors (benign or malignant). Enlargement may also appear in hyperthyroidism, especially Graves' disease.

gout: Gout represents a heterogeneous group of metabolic disorders marked by an elevated level of serum uric acid and the deposition of urate crystals in the joints, soft tissues, and kidneys. Primary gout refers to hyperuricemia in the absence of other disease. Secondary gout refers to hyperuricemia resulting from an antecedent disease.

grand mal seizure: Grand mal or tonic-clonic seizure is the archetypal seizure, which means total loss of control. The seizure begins with a sudden loss of consciousness, generalized rigidity (tonic) followed by jerking movements (clonic), incontinence of bowel and bladder. In the tonic phase, respiration can cease briefly.

Graves' disease: Hyperthyroidism, the excess secretion of thyroid hormone, creates a generalized elevation of body metabolism that is manifested in almost every system. Graves' disease, which increases T4 production, accounts for 85% of hyperthyroidism. The classic symptoms of Graves' disease are mild symmetrical enlargement of the thyroid (goiter), nervousness, heat intolerance, weight loss despite increased appetite, sweating, diarrhea, tremor, and palpitations.

Guillain-Barré syndrome (GBS): Guillain-Barré syndrome, also called *acute inflammatory demyelinating polyradiculoneuropathy* (AIDP), which describes the syndrome, is an immune-mediated disorder. Viral and bacterial infections, surgery, and vaccinations have been associated with AIDP. There is increased sensitivity response in the peripheral nervous system and inflammation of the spinal nerve roots, peripheral nerves, and occasionally the cranial nerves. It also results in rapid paralysis of the limbs, accompanied by sensory loss and muscle atrophy.

Gulf War syndrome: Occurring in individuals who served in the Persian Gulf War, symptoms include fatigue, skin rash, headache, muscle and joint pain, memory loss, shortness of breath, sleep disturbances, diarrhea and other gastrointestinal symptoms, and depression. There is no known cause, but possible causes include chemical or biologic weapons, insecticides, Kuwaiti oil well fires, parasites, pills protecting against nerve gas, and inoculations against petrochemical exposure.

heart block: *See* arrhythmias.

heartburn: A burning sensation in the esophagus usually felt in the midline below the sternum in the region of the heart. It is often a symptom of indigestion and occurs when acidic contents of the stomach move backward or regurgitate into the esophagus. Also called *dyspepsia*, *pyrosis*, or *indigestion*.

hemophilia: A bleeding disorder inherited as a sex-linked autosomal recessive trait in two-thirds of all cases. It is a coagulation (blood-clotting) disorder and caused by an abnormality of plasma-clotting proteins necessary for blood coagulation.

hemorrhoids: Hemorrhoids, or piles, are varicose veins in the perianal region and may be internal or external.

hemostasis: The arrest of bleeding after blood vessel injury involving the interaction between the blood vessel wall, the platelets, and the plasma coagulation proteins. Disorders of hemostasis are caused by defects in platelet number or function or problems in the formation of a blood clot, resulting in a bleeding or clotting disorder.

hemothorax: Blood in the pleural cavity following chest trauma.

hepatic encephalopathy: Also termed *hepatic coma*, it refers to a variety of neurologic signs and symptoms in persons with chronic liver failure or in whom portal circulation is impaired.

hepatitis: An acute or chronic inflammation of the liver caused by a virus, a chemical, a drug reaction, or alcohol abuse.

hernia: An acquired or congenital abnormal protrusion of part of an organ or tissue through the structure normally containing it.

herpes simplex: An acute virus disease marked by groups of watery blisters on the skin; mucous membranes, such as the borders of the lips or the nose; or the mucous surface of the genitals. It often accompanies fever. Also known as *cold sores.*

herpes zoster: Also called *shingles*, it is a local disease brought about by the reactivation of the same virus that causes the systemic disease called *varicella* (chickenpox). The disease is brought on by an immunocompromised state.

hiatal hernia: A hiatal or diaphragmatic hernia occurs when the cardiac (lower esophagus) sphincter becomes enlarged, allowing the stomach to pass through the diaphragm into the thoracic cavity.

hip dysplasia: *See* congenital hip dysplasia.

Hodgkin's disease: A neoplastic disease of lymphoid tissue with the primary histologic finding of giant Reed-Sternberg cells in the lymph nodes. These cells are part of the tissue macrophage system and have twin nuclei and nucleoli that give it the appearance of "owl eyes."

Horner's syndrome: Horner's syndrome includes ptosis (drooping of the upper eyelid), miosis (constriction of the pupil), and loss of sweating over the ipsilateral side of the face following an anterior inferior cerebellar artery stroke.

human immunodeficiency virus (HIV): A retrovirus that predominantly infects human T4 (helper) lymphocytes, the major regulators of the immune response, and destroys or activates them (*see also* acquired immunodeficiency syndrome [AIDS]).

Huntington's disease (HD): A progressive hereditary disease of the basal ganglia characterized by abnormalities of movement, abnormal posture, postural reactions, trunk rotation, distribution of tone, extraneous movements, personality disturbances, and progressive dementia. Often associated with choreic movement, which is brief, purposeless, involuntary, and random. The disease slowly progresses, and death is usually due to an intercurrent infection. Also called *Huntington's chorea*.

hyaline membrane disease: A respiratory disease of unknown cause in newborn infants, especially if premature, characterized by an abnormal membrane of protein lining the alveoli of the lungs.

hydrocephalus: The increased accumulation of cerebrospinal fluid within the ventricles of the brain. Results from interference with normal circulation and with absorption of fluid, and especially, from destruction of the foramina of Magendie and Luschka.

hyperparathyroidism: A metabolic disorder caused by overactivity of one or more of the four parathyroid glands that disrupts calcium, phosphate, and bone metabolism.

hyperpituitarism: An oversecretion of one or more of the hormones secreted by the pituitary gland, especially growth hormone, resulting in gigantism or acromegaly. It is primarily caused by a hormone-secreting pituitary tumor, typically a benign adenoma. Other syndromes associated with hyperpituitarism include Cushing's disease, amenorrhea (absence of the menstrual cycle), and hyperthyroidism.

hypersensitivity disorder: An exaggerated or inappropriate immune response, overreaction to a substance, or hypersensitivity, this disorder is often referred to as an *allergic response*. Although the term *allergy* is widely used, the term *hypersensitivity* is more appropriate. Hypersensitivity designates an increased immune response to the presence of an antigen that results in tissue destruction.

hypertension (HTN): Hypertension, or high blood pressure, is defined by the World Health Organization (WHO) as a persistent elevation of systolic blood pressure above 140 mmHg and of diastolic pressure above 90 mmHg measured on at least two separate occasions at least 2 weeks apart.

hyperthyroidism: An excessive secretion of thyroid hormone. It is sometimes referred to as *thyrotoxicosis*, a term used to describe the clinical manifestations that occur when the body tissues are stimulated by increased thyroid hormone. Excessive thyroid hormone creates a generalized elevation of body metabolism, the effects of which are manifested in almost every system.

hypochondriasis: A marked preoccupation with one's health; exaggeration of normal sensations and minor complaints into a serious illness.

hypoparathyroidism: Hyposecretion, hypofunction, or insufficient secretion of the parathyroid hormone (PTH) results in hypocalcemia, as the parathyroid's primary role is to regulate calcium balance. The most significant clinical consequence is neuromuscular irritability producing tetany.

hypopituitarism: Also called *panhypopituitarism* and *dwarfism*, it results from decreased or absent hormonal secretion by the anterior pituitary gland. It is a generalized condition in which all six of the pituitary's vital hormones (adrenocorticotropic hormone, thyroid-stimulating hormone, luteinizing hormone, follicle-stimulating hormone, human growth factor, and prolactin) are inadequately produced or absent.

hypotension: Decrease of systolic and diastolic blood pressure below normal due to a deficiency in tonus or tension (*see also* orthostatic hypotension).

hypothyroidism: Refers to a deficiency of thyroid hormone that results in a generalized slowed body metabolism. In primary hypothyroidism, the loss of thyroid tissue leads to a decreased production of thyroid hormone, and the thyroid gland responds by enlarging to compensate for the deficiency (*see* goiter). Secondary hypothyroidism is most commonly the result of failure of the pituitary to synthesize adequate amounts of thyroid-stimulating hormone (TSH).

iatrogenic immunodeficiency: A condition induced by immunosuppressive drugs, radiation therapy, or splenectomy in which the immune system is weakened by the intervention.

ichthyosis: A group of skin disorders characterized by dryness, roughness, and scaliness of the skin, resulting in thickening of the skin. It is sometimes referred to as *alligator skin*, *fish skin*, *crocodile skin*, or *porcupine skin*.

immune complex disease: Normally, excessive circulating antigen-antibody complexes called *immune complexes* are effectively cleared by the reticuloendothelial system. When circulating immune complexes successfully deposit in tissue around small blood vessels, they activate the complement cascade and cause acute inflammation and local tissue injury. This results in vasculitis, which can affect skin, causing an allergic reaction; synovial joints, such as in rheumatoid arthritis; kidneys, causing nephritis; the pleura, causing pleuritis; and the pericardium, causing pericarditis.

impotence: Impotence is a general term that expresses a problem with libido, penile erection, ejaculation, or orgasm. The contemporary diagnostic term is erectile dysfunction.

incontinence: Inability to retain urine, semen, or feces through loss of sphincter control (s*ee also* fecal incontinence and urinary incontinence).

infection: A process in which an organism establishes a parasitic relationship with its host. This invasion and multiplication of microorganisms produce signs and symptoms, as well as an immune response.

infectious diseases: Clinical manifestations of infectious disease are many and varied depending upon the etiologic agent (eg, viruses, bacteria, etc) and the system affected (eg, respiratory, central nervous system, gastrointestinal, genitourinary, etc).

Systemic symptoms can include fever and chills, sweating, malaise, and nausea and vomiting. There may be changes in blood composition, such as an increased number of white blood cells (ie, leukocytes).

inflammatory bowel disease (IBD): Refers to 2 inflammatory conditions: Crohn's disease (CD) and ulcerative colitis (UC) (*see* Crohn's disease and ulcerative colitis).

insulin resistance syndrome: A syndrome of insulin resistance that is associated with hypertension, carbohydrate intolerance, abdominal obesity, dyslipidemia, and accelerated atherosclerosis associated with noninsulin dependent diabetes mellitus (NIDDH).

internal carotid artery syndrome: The clinical picture of internal carotid occlusion varies, depending on whether the cause of ischemia is thrombus, embolus, or low flow. The cortex supplied by the middle cerebral territory is most often affected (*see* middle cerebral artery syndrome). Occasionally, the origins of both the anterior (*see* anterior cerebral artery syndrome) and middle cerebral arteries are occluded at the top of the carotid artery. Symptoms consistent with both syndromes result.

intestinal ischemia: Results from embolic occlusions of the visceral branches of the abdominal aorta, generally in people with valvular heart disease, atrial fibrillation, or left ventricular thrombus. Symptoms include acute abdominal cramps or steady epigastric or periumbilical abdominal pain combined with high leukocyte count. It is sometimes called *intestinal angina* as it is the result of atherosclerotic plaque-induced ischemia. Intermittent back pain at the thoracolumbar junction, particularly with exertion, is also a common complaint.

intracerebral hemorrhage: It is bleeding from an arterial source into brain parenchyma (therefore is often referred to as an *interparenchymal hemorrhage*) and is widely regarded as the most deadly of stroke subtypes. It is characterized by spontaneous bleeding in the absence of an identifiable precipitant and usually associated with hypertension and/or aging.

irritable bowel syndrome (IBS): A group of symptoms that represent the most common disorder of the gastrointestinal system. IBS is referred to as *nervous indigestion*, *functional dyspepsia*, *spastic colon*, *nervous colon*, and *irritable colon*, but because of the absence of inflammation, it should not be confused with colitis or other inflammatory diseases of the intestinal tract. IBS is a functional disorder of motility as a response to diet or stress.

ischemic heart disease: Narrowing or blockage of the coronary arteries causing ischemia in the heart muscle supplied by that artery. Infarction may result (*see also* coronary heart [artery] disease).

Kaposi's sarcoma (KS): A malignancy of angiopoietic tissue that presents as a skin lesion. Growth of this tumor is promoted with a suppressed immune system and is an opportunistic infection associated with AIDS. It is characterized by raised, nontender, purplish lesions.

Kawasaki disease: A cardiovascular pathology also known as *mucocutaneous lymph node syndrome*, it is an acute systemic vasculitis that can occur in any ethnic group but seems most prevalent in Asian populations. There is extensive inflammation of the arterioles, venules, and capillaries initially, then progressing to the main coronary arteries and larger veins.

Vessels develop scarring, intimal thickening, calcification, and formation of thrombi. This syndrome is characterized by high fever, swollen lymph nodes in the neck, rashes, irritated eyes and mucous membranes, with damage to the cardiovascular system. *Synonym*: Kawasaki's syndrome.

keratitis: Inflammation of the cornea.

Klebsiella pneumoniae: An organism closely similar to *Aerobacter aerogenes*, but occurring in patients/clients with lobar pneumonia and other infections of the respiratory tract.

Klinefelter's syndrome: Syndrome characterized by the presence of an extra X chromosome in males causing failure to develop secondary sex characteristics, enlarged breasts, poor musculature development, and infertility.

Klippel-Feil syndrome: Condition in which one or more vertebrae are fused together in the neck area, causing shortening of the cervical spine.

Korsakoff's psychosis: A chronic subcortical disorder caused by prolonged vitamin B_1 deficiency, which is usually caused by alcoholism.

kyphoscoliosis: Also called *Scheuermann's disease*, *juvenile kyphosis*, and *vertebral epiphysitis*, it is a condition of anteroposterior curvature of the spine affecting adolescents between the ages of 12 and 16. Growth retardation or vascular disturbance in the vertebral epiphyses are the two most common theories of pathogenesis of this structural deformity. This condition can also develop with advancing age and is associated with osteoporosis, endocrine disorders, Paget's disease, tuberculosis, poor posture, osteochondritis, and disk degeneration.

lacunar syndrome: Lacunar syndrome appears when a stroke (CVA) occurs in the deep areas of the brain and is representative of the area of infarct in which the lacunae are predominant. If the posterior limb of the internal capsule is affected, a pure motor deficit may result; in the anterior limb of the internal capsule, weakness of the face and dysarthria may occur. If the posterior thalamus is affected, there is a pure sensory stroke. When the lacunae occur predominantly in the pons, ataxia, clumsiness, and weakness may be seen.

Laënnec's cirrhosis: Alcoholic cirrhosis (*see* cirrhosis).

Landau-Kleffner syndrome: Acquired epileptic aphasia characterized by an acquired aphasia secondary to epileptic seizures in the absence of other neurological abnormalities.

lateral sclerosis: A rare form of involvement in ALS that results in neuronal loss in the cortex. Signs of corticospinal tract involvement include hyperactivity of tendon reflexes with spasticity causing difficulty in active movement. Weakness and spasticity of specific muscles represent the level and progression of the disease along the corticospinal tracts. There is no muscle atrophy, and fasciculations are not present.

Legg-Calvé-Perthes disease: Also known as *coxa plana* and *osteochondritis deformans juvenilis*, this disease is avascular necrosis of the proximal femoral epiphysis with flattening of the head of the femur caused by vascular interruption and ischemic necrosis (affects boys aged 3 to 12).

legionnaires' disease: An acute respiratory infection, often with pneumonia, caused by bacteria (*Legionella pneumophila*) that may contaminate water or soil. It was named after an outbreak of the illness at an American Legion convention in July 1976.

Lennox-Gastaut syndrome: A syndrome that occurs with epilepsies of infancy and childhood usually between ages 1 and 6 years of age. The most common seizures are atonic-akinetic, resulting in loss of postural tone. Violent falls occur suddenly with immediate recovery and resumption of activity, the attack lasting less than 1 second. Tonic attacks consist of sudden flexion of the head and trunk and consciousness is clouded.

leukemia: A malignant neoplasm of the blood-forming cells, specifically replacement of the bone marrow by a malignant clone (genetically identical cell) of lymphocytic or granulocytic cells. Acute leukemia is an accumulation of neoplastic, immature lymphoid, or myeloid cells in the bone marrow and peripheral blood; tissue invasion by these cells; and associated bone marrow failure. Chronic leukemia is a neoplastic accumulation of mature lymphoid or myeloid elements of the blood that usually progresses more slowly than an acute leukemic process.

leukocytosis: A condition in which there is an increase in number of leukocytes (above $10,000/mm^3$) in the blood, generally caused by the presence of infection. Leukocytosis may occur in response to bacterial infections, inflammation or tissue necrosis, metabolic intoxication, neoplasms, acute hemorrhage, splenectomy, acute appendicitis, pneumonia, intoxication by chemicals, or acute rheumatic fever. It may also occur as a normal protective response to physiologic stressors, such as strenuous exercise; emotional changes; temperature changes; anesthesia; surgery; pregnancy; and some drugs, toxins, and hormones.

leukopenia: A reduction of the number of leukocytes in the blood (below 5000/µL), which is caused by a variety of factors, such as anaphylactic shock and systemic lupus erythematosus, bone marrow failure associated with radiation therapy, dietary deficiencies, and in autoimmune diseases.

limbic lobe syndrome: Central nervous system disorder involving primary emotions (ie, those associated with pain, pleasure, anger, and fear).

lupus erythematosus: A chronic inflammatory disorder of connective tissues. It can result in several forms, including discoid lupus erythematosus (DLE), which affects only the skin, and systemic lupus erythematosus (SLE), which affects multiple organ systems, including the skin, and can be fatal (*see* discoid lupus erythematosus and systemic lupus erythematosus).

Lyme disease: An infectious multisystemic disorder caused by a spiral-shaped form of bacteria. It is carried by a deer tick. Initially, flu-like symptoms accompanied by a rash appear, followed by skin lesions that resemble a raised, red circle with a clear center, called *erythema migrans* or *bull's-eye rash*, often at the site of the tick bite. Within a few days the infection spreads, more lesions erupt, and a migratory, ring-like rash, conjunctivitis, or diffuse urticaria (hives) occur. Malaise and fatigue are constant and symptoms include headache, fever, chills, achiness, and regional lymphadenopathy. Lyme disease can progress to include neurologic abnormalities (meningoencephalitis with peripheral and cranial neuropathy, abnormal skin sensations, insomnia and sleep disorders, memory loss, difficulty concentrating, and hearing loss) and cardiac involvement (fluctuating atrioventricular heart block; irregular, rapid, or slowed heart beat; chest pain; fainting; dizziness; and shortness of breath).

Ultimately, the end stage leads to joint changes characteristic of rheumatoid arthritis.

lymphedema: This is not a disease but a symptom of lymphatic transport malfunction that results in an accumulation of lymphatic and edema fluid. Primary lymphedema is defined as impaired lymphatic flow owing to congenital malformation of the lymphatic vessels. Secondary lymphedema is acquired and most common, resulting from surgical removal of the lymph nodes, fibrosis secondary to radiation, and traumatic injury to the lymphatic system.

malabsorption syndrome: This is a group of disorders (celiac disease, cystic fibrosis, Crohn's disease, chronic pancreatitis, pancreatic carcinoma, pernicious anemia) characterized by reduced intestinal absorption of dietary components and excessive loss of nutrients in the stool.

malignant melanoma: A neoplasm of the skin originating from melanocytes or cells that synthesize the pigment melanin. The melanomas occur most frequently in the skin but can also be found in the oral cavity, esophagus, anal canal, vagina, meninges, or within the eye.

Mallory-Weiss syndrome: A laceration of the lower end of the esophagus associated with bleeding. The most common cause is severe retching and vomiting as a result of alcohol abuse; eating disorders, such as bulimia; or in the case of a viral syndrome.

manic depressive disorder: Also called *bipolar disorder*, it is characterized by cyclical mood swings that often include intense outbursts of high energy and activity, elevated mood, a decreased need for sleep, and a flight of ideas (mania) followed by extreme depression. The cause is a biochemical dysfunction.

Marfan syndrome: A hereditary disorder characterized by abnormalities of the blood circulation and the eyes, abnormally long bones of the limbs, and very mobile joints.

Meniere's disease: A disorder of the labyrinth of the membranous inner ear function that can cause devastating hearing and vestibular symptoms. Deficits are related to volume and pressure changes within closed fluid systems. It leads to progressive loss of hearing, characterized by ringing in the ear, dizziness, nausea, and vomiting.

meningitis: Infection of the cerebrospinal fluid within the cranium and spinal cord; meninges of the brain and spinal cord become inflamed. Early features include fever and headache. The cardinal signs are a stiff and painful neck with pain in the lumbar areas and posterior aspects of the thigh. Meningitis may produce damage to the cerebral cortex, which may affect motor function, sensation, and perception, as well as other areas of the central nervous system. Meningitis is almost always a complication of another infection and can be caused by a wide variety of organisms.

meningocele: Hernial protrusion of the meninges through a defect in the vertebral column; a form of spina bifida consisting of a sac-like cyst of meninges filled with spinal fluid. External protrusion of the meninges due to failure of neural tube closure of the spine.

meningomyelocele: Hernial protrusion of a sac-like cyst of meninges, spinal fluid, and a portion of the spinal cord with its nerves through a defect in the vertebral column.

middle cerebral artery syndrome (MCA): A syndrome related to occlusion of the middle cerebral artery that results in contralateral hemiplegia and hemianesthesia, or loss of movement and sensation on one half of the body. If the dominant hemisphere is affected, global aphasia, or the loss of fluency, ability to name objects, comprehend auditory information, and repeat language, is the result.

migraine: A throbbing, episodic headache that is usually confined to one side of the head. The pain associated with migraine is associated with a change in the vasculature in the brain. The pain appears to come from a complex inflammatory process of the trigeminal and cervical dorsal nerve roots that innervate the cephalic arteries and venous sinuses.

mitral regurgitation (MR): There are many possible causes of MR, but mitral valve prolapse accounts for approximately half of all cases. Regurgitation occurs when the valve does not close properly, causing blood to flow back into the heart chamber.

mitral stenosis (MS): A narrowing or constriction of the mitral valve of the heart that prevents the valve from opening fully. It may be caused by scars or abnormal deposits on the leaflets. It causes obstruction to blood flow so the left atrium must work harder to sustain cardiac output. Because the mitral valve is thickened, it opens early during diastole with a "snap" that is audible on auscultation, then closes slowly with a resultant murmur.

mitral valve prolapse (MVP): Prolapse of the mitral valve occurs when enlarged leaflets bulge backward into the left atrium. It is also called *floppy valve syndrome*, *Barlow's syndrome*, and *click-murmur syndrome*. Mitral valve prolapse appears to be the result of connective tissue abnormalities in the valve leaflets.

mononeuropathy: Injury to a single nerve; commonly a result of trauma.

multiple myeloma: Also called *plasma cell myeloma*, it is a primary malignant neoplasm of plasma cells arising most often in bone marrow. Malignant plasma cells arise from B cells that produce abnormally large amounts of one class of immunoglobulin (usually IgG, occasionally IgA). The abnormal immunoglobulin produced by the malignant transformed plasma cell is called the *M-protein*. Bone pain is the most prominent symptom.

multiple organ dysfunction syndrome: Often the final complication of critical illness. It is the progressive failure of 2 or more organ systems after a serious illness or injury.

multiple sclerosis (MS): A virus-induced autoimmune disease mediated by lymphocytes and macrophages, which are the cells of the immune system that trigger the demyelination of the central nervous system. It is primarily the white matter that is damaged, but lesions of the gray matter have also been found. Characterized by local inflammation, edema, and demyelination, the disease causes a significant decrease in the conduction rate of the axon.

muscle tension headache: Tension headache associated with muscle contraction occurring in response to stress.

muscular dystrophy (MD): A group of inherited, progressive neuromuscular disorders with a genetic origin characterized by ongoing symmetrical muscle wasting without neural or sensory deficits but with increasing weakness, atrophy, deformity, and disability. Paradoxically, the wasted muscles tend to hypertrophy because of connective tissue and fat deposits.

There are 4 types: Duchenne's (pseudohypertrophic), Becker's (benign pseudohypertrophic), facioscapulohumeral (Landouzy-Dejer-ine), and limb-girdle dystrophy.

myalgia: Tenderness or pain in the muscles; often called *muscular rheumatism.*

myasthenia gravis (MG): Chronic progressive autoimmune disorder of striated muscles that leads to weakness in the voluntary muscles, particularly those innervated by the bulbar nucleus. A disorder of neuromuscular transmission characterized by fluctuating weakness and fatigability of skeletal muscle. It is a fundamental defect of the neuromuscular junction in which the number of acetylcholine receptors are decreased and those that remain are flattened, which results in decreased efficiency of neuromuscular transmission.

myelodysplasia: A general term used to describe defective development of any part of the spinal cord but especially of the lower spinal cord levels.

myelomeningocele: Protrusion of the meninges and spinal cord due to failure of neural tube closure.

myocardial infarction (MI): Also known as a *heart attack* or *coronary*, it is the development of ischemia with resultant necrosis of myocardial tissue. Any prolonged obstruction depriving the heart muscle of oxygen can cause an MI.

myocarditis: A relatively uncommon inflammatory condition of the muscular walls of the heart most often the result of bacterial or viral infection.

myofascial pain dysfunction: A condition marked by the presence of tender myofascial trigger points. The trigger point is viewed as more of a clinical entity than a pathologic entity.

myopathy: Involvement of muscle typically reflected by proximal weakness, wasting, and hypotonia without sensory impairment.

myositis: A rare but potentially life-threatening entity characterized by severe pain and inflammation in the affected muscle. Inflammation is the result of a streptococcal infection and is often referred to as *streptococcal myositis*.

neurapraxia: Involves segmental demyelination, which slows or blocks conduction of the action potential at the point of demyelination on a myelinated nerve. Often occurs following nerve compression that induces mild ischemia in nerve fibers.

neuropathy: Any disease of the nerves (s*ee* peripheral neuropathies).

neurotmesis: The complete severance of nerve fiber and its supporting endoneurium, also producing axonal loss in which the connective tissue coverings are disrupted at the site of injury (eg, gunshot or stab wounds or avulsion injuries that disrupt a section of the nerve).

neutropenia: A condition associated with a reduction in circulating neutrophils (less than 2000/mL). This may occur in severe, prolonged infections when production of granulocytes cannot keep up with demand. Neutropenia may also occur in the presence of decreased bone marrow production, such as happens with radiation, chemotherapy, leukemia, and aplastic anemia.

non-insulin-dependent diabetes mellitus (NIDDM): Diabetes associated with obesity through a negative feedback mechanism in which excessive insulin levels decrease the number of insulin receptor sites on adipose cells. The decrease in insulin receptor sites decreases the amount of glucose that can enter cells. This promotes high blood glucose levels.

obesity: A medically defined weight greater than 20% of desirable weight for adults of a given sex, body structure, and height.

orchitis: Inflammation of the testis that can be acute or chronic and associated with epididymitis.

orthostatic hypotension: The term *orthostatic* (postural) *hypotension* signifies a decrease of 20 mmHg or greater in systolic blood pressure or a drop of 10 mmHg or more of both systolic and diastolic arterial blood pressure with a concomitant pulse increase of 15 beats/min or more on standing from a supine or sitting position.

Osgood-Schlatter disease: Also called *osteochondrosis*, it results from fibers of the patellar tendon pulling small bits of immature bone from the tibial tuberosity. Osgood-Schlatter disease is considered a form of tendonitis of the patellar tendon rather than a degenerative disease.

osteoarthritis (OA): A degenerative joint disease that is a slow, progressive degeneration of joint structures due to mechanical stresses, which results in loss of mobility, chronic pain, deformity, and loss of function. Joint degeneration results from periods of inflammation of the joints in response to wear and tear stresses.

osteoblastoma: A benign tumor of the bone similar to osteoid osteoma, only larger, with a tendency to expand.

osteochondroma: The most common primary benign neoplasm of bone.

osteogenesis imperfecta: Autosomal dominant disorder that occurs in one of 30,000 births. It is characterized by increased susceptibility to fractures.

Normal intelligence and possible hearing loss are associated. Sometimes referred to as *brittle bones*, it is a rare congenital disorder of collagen synthesis affecting bones and connective tissue. Clinically, occasional fractures result from brittle bone with growth retardation and long bone deformities.

osteoid osteoma: A benign vascular osteoblastic lesion that is often found in the cortex of long bones, such as the femur, near the end of disphysis. Pathologic study shows areas of immature bone surrounded by prominent osteoblasts and osteoclasts. The lesion is vascular, but no cartilage is present. The tumor can lead to joint pain and dysfunction.

osteomalacia: Softening of bone without loss of bone matrix. It is a generalized bone condition in which insufficient mineralization (deficient bone calcification) of bone matrix results from calcium and/or phosphate deficiency. Sometimes referred to as the adult form of "rickets."

osteomyelitis: An inflammation of bone caused by an infectious organism. Acute osteomyelitis is a rapidly destructive pyogenic infection. Chronic osteomyelitis is a recognized complication of treatment of open fractures.

osteonecrosis: The term *osteonecrosis* refers to the death of bone and bone marrow cellular components in the absence of infection. Avascular necrosis and aseptic necrosis are synonyms for this condition. The femoral head is most commonly affected.

osteopenia: A condition that results in the loss of bone mass, usually in isolated areas. When this condition of demineralization progresses to include the entire skeletal system, it is termed *osteoporosis.*

osteoporosis: A reduction of bone mass per unit of bone volume. Reduction in bone mass associated with loss of bone mineral and matrix occurring when bone resorption is greater than formation; found in sedentary, postmenopausal women or following steroidal therapy.

osteosarcoma: Tumors, with malignant properties, that are usually destructive lesions with abundant sclerosis both from the tumor itself and from reactive bone formation. A characteristic of osteosarcoma is the production of osteoid by malignant, neoplastic cells.

Paget's disease: Paget's disease, or osteitis deformans, is a progressive disorder of abnormal bone remodeling. Initially, excessive bone resorption occurs followed by disorganized and excessive bone formation. The disease is characterized by a greatly accelerated remodeling process in which osteoclastic resorption is massive and osteoblastic bone formation is extensive. As a result, there is an irregular thickening and softening of the bones of the skull, pelvis, and extremities. It rarely occurs in those younger than 50 years of age.

pancreatitis: A potentially serious inflammation of the pancreas that may result in autodigestion of the pancreas by its own enzymes. Acute pancreatitis is thought to result from the "escape" of activated pancreatic enzymes from acinar cells into surrounding tissues. The pathogenesis is unknown, but it may include edema or obstruction of the ampulla of Vater with resultant reflux of bile into pancreatic ducts or direct injury to the acinar cells, which allows leakage of pancreatic enzymes into pancreatic tissue.

paraneoplastic syndromes: Neurologic complications in cancer caused by 3 phenomena: tumor metastases to the brain; endocrine, fluid, and electrolyte abnormalities; and paraneoplastic syndromes. When tumors produce signs and symptoms at a site distant from the tumor or its metastasized sites, these "remote effects" of malignancy are collectively referred to as *paraneoplastic syndromes*. Symptoms include anorexia, malaise, diarrhea, weight loss, and fever (non-specific symptoms); necrotizing vasculitis, Raynaud's disease, arthralgia, neurologic symptoms, nephrotic syndrome, palmar fasciitis and polyarthritis, scleroderma-like changes, enteric bacteria cultured from joints, bone pain, stress fractures, digital necrosis, and subcutaneous nodules.

Parkinson's disease: A chronic progressive disease of the motor component of the central nervous system characterized by rigidity, tremor, and bradykinesia. It is a degenerative disease of the substantia nigra in the basal ganglia. Abnormal functioning in the area of the basal ganglia in the brain is referred to as *parkinsonism*. Parkinson's disease usually affects the elderly population.

pediculosis: An infestation by *Pediculus humanus*, a very common parasite infecting the head, body, and genital area. More commonly referred to as lice.

peptic ulcer disease (PUD): A break in the protective mucosal lining exposing submucosal areas to gastric secretions. The word *peptic* refers to pepsin, a proteolytic enzyme, the principal digestive component of gastric juice, which acts as a catalyst in the chemical breakdown of protein.

pericarditis: Inflammation of the pericardium.

peripheral neuropathies: Trauma, inherited disorders, environmental toxins, and nutritional disorders may affect the myelin (myelinopathy), axon (axonopathy), or cell body of a peripheral nerve, leading to loss of sensation and subsequent loss of muscle function. Symptoms occur related to the affected nerves, or in many conditions, such as diabetic neuropathy, the pattern of loss is distal and in a sock-like or glove-like pattern.

peripheral vascular disease: Diseases affecting the peripheral blood vessels, including inflammatory diseases (eg, polyarteritis, arteritis, allergies, Kawasaki's disease, Buerger's disease), occlusive disorders (eg, arteriosclerosis, thromboangiitis obliterans, arterial thrombosis or embolism), venous disorders (eg, thrombophlebitis, varicose veins, chronic venous insufficiency), and vasomotor dysfunction (eg, Raynaud's disease, reflex sympathetic dystrophy).

peritonitis: Inflammation of the serous membrane lining the walls of the abdominal cavity caused by a number of situations that introduce microorganisms into the peritoneal cavity.

pervasive developmental disorder (PDD): Severe and pervasive impairment in the development of reciprocal social interaction or verbal and nonverbal communication skills, or when stereotyped behavior, interest, and activities are present, but the criteria do not allow to categorize features under autistic, Rett, childhood disintegrative, or Asperger's disorders.

phenylketonuria (PKU): Disorder in which a metabolic error occurs when an enzyme fails to convert phenylalanine to tyrosine, resulting in the accumulation of phenylalanine in the blood, causing mental retardation.

Pick's disease: A rare form of dementia involving the frontal and temporal regions of the cortex. Symptoms include prominent apathy, as well as memory disturbances, increased carelessness, poor personal hygiene, and decreased attention span. Often severe emotional displays of anxiety and agitation accompany this disease of the brain.

pickwickian syndrome: The complex of exogenous obesity, somnolence, hypoventilation, and erythrocytosis. Named after an obese character in a Dickens novel.

pleural effusion: The collection of fluid in the pleural space (between the membrane encasing the lung and the membrane lining the thoracic cavity) where there is normally only a small amount of fluid to prevent friction as the lung expands and deflates.

pleurisy: An inflammation of the pleura caused by infection, injury (eg, rib fracture), or tumor. It is often a complication of pneumonia but can also be secondary to tuberculosis, lung abscesses, influenza, systemic lupus erythematosus, rheumatoid arthritis, or pulmonary infarction.

pneumoconiosis: A group of lung diseases resulting from inhalation of particles of industrial substances, particularly inorganic dusts such as that of iron ore or coal with permanent deposition of substantial amount of such particles in the lung ("dusty lungs"). Common pneumoconiosis include coal worker's pneumoconiosis, silicosis, and asbestosis. Other types of pneumoconiosis include talc, beryllium lung disease, aluminum pneumoconiosis, cadmium's worker's disease, and siderosis (inhalation of iron or other metallic particles).

***Pneumocystis carinii* pneumonia:** A progressive, often fatal pneumonia that represents the most frequently occurring opportunistic infection in persons with AIDS.

pneumonia: An inflammation affecting the parenchyma of the lungs. It can be caused by bacterial, viral, or mycoplasmal infection; inhalation of toxic or caustic chemicals, smoke, dusts, or gases; or aspiration of food, fluids, or vomitus. It often follows influenza.

pneumothorax (Ptx): An accumulation of air or gas in the pleural cavity caused by a defect in the visceral pleura or chest walls. The result is the collapse of the lung on the affected side.

poliomyelitis: Inflammation of the gray matter of the spinal cord resulting in paralysis, atrophy of muscles, and deformities.

polyarteritis nodosa: Refers to a condition consisting of multiple sites of inflammatory and destructive lesions in the arterial system; the lesions are small masses of tissue in the form of nodes or projections (nodosum). The cause is unknown, although hepatitis B is present in 50% of cases, and polyarteritis occurs more commonly among intravenous drug abusers and other groups who have a high prevalence of hepatitis B.

polycythemia vera: Also known as *erythrocytosis*, it is a neoplastic disease of the bone marrow stem cell primarily affecting the erythroid cells, which produce erythrocytes, but causing overproduction of all three hematopoietic cell lines. It is characterized by an excessive number of erythrocytes, leading to an increased concentration of hemoglobin, increased hematocrit (measure of the volume of packed RBCs), and an increased hemoglobin level.

polymyalgia rheumatica: A disorder marked by diffuse pain and stiffness that primarily affects the shoulder and pelvic girdle musculature.

polymyositis: A diffuse, inflammatory myopathy that produces symmetrical weakness of striated muscle, primarily the proximal muscles of the shoulder and pelvic girdle, neck, and pharynx.

polyneuropathy: *See* peripheral neuropathies. Indicates involvement of several peripheral nerves.

polyp: A growth or mass protruding into the intestinal lumen from any area of mucous membrane.

polyradiculitis: Injury that affects several nerve roots and occurs when infections create an inflammatory response.

polyradiculoneuropathy: Inflammatory breakdown of myelin usually associated with motor and sensory deficits (*see* Guillain-Barré syndrome).

polyuria: A cardinal sign of diabetes, polyuria is excessive urination. The pathophysiologic basis is that water is not reabsorbed from renal tubules because of osmotic activity of glucose in the tubules.

portal hypertension: An abnormally high blood pressure in the portal venous system of the liver, occurring commonly in conditions such as cirrhosis, as a result of obstruction of portal blood flow.

posterior cerebral artery syndrome (PCA): When the proximal posterior cerebral artery is occluded, including penetrating branches, the area of the brain that is affected is the subthalamus, medial thalamus, and ipsilateral (same side) cerebral peduncle and midbrain. Signs include thalamic syndrome, including loss of pain and temperature (superficial sensation) and proprioception and touch (deep sensation). This may develop into intractable, searing pain, which can be incapacitating.

posterior cord syndrome: This is an extremely rare syndrome secondary to injury of the spinal cord. Motor function, pain, and light touch sensation are preserved. There is loss of proprioception below the level of the lesion, leading to a wide-based steppage gait.

posterior inferior cerebellar artery syndrome (PICA): Blood supply to the brainstem, medulla, and cerebellum is provided by the vertebral and posterior cerebellar arteries. When infarction occurs in the posterior inferior cerebellar artery, the lateral medulla and the posteroinferior cerebellum are affected, resulting in Wallenberg's syndrome, which is characterized by vertigo, nausea, hoarseness, and dysphagia (difficulty swallowing). Other symptoms include ipsilateral ataxia (ie, uncoordinated movement), ptosis (ie, eyelid droop), and impairment of sensation in the ipsilateral portion of the face and contralateral portion of the torso and limbs.

postpolio syndrome (PPS): Refers to new neuromuscular symptoms that occur decades after recovery from the acute paralytic episode (average postpolio interval is 25 years).

post-traumatic stress disorder (PTSD): Development of characteristic symptoms following exposure to an extreme traumatic stressor involving direct personal experience of an event that involves actual or threatened death or serious injury, or other threat to one's physical integrity; or witnessing an event that involves death, injury, or threat to someone else. Symptoms include intense fear, helplessness, or horror.

Pott's disease: Vertebral tuberculosis (TB).

Prader-Willi syndrome: Characterized by severe obesity; mental retardation; and small hands, feet, and genitalia. In infancy, problems with poor tone, feeding, and body temperature control are common. Over 50% of Prader-Willi children have a deletion of a chromosome.

pressure ulcer: A lesion caused by unrelieved pressure resulting in damage to the underlying tissue. Pressure ulcers usually occur over bony prominences and are graded or staged to classify the degree of tissue damage observed.

primary ciliary dyskinesia (PCD): PCD is an inherited, relatively rare condition associated with an abnormality of cilia, which may affect the lungs, sinuses, and ears. The mainstay of treatment is chest physical therapy. The condition involves recurrent infections of nose, ears, sinuses, and lungs. If untreated, it can lead to bronchiectasis, sinusitis, dextrocardia, and situs inversus.

prostatitis: Inflammation of the prostate gland, which can be acute or chronic and bacterial or nonbacterial.

pseudobulbar palsy: *See* amyotrophic lateral sclerosis (ALS).

psoriasis: A chronic, inherited recurrent inflammatory dermatosis characterized by well-defined erythematous plaques covered with a silvery scale.

psoriatic arthritis: A form of arthritis that differs from rheumatoid arthritis in that it more frequently involves the distal interphalangeal joints, asymmetrical distribution, and the presence of spondyloarthropathy. Joints are less tender, although pain and stiffness are increased by periods of immobility.

pulmonary edema: Also called *pulmonary congestion*, it is an excessive fluid build-up in the lungs, which may accumulate in the interstitial tissue, in the air spaces (alveoli), or in both. Pulmonary edema is a complication of many disease processes.

pulmonary embolism: The lodging of a blood clot in a pulmonary artery with subsequent obstruction of blood supply to the lung parenchyma.

pulmonary fibrosis: An excessive amount of fibrous or connective tissue in the lung, predominantly fibroblasts and small blood vessels, that progressively remove and replace normal tissue. Categorized as a restrictive lung disease.

pulmonary hypertension: High blood pressure in the pulmonary arteries defined as a rise in pulmonary artery pressure of 5 to 10 mmHg above normal (normal is 15 to 18 mmHg).

pyelonephritis: An infectious, inflammatory disease involving the kidney parenchyma and renal pelvis. Typically related to a bacterial infection.

pyloric stenosis: An obstruction at the pyloric sphincter (ie, the sphincter at the distal opening of the stomach into the duodenum).

pyoderma: Any purulent (containing or forming pus) skin disease.

rachischisis: Congenital fissure of the vertebral column; seen in spina bifida.

radiculoneuropathy: Indicates involvement of the nerve root as it emerges from the spinal cord.

Raynaud's disease/phenomenon: Intermittent episodes of small artery or arteriole constriction of the extremities causing temporary pallor and cyanosis of the digits and changes in skin temperature is called *Raynaud's phenomenon*. These episodes occur in response to cold temperature or strong emotions, such as anxiety or excitement. When this condition is a primary vasospastic disorder, it is called *Raynaud's disease*. If the disorder is secondary to another disease or underlying cause, the term *Raynaud's phenomenon* is used.

rectocele: Herniation of the rectum into the vagina.

reflex sympathetic dystrophy (RSD): Differentiation syndrome with autonomic nerve changes. Sympathetic dysfunction of the extremity following trauma, nerve injury, or central nervous system disorder; usually occurs secondary to a preexisting condition. For instance, adhesive capsulitis in the shoulder is often accompanied by vasomotor instability of the hand and known as *reflex sympathetic dystrophy* (formerly known as *shoulder-hand syndrome*). This condition is characterized by severe pain, swelling, and trophic skin changes of the hand (eg, thinning and shininess of the skin with loss of wrinkling, sometimes with increased hair growth). Skin and subcutaneous tissue atrophy and tendon flexion contractures develop.

Reiter's syndrome: One of the most common reactive arthritic conditions. Reactive arthritis is defined as a sterile inflammatory arthropathy distant in time and place from the initial inciting infectious process. Reiter's syndrome usually follows venereal disease or an episode of bacillary dysentery and is associated with typical extra-articular manifestations of arthritis.

renal calculi: Urinary stone disease is a common urinary tract disorder and can result from sex, age, geography, climate, diet, genetics, and environmental factors. Pathologically, there is an increased risk of stone formation due to the urine being supersaturated with calcium, salts, uric acid, magnesium ammonium phosphate, or cystine.

renal cystic disease: A renal cyst is a cavity filled with fluid or renal tubular elements making up a semisolid material. The presence of these cysts can lead to degeneration of renal tissue and obstruction of tubular flow.

renal failure: *See* chronic renal failure.

restrictive lung disease: A major category of pulmonary problems including any condition that limits lung expansion. Pulmonary function tests are characterized by a decrease in lung volume or total lung capacity.

Rett syndrome: Disorder characterized by the development of multiple specific deficits following a period of normal functioning at birth. There is a loss of previously acquired purposeful hand skills between ages 5 and 30 months, with the subsequent development of characteristic stereotyped hand movements resembling hand wringing or hand washing. Problems develop in the coordination of gait or trunk movements. There is also severe impairment in expressive and receptive language development, with severe psychomotor retardation.

Reye's syndrome: Illness that occurs following a viral infection. It is characterized by vomiting and brain dysfunction, such as disorientation, lethargy, and personality disorder, and may progress into coma. It usually affects children and teenagers.

rheumatic fever: One form of endocarditis (ie, infection of the heart) caused by streptococcal group A bacteria. It can be fatal or may lead to rheumatic heart disease, a chronic condition caused by scarring and deformity of the heart valves. It is called rheumatic fever because the 2 most common symptoms are fever and joint pain.

rheumatoid arthritis (RA): A chronic, systemic inflammatory disease of the joints. Chronic polyarthritis perpetuates a gradual destruction of joint tissues and can result in severe deformity and disability. Pathologically, the indicator of rheumatoid arthritis is a positive rheumatoid factor (antibodies that react with immunoglobulin antibodies found in the blood and in the synovium). Interaction between rheumatoid factor and the immunoglobulin triggers events that initiate an inflammatory reaction. It typically involves the joints of the fingers, hands, wrists, and ankles. Often the hips, knees, and shoulders are severely affected. As a systemic disease, it can affect the juncture at any articulation (eg, ribs to vertebrae, scapula to clavicle). The joints are affected symmetrically, and there is a considerable range of severity.

rickets: Condition affecting children characterized by soft and deformed bones resulting from inadequate calcium metabolism due to vitamin D deficiency.

right hemisphere syndrome: This syndrome, following a stroke, represents the inability to orient the body within external space and generate the appropriate motor responses. Hemineglect is a common feature of right hemisphere involvement. The individual does not respond to sensory stimuli on the left side.

sarcoidosis: A systemic disease of unknown origin involving any organ. Sarcoidosis is characterized by granulomatous inflammation present diffusely throughout the body. The lungs and lymph nodes are most commonly affected. Secondary sites include skin, eyes, liver, spleen, heart, and small bones in the hands and feet. Symptoms include dyspnea, cough, fever, malaise, weight loss, skin lesions, and erythema nodosum (multiple, tender, nonulcerating nodules).

sarcoma: Refers to a malignant tumor of mesenchymal origin.

Saturday night palsy: This is a radial nerve compression at the spiral groove of the humerus. Compression of the nerve causes segmental demyelination. Paralysis of upper extremity musculature and sensory loss is associated with the level of compression. It is also referred to as *crutch palsy*.

scabies: This is a skin eruption caused by a mite, *Sarcoptes scabiei*. The mite burrows into the skin and deposits eggs, which hatch, causing the skin eruption.

scapuloperoneal muscular dystrophy: This is a variation of facioscapulohumeral dystrophy (*see* muscular dystrophy) with involvement of the distal muscles of the lower extremities instead of the face and proximal muscles of the shoulder girdle.

Scheuermann's disease: *See* kyphoscoliosis.

sciatica: Radiculopathy in which the nerve root of the sciatic nerve is affected, most typically caused by compression. It results in low back pain with potential radiation down the back of the lower extremity consistent with the innervation of the sciatic nerve.

scleroderma: Systemic sclerosis (SS), or scleroderma, is an autoimmune disease of connective tissue characterized by excessive collagen deposition in the skin and internal organs.

scoliosis: An abnormal lateral curvature of the spine. The curvature of the spine may be to the right (more common in thoracic curves) or left (more common in lumbar curves). Rotation of the vertebral column around its axis occurs and may cause rib cage deformity. Scoliosis is often associated with kyphosis and lordosis.

septic arthritis: Osteomyelitis is one type of infection that is capable of extending into a joint and causing infection (ie, sepsis). Bacteria, viruses, and fungi can also affect the joints. Infection in the joint causes erosion of the joint capsule, leading to arthritic changes in the septic joint.

shoulder-hand syndrome: *See* reflex sympathetic dystrophy.

sickle cell anemia: A hereditary, chronic form of hemolytic anemia in which the rupture of erythrocytes (forming sickle cells) releases hemoglobin prematurely into the plasma, thereby reducing the delivery of oxygen to tissues.

sick sinus syndrome: Also called *brady-tachy syndrome*, it is a complex cardiac arrhythmia associated with coronary artery disease or drug therapy (eg, digitalis, calcium channel blockers, ß-blockers, antiarrhythmics). Sick sinus syndrome as a result of degeneration of conductive tissue necessary to maintain normal heart rhythm occurs most often among the elderly.

sleep apnea syndrome: Defined as episodes of cessation of breathing occurring at the transition from nonrapid eye movement (NREM) to rapid eye movement (REM) sleep, with repeated wakening and excessive daytime sleepiness.

somatoform disorder: The presence of physical symptoms that suggest a medical condition causing significant impairment in social, occupational, or other areas of functioning. The physical symptoms associated with somatoform disorders are not intentional or under voluntary control. It is a psychophysiologic disorder in which emotional problems or conflicts may develop physical symptoms as a means of coping.

spina bifida: Congenital malformation of the spine in which the walls of the spinal canal do not develop typically due to the lack of union between vertebrae; the degree of impairment depends on the location of the malformation. A term used to describe various forms of myelodysplasia. A defective closure of the bony encasement of the spinal cord (ie, the bony vertebral column is divided into two parts through which the spinal cord and meninges may or may not protrude). If the anomaly is not visible, the condition is called *spina bifida occulta*. If there is an external protrusion of the saclike structure, it is called *spina bifida cystica*, which is further classified according to the extent of involvement (eg, meningocele, meningomyelocele, or myelome-ningocele).

spinal cord injury (SCI): Injury to the spinal cord that results in temporary or permanent paralysis of the muscles of the limbs and the autonomic nervous system. SCI is categorized into traumatic and nontraumatic injuries. Traumatic injury is the most common and is due to a concussion, contusion, or laceration. The spinal cord is violently displaced or compressed. A concussion is an injury caused by a blow or violent shaking and results in temporary loss of function.

Contusions are bruises with hemorrhage beneath the unbroken skin often associated with fractured bone segments striking the spinal cord. Laceration (ie, disruption of tissue) results from complete transection of the cord. Nontraumatic SCI is the result of tumors, infection, or bony changes in the spinal column.

spinal muscular atrophy: Also known as *Werdnig-Hoffmann disease*, it is a progressive infantile spinal muscular atrophy, and floppy infant syndrome. It is characterized by progressive weakness and wasting of muscles and is the second most common fatal autosomal recessive disorder after cystic fibrosis.

splenomegaly: The spleen's involvement in the lymphopoietic and mononuclear phagocyte systems predisposes it to multiple conditions, causing splenomegaly. The spleen becomes enlarged by an increase in the number of cellular elements, by the deposition of extracellular material, or in the presence of extracellular hemopoiesis that accompanies reactive bone marrow disorders and neoplasm.

spondylitis: *See* ankylosing spondylitis.

squamous cell carcinoma: The second most common skin cancer usually arising in sun-damaged skin, such as the rim of the ear, face, lips and mouth, and the dorsa of the hands.

staphylococcal infection: *Staphylococcus aureus* is one of the most common bacterial pathogens normally residing on the skin and easily inoculated into deeper tissues where it causes suppurative (pus formation) infections. "Staph" infections are associated with bacteremia, pneumonia, enterocolitis, osteomyelitis, food poisoning, and skin infections.

Still's disease: A form of juvenile rheumatoid arthritis characterized by systemic manifestations, including fever and rash. The rash typically appears on the trunk and extremities, leaving palms and soles unaffected. Inflammatory arthritis typically develops at some point.

streptococcal infection: *Streptococcus pyogenes* is one of the most frequent bacterial pathogens of humans and causes many diseases of diverse organ systems ranging from skin infections, to acute pharyngitis, to major-illnesses such as rheumatic fever, scarlet fever, pneumococcal pneumonia, otitis media, meningitis, and endocarditis.

stroke: Stroke, or cerebrovascular accident (CVA), is the result of thrombosis and/or embolic occlusion of a major artery in the brain, causing ischemia and death of brain tissue. An array of neurologic syndromes can result dependent on the artery occluded and the area of the brain affected (s*ee* middle cerebral artery syndrome, anterior cerebral artery syndrome, internal artery syndrome, posterior cerebral artery syndrome, vertebral and posterior inferior cerebellar artery syndrome, basilar artery syndrome, superior cerebellar artery syndrome, anterior inferior cerebellar artery syndrome, and lacunar syndrome). These syndromes reflect the dysfunction associated with disruption of blood flow in specific areas of the brain. The syndromes are named according to the arteries that feed the specific area.

substance abuse: Defined as the excessive use of mood-affecting chemicals that are a potential or real threat to either physical or mental health.

sudden infant death syndrome (SIDS): Rare form of death in infants ages 2 to 6 months in which the child dies mysteriously without cause.

superior cerebellar artery syndrome: Occlusion of the superior cerebellar artery results in severe ipsilateral cerebellar ataxia, nausea and vomiting, and dysarthria, which is a slurring of speech. Loss of pain and temperature in the contralateral extremities, torso, and face occurs. Dysmetria, characterized by the inability to place an extremity at a precise point in space, affects the ipsilateral upper extremity.

systemic lupus erythematosus (SLE): Sometimes referred to as *lupus*, it is a chronic inflammatory autoimmune disorder. The cause of SLE remains unknown, but evidence points to interrelated immunologic, environmental, hormonal, and genetic factors. The central immunologic disturbance is autoantibody production, which destroy the body's normal cells. Arthralgias and arthritis constitute the most common presenting manifestations.

systemic sclerosis: A diffuse connective tissue disease that causes fibrosis of the skin, joints, blood vessels, and internal organs. It is an autoimmune disorder (*see also* scleroderma).

Tay-Sachs disease: Genetic progressive disorder of the nervous system that causes profound mental retardation, deafness, blindness, paralysis, and seizures; life expectancy is 5 years.

temporal lobe syndrome: Temporal lobe syndrome involves the primary emotions (ie, those associated with pain, pleasure, anger, and fear). In this syndrome these emotions are amplified.

tendonitis: Inflammation of any tendon.

tenosynovitis: A rheumatologic condition found most often in diabetics. The is caused by accumulation of fibrous tissue in the tendon sheath and can cause aching, nodularity along the tendons, and contracture. It is most frequently associated with the flexor tendons.

thalassemia: A group of inherited chronic hemolytic anemias predominantly affecting people of Mediterranean or southern Chinese ancestry (thalassa means "sea," referring to early cases of sickle cell disease reported around the Mediterranean). Thalassemia is a sickle cell trait with clinical manifestations inclusive of defective synthesis of hemoglobin, structurally impaired RBCs, and shortened life span of erythrocytes.

thoracic outlet syndrome (TOS): A nerve entrapment syndrome caused by pressure from structures in the thoracic outlet on fibers of the brachial plexus; in addition, vascular symptoms can occur because of pressure on the subclavian artery. Chronic compression of nerves and arteries between the clavicle and first rib or impinging musculature results in edema and ischemia in the nerves. It initially creates a neurapraxia and segmental demyelination of the nerve.

thromboangiitis obliterans: *See* Buerger's disease.

thrombocytopenia: A decrease in the platelet count below $150,000/mm^3$ of blood caused by inadequate platelet production from the bone marrow, increased platelet destruction outside the bone marrow, or splenic sequestration.

Thrombocytopenia is a common complication of leukemia or metastatic cancer (bone marrow infiltration) and aggressive cancer chemotherapy (cytotoxic agents). Presenting symptoms are aplastic anemia and primary bleeding sites in the bone marrow and spleen and secondary bleeding occurring from small blood vessels in the skin, mucosa, and brain. Other symptoms include petechiae and/or purpura in the skin and mucosa, easy bruising, epistaxis, melena, hematuria, excessive menstrual bleeding, and gingival bleeding.

thrombocytosis: An increase in the number of circulating platelets greater than $400,000/\text{mm}^3$. Overproduction of platelets is associated with conditions such as chronic nonlymphoblastic leukemia, polycythemia vera, and myelofibrosis (replacement of hematopoietic bone marrow with fibrous tissue). Blood viscosity is increased, leading to an increased risk of thrombosis or emboli.

thrombophlebitis: A partial or complete occlusion of a vein by a thrombus (clot) with secondary inflammatory reaction in the wall of the vein. It may affect the deep superficial veins.

torticollis: Torticollis means "twisted neck" and is a contracted state of the sternocleidomastoid muscle producing a bending of the head to the affected side with rotation of the chin to the opposite side.

traumatic brain injury (TBI): A closed head injury occurring when the soft tissue of the brain is forced into contact with the hard, bony, outer covering of the brain, the skull. The long-term effects associated with closed head injury vary, depending on the severity of the injury. A mild head injury occurs when there is no skull fracture or laceration of the brain. There is an altered state of consciousness though loss of consciousness does not always occur.

Usually, neurologic examination is normal, though postconcussive syndrome may develop, which severely limits an individual's ability to perform activities of daily living. Severe head injuries result from significant bruising and bleeding within the brain. Permanent disability cognitively and physically is often the consequence.

traumatic spinal cord injury: *See* spinal cord injury.

tricuspid atresia: A congenital heart disease in which there is a failure of the tricuspid valve to develop with a lack of communication from the right atrium to the right ventricle. Blood flows through an atrial septal defect or a patent ductus ovale to the left side of the heart and through a ventricular septal defect to the right ventricle and out to the lungs. There is complete mixing of unoxygenated and oxygenated blood in the left side of the heart, resulting in systemic desaturation and varying amounts of pulmonary obstruction.

tricuspid stenosis: Tricuspid stenosis occurs in people with severe mitral valve disease (usually rheumatic in origin) and is rare. A secondary complication is tricuspid regurgitation, which is associated with carcinoid syndrome, SLE, infective endocarditis, and in the presence of mitral valve disease. Surgical repair is more common than valvular replacement.

tuberculosis (TB): Respiratory disease caused by the tubercle bacilli. Formerly known as *consumption*, TB is an infectious, inflammatory systemic disease that affects the lungs and may disseminate to involve lymph nodes and other organs. It is caused by infection with *Mycobacterium tuberculosis* and is characterized by granulomas, caseous (resembling cheese) necrosis, and subsequent cavity formation.

Turner's syndrome: Absence of an X chromosome in females, resulting in lower amounts of estrogen and tendencies to be shorter in height, have fertility problems, and mild mental retardation or learning difficulties.

ulcerative colitis: An inflammatory intestinal tract disease with prominent erythema and ulceration affecting the colon and rectum. Inflammation and ulceration affect mucosal and submucosal layers. It is associated with mild to severe abdominal pain; chronic, severe diarrhea; bloody stools; mild to moderate anorexia; and mild to moderate joint pain.

urinary incontinence: The involuntary loss of urine that is sufficient to be a social and/or hygiene problem. There are 5 categories of urinary incontinence: stress incontinence is the loss of urine during activities that increase the intra-abdominal pressure, such as coughing, laughing, lifting; urge incontinence is the uncontrolled loss of urine that is preceded by an unexpected, strong urge to void; mixed or total incontinence is a combination of stress and urge incontinence; overflow incontinence is the uncontrolled loss of urine when intravesicular pressure exceeds outlet resistance, usually the result of a obstruction (eg, tumor) or neurologic symptoms; and functional incontinence, which is the functional inability to get to the bathroom or manage the clothing required to go to the bathroom.

urinary tract infection (UTI): An example of urinary tract infection affecting the lower urinary tract (ie, ureter, bladder, urethra) is cystitis. An example of urinary tract infection involving the upper urinary tract (ie, kidneys) is pyelonephritis (*see* pyelonephritis).

Elderly individuals have a higher risk for this due to inactivity or immobility, which causes impaired bladder emptying; bladder ischemia resulting from urine retention; urinary overflow obstruction from renal calculi and prostatic hyperplasia; senile vaginitis; constipation; and diminished bactericidal activity of prostatic secretions. UTI is a bacterial infection with a bacteria count of greater than 100,000 organisms per mL of urine.

urticaria: An eruption of itching wheals (hives); a vascular reaction of the skin with the appearance of slightly elevated patches that are redder or paler than the surrounding skin.

uterine prolapse: The bulging of the uterus into the vagina.

varicose veins: Abnormal dilation of veins, usually the saphenous veins of the lower extremities, leading to tortuosity (twisting and turning) of the vessel, incompetence of the valves, and propensity to thrombosis.

vertebral cerebellar artery syndrome: Blood supply to the brainstem, medulla, and cerebellum is provided by the vertebral and posterior cerebellar arteries. An occlusion of the vertebral artery leading to a medial medullary infarction of the pyramid can result in contralateral hemiparesis of the arm and leg, sparing the face. If the medial lemniscus and the hypoglossal nerve fibers are involved, loss of joint position sense and ipsilateral tongue weakness can occur. The edema associated with cerebellar infarction can cause sudden respiratory arrest due to raised intracranial pressure in the posterior fossa. Gait unsteadiness, dizziness, nausea, and vomiting may be the only early symptoms.

vestibular dysfunction: Lesions of the vestibular system that cause dizziness, lightheadedness, disequilibrium, nystagmus (rhythmic eye movements), abnormalities of saccadic eye movements (fast eye movements), oscillopsia (illusion of environmental movement), and diminished vestibulospinal reflexes. Lesions of the vestibular system can be broadly categorized into 5 anatomic sites: the vestibular end organ and vestibular nerve terminals, the vestibular ganglia and nerve within the internal auditory canal, the cerebellopontine angle, the brainstem and cerebellum, and the vestibular projections to the cerebral cortex. The causes are varied and include bacterial infection, viral infection, vascular disease, neoplasia, trauma, metabolic disorders, and toxic drugs.

Vogt's disease: *See* athetoid cerebral palsy.

von Recklinghausen's disease: Multiple neurofibromata of nerve sheaths that occur along peripheral nerves and on spinal and cranial nerve roots. The area over the tumor may be hyperpigmented. Symptoms may be completely absent or may be those of pain due to pressure on spinal cord and nerves.

Wallenberg's syndrome: *See* posterior inferior cerebellar artery syndrome.

wallerian degeneration: Anterograde (distal) degeneration of the axon (unlike segmental demyelination which leaves the axon intact as myelin breaks down).

Weber's syndrome: When a third cranial nerve palsy occurs with contralateral hemiplegia. Paralysis of oculomotor nerve on one side with contralateral spastic hemiplegia is referred to as *Weber's paralysis*.

Wernicke's aphasia: Infarct to a specific area of the brain that severely affects the person's level of comprehension. The person is able to visualize but is frequently nonfunctional. Usually involves a vitamin deficiency of vitamin B_1 and vitamin B_{12}.

Williams syndrome: Syndrome caused by a genetic defect, characterized by cardiovascular problems, high blood calcium levels, mental retardation, developmental delays, and a "little pixie face" with puffy eyes and a turned-up nose.

Wilms' tumor: Wilms' tumor is a nephroblastoma and is the most common malignant neoplasm in children. The tumor appears to be fleshy but may have areas of necrosis that lead to cavity formation. The most common presenting feature is a large abdominal mass and abdominal pain. Hematuria may occur, as well as hypertension, anorexia, nausea, and vomiting.

Wilson's disease: Also known as *hepatolenticular degeneration*, it is a progressive disease inherited as an autosomal recessive trait that produces a defect in the metabolism of copper, with accumulation of copper in the liver, brain, kidney, cornea, and other tissues. The disease is characterized by the presence of Kayser-Fleischer rings around the iris of the eye (from copper deposition), cirrhosis of the liver, and degenerative changes in the brain, particularly the basal ganglia.

xeroderma: A mild form of ichthyosis; excessive dryness of the skin.

REFERENCES

American Physical Therapy Association. Guide to physical therapy practice. *J Am Phys Assoc.* 1997;77(11).

Bottomley JM, Lewis CB. *Geriatric Rehabilitation: A Clinical Approach.* 2nd ed. Upper Saddle River, NJ: Prentice Hall Publishers; 2003.

Goodman CC, Boissonnault WG. *Pathology: Implications for the Physical Therapist.* Philadelphia, Pa: WB Saunders; 1998.

International Classification of Diseases: Clinical Modification. 9th rev. New York, NY: World Health Organization; 1997.

Tan JC. *Physical Medicine and Rehabilitation: Diagnostics, Therapeutics, and Basic Problems.* St. Louis, Mo: Mosby-Year Book; 1998.

Thomas CL. *Taber's Cyclopedic Medical Dictionary.* 18th ed. Philadelphia, Pa: FA Davis; 1997.

Licensure by State

For a list of licensed and unlicensed states consult any *Massage Magazine*. For additional state licensing information consult www.massageregister.com.

State, local, and national legislation can affect the scope of practice of a massage therapist. It is the massage therapist's responsibility to know of those legislative madates.

UNITED STATES MASSAGE THERAPY LICENSURE

Alabama   Massage Therapist License
334-269-9990 x7
Alabama Licensing Board
610 S. McDonough St.
Montgomery, AL 36104
www.almtbd.state.al.us

Alaska   Unlicensed
Consult with: www.amtamassage.org
www.abmp.com

Arizona   Massage Therapist License
602-542-8604
Massage Therapy Board
1400 W. Washington Room 230
Phoenix, AZ 85007
info@massageboard.gov
www.massageboard.az.gov

Arkansas	Massage Therapist License
	501-623-0444
	Master Massage Therapist
	State Board of Massage Therapy
	103 Airways
	PO Box 20739
	Hot Springs, AR 71903
	www.state.ar.us/directory
California	Regulated by city or county
	Consult with: www.amtamassage.org
	www.abmp.com
Colorado	Unlicensed
	Consult with: www.amtamassage.org
	www.abmp.com
Connecticut	Massage Therapist License
	860-509-7570
	State of Connecticut
	Dept. of Public Health
	410 Capital Ave. MS12MQA
	Hartford, CT 06134-0308
	www.ct-clic.com/ detail.asp?code =1730
Delaware	Massage/Bodywork Therapist License
	302-739-4522 x205
	Certified TechnicianCertification
	Division of Professional Regulation
	861 Silver Lake Blvd., Suite 203
	Dover, DE 19904
	www.professionallicensing.state. de.us

Florida	Massage Therapist License 850-488-0595 Ext. 3 Florida Dept. of Health Division of Medical Quality Assurance Board of Massage Therapy 4052 Bald Cypress Way - BIN # C06 Tallahassee, FL 32399-3259 www.doh.state.fl.us/mqa/ massage/ma_consumer.html
Georgia	Unlicensed Consult with: www.amtamassage.org www.abmp.com
Hawaii	Massage Therapist License/ Massage Apprentice Permit 808-586-3000 Dept. of Commerce & Consumer Affairs State Board of Massage PO Box 3469 1010 Richards Street Honolulu, HI 96801 www.hawaii.gov/dcca/pvl/ areas_massage.html
Idaho	Unlicensed Consult with: www.amtamassage.org www.abmp.com

Illinois	Massage Therapist License
	Licensure begins on Jan. 1, 2005
	217-782-8556
	Illinois Dept. of Professional
	Regulation
	320 West Washington St., 3rd Floor
	Springfield, IL 62786
	www.ildpr.com/who/masst.asp
Indiana	Unlicensed
	Consult with: www.amtamassage.org
	www.abmp.com
Iowa	Massage Therapist License
	515-281-6959
	Bureau of Professional Licensure
	Board of Massage Therapy Examiner
	Lucas State Office Building
	321 E. 12th St.
	Des Moines, IA 50319-0075
	www.idph.state.ia.us/licensure
Kansas	Unlicensed
	Consult with: www.amtamassage.org
	www.abmp.com
Kentucky	Massage Therapist License
	Effective 2005
	502-564-3296 Ext. 240
	Massage Therapist
	Division of Occupations &
	Professions
	PO Box 1360
	Frankfort, KY 40602
	occupations.ky.gov/
	massagetherapists/index.htm

Louisiana	Massage Therapist License 225-771-4090 Louisiana Board of Massage Therapy 12022 Plank Rd. Baton Rouge, LA 70811 www.lsbmt.org
Maine	Massage Therapist License 207-624-8613 State of Maine Dept. of Professional & Financial Regulations Office of Licensing and Registration 35 State House Station Augusta, ME 04333-0035 www.state.me.us/pfr/olr/categories/cat26.htm
Maryland	Massage Therapist Certification 410-764-4738 Maryland Dept. of Health & Mental Hygiene Massage Therapy Program 4201 Patterson St. Baltimore, MD 21215-2299 www.mdmassage.org
Mass.	Unlicensed Consult with: www.amtamassage.org www.abmp.com
Michigan	Unlicensed Consult with: www.amtamassage.org www.abmp.com

Minnesota   Regulated by city or county
             Consult with: www.amtamassage.org
             www.abmp.com

Mississippi Registered Massage Therapist
             601-856-2127
             State Board of Massage
             PO Box 12489
             Jackson, MS 39236-2489
             www.msbmt.state.ms.us

Missouri   Massage Therapist License
             573-751-0293
             Missouri State Board of Therapeutic
             Massage
             3605 Missouri Blvd.
             PO Box 1335
             Jefferson, MO 65102-1335
             www.ecodev.state.mo.us/pr

Montana   Unlicensed
             Consult with: www.amtamassage.org
             www.abmp.com

Nebraska   Massage Therapist License
             402-471-2115
             HHSR&L Credentialing Division
             PO Box 94986
             Lincoln, NE 68509
             www.sos.state.ne.us/crl/mhcs/mass/
             massage.htm

Nevada   Unlicensed
             Consult with:www.amtamassage.org
             www.abmp.com

New
Hampshire
Massage Therapist License
603-271-4814
New Hampshire Dept. Of Health &
Human Services
129 Pleasant St.
Concord, NH 03301-3857
www.dhhs.state.nh.us/DHHS/LRS
/eligibility/default.htm

New Jersey   Massage Therapist Certification
973-504-6200
Board of Nursing
PO Box 45010
Newark, NJ 07101
www.state.nj.us/lps/ca/nursing/
mass.htm

New Mexico Massage Therapist License
505-476-4870
State of New Mexico
Massage Therapy Board
2550 Cerrillos Rd.
Sante Fe, NM 87504
www.rld.state.nm.us/b&c/massage

New York   Massage Therapist License
518-474-3817 Ext. 270
New York State Education Dept.
Office of Professions
Division of Professional Licensing
Services
89 Washington Ave.
Albany, NY 12234
www.op.nysed.gov/massage.htm

North Carolina	Massage and Bodywork Thereapist License 919-546-0050 North Carolina Board of Massage & Bodywork Therapy PO Box 2539 Raleigh, NC 27602 www.bmbt.org
North Dakota	Massage Therapist License 701-225-3906 State Board of Massage 119 Victoria Court Grand Forks, ND 58201 www.health.state.nd.us
Ohio	Massage Therapist License 614-466-3934 State Medical Board of Ohio Massage Licensing Division 77 S. High St., 17th Floor Columbus, OH 43215-6127 www.state.oh.us./med
Oklahoma	Unlicensed Consult with: www.amtamassage.org www.abmp.com
Oregon	Massage Therapist License 503-365-8657 Oregon Board of Massage Therapy 746 Hawthorne Ave. NE Salem, OR 97301 www.oregonmassage.org

Penn.	Unlicensed Consult with: www.amtamassage.org www.abmp.com
Rhode Island	Massage Therapist License 401-222-2827 State of Rhode Island Division of Health Services Regulation 3 Capitol Hill - Room 105 Providence, RI 02908 www.health.state.ri.us/hsr/ professions/massage.php
South Carolina	Massage and Bodywork Therapist License 803-896-4490 South Carolina Dept. of Labor, Licensing and Regulation PO Box 11329 Columbia, SC 2921-1329 www.llr.state.sc.us/POL/massageth erapy
South Dakota	Unlicensed Consult with: www.amtamassage.org www.abmp.com
Tennessee	Massage Therapist License 800-778-4123 Massage Licensure Bd. Cordell Hull Bldg., 1st. Floor 425 5th Ave. North Nashville, TN 37247-1010 www2.state.tn.us/health/ Boards/Massage

Texas	Massage Therapist Registration 512-834-6616 Dept. of State Health Services Massage Therapy Registration Program 1100 W. 49th St. Austin, TX 78756-3183 www.tdh.state.tx.us/hcqs/plc/massage.htm
Utah	Massage Therapist and Apprentice License 801-530-6628 Division of Occupational and Professional Licensing Board of Massage Therapy 160 East 300 South Salt Lake City, UT 84144-6741 www.dopl.utah.gov/licensing/massage.html
Vermont	Unlicensed Consult with: www.amtamassage.org www.abmp.com
Virginia	Massage Therapist Certification 804-662-9909 Department of Health Professions Board of Nursing 6603 W. Broad St., 5th Floor Richmond, VA 23230-1712 www.dhp.state.va.us/nursing/nursing_laws_regs.htm

Washington   Massage Practitioner License
             360-236-4866
             Washington State Dept. of Health
             Health Professions Quality
             Assurance
             Board of Massage
             PO Box 47865
             Olympia, WA 98504-7868
             https://fortress.wa.gov/doh/hpqa1
             hps3/Massage_Therapy/default.htm

Wash., DC   Massage Therapist License
             202-442-9200
             Board of Massage Therapy
             825 N. Capitol St. NE,
              2nd Floor # 2224
             Washington, DC 20002
             www.dchealth.dc.gov/prof_license/
             services/boards_main.asp

W. Virginia Massage Therapist License
             Reciprocal LMT License
             304-487-1400
             Massage Therapy Licensure Board
             200 Davis St. #1
             Princeton, WV 24740-7430
             http://wvmassage.org

Wisconsin	Massage Therapist or Bodyworker Registration 608-266-2112 State of Wisconsin Department of Regulation & Licensure Massage Therapy and Bodywork PO Box 8935 Madison, WI 53708-8935 http://drl.wi.gov/prof/mass/def.htm
Wyoming	Unlicensed Consult with: www.amtamassage.org www.abmp.com

Canada Licensure by Province

CANADIAN MASSAGE THERAPY LICENSURE

Alberta   Self-Regulating
                403-340-1913
                Massage Therapist Association of
                Alberta
                Box 24031 RPO Plaza Centre
                Red Deer, AB T4N 6X6
                http://209.61.238.11/~admin18/con
                tact_us.html

British
Columbia   Massage Therapist License
                604-736-3404
                College of Massage Therapists of
                British Columbia
                Ste. 103, 1089 W. Broadway St.
                Registered Massage Practitioner
                Vancouver, BC V6H 1E5
                www.cmtbc.bc.ca

Manitoba	Massage Therapist Licensed by city
	204-254-0406
	Massage Therapy Association of
	Manitoba, Inc.
	Box 65026 Elmwood
	355 Henderson Highway
	Winnipeg, MB R2L 1M0
	www.mtam.mb.ca

New
Brunswick   No designation - Self-Regulated
506-459-5788
New Brunswick Massotherapy
Association, Inc.
PO Box 21009
Fredericton, NB E3B 7A3
info@masssagemassotherapie.nb.ca

Newfoundland Massage Therapy Registration
NMLA
PO Box 23212, Churchill Square
St. John's, NL A1B4J9
Or
NMLTB
Rawlins Cross, PO Box 60502
St. John's, NL A1C 1V0
www.nlmta.ca

Northwest
Territories   No designation - Self-Regulated
Northwest Territories Massage
Therapy Association
#7-5102 50th Ave.
Yellowknife, NT X1A 3S8
rbeatch@tamarack.nt.ca

Nova Scotia	Massage Therapist Legislation Pending
	902-429-2190
	College of Massage Therapists of Nova Scotia
	PO Box 9410 Stn. A
	Halifax, NS B3K 5S3
	association@pathfinder-group.com
Ontario	Massage Therapist Licensure
	416-489-2626
	College of Massage Therapists of Ontario
	1867 Yonge St., Suit 810
	Toronto, Ontario M4S 1Y5
	www.cmto.com
Quebec	No designation - Self-Regulated
	Severine Jacquart
	Directrice Generale Adjointe
	Federation Quebecoise des Massotherapeutes
	514-597-0505 poste 232
Saskatchewan	Massage Therapist
	New legislation
	306-384-7077
	Massage Therapist Association of Saskatchewan
	230 Ave. R South Room 327
	Old Nurses Residence
	Saskatchwan, SK S7M 2Z1
	www.gpfn.sk.ca/health/groups/mtas.html

Medical Codes for Massage Therapy

DIAGNOSTIC CODES (ICD CODES)

The history of medical coding began in the 17th century. In the late 1600s in England, statistical information was collected by John Graunt in an attempt to predict the number of children who would die of specific illnesses before the age of 6. The data collected was used to predict that 36% would die before the age of 6.

- Francois Bossier de Lacroix (1706-1777) is credited with creating the first system devised to track diseases and mortality.
- Britain's William Cullen (1710-1790) published a system in 1785.
- In 1837 the General Registry Office of England and Wales hired their first medical statistician, William Farr (1807-1883). Farr improved the Cullen system and created international uniformity in its use.
- Farr and Marc d'Espine of Geneva, Switzerland were hired to create a new system of classification.
- A compromise system using 138 classifications was created. This system was revised in 1864, 1874, 1880, and 1886.
- In 1891, Jacques Bertillon (1851-1922) headed a committee that prepared a document titled *International List of Causes of Death*. This was published by the International Statistical Institute of Chicago, Ill.

- The American Public Health Association recommended the adoption of the Bertillion format in 1898. This document underwent revisions in 1900, 1910, and 1920.

- Bertillion passed away in 1922. Further revisions are made in 1929 and then in 1938.

- In 1946, the World Health Organization (WHO) took over the task of yearly publication of the *International List of Causes of Death* renaming it as *The International Causes of Disease.* The 6th revision added non-fatal conditions and by the 8th revision the system was firmly entrenched in medical computers worldwide.

- In 1969 the WHO held a conference that led to the publication of the 9th revision. The document published was titled *The International Classification of Disease.*

- By 1975 the 9th revision was modified to include clinical considerations. The new manual was then called *The International Classification of Disease, 9th Revision, Clinical Modification* (ICD 9 CM). At the time this text was printed the ICD 9 CM manual was still in use in the United States.

- ICD 10 CM has been created and is in use in Canada, Australia, and numerous other countries. The United States will convert to ICD 10 CM over a 2 year period. As of the publication of this manual the implementation period had not been released.

ICD Codes are 3 to 5 digit codes in widespread use internationally.

- 812: Fracture of humerous—General
- 812.0: Upper end, closed—More specific
- 812.01: Surgical neck—Most specific

Because only those licensed to diagnose may identify the cause of illness, massage therapists may not select ICD codes for general use. There are 3 sources of the ICD codes that a massage therapist may use:

- The physician's script
- A call to the physician's office
- The superbill (receipt) provided to a client after diagnosis

The ICD 9 CM code is used in conjunction with CPT codes and the universal insurance form identified as the CMS 1500 (also known as the HCFA 1500) to submit bills to insurance companies and Worker's Compensation for reimbursement for massage therapy services.

CURRENT PROCEDURAL TERMINOLOGY CODES (CPT)

- The CPT manual was first published in 1966 by the American Medical Association. It is a manual written for physicians for the purpose of identifying codes and listing descriptive terms for reporting medical services performed.

- The 2004, 4th edition, CPT manual has been revised 4 times. The CPT manual is published annually with additions of new codes, modifications of current codes, and deletions of codes. Because codes may be deleted or added each year, a therapist must purchase a new manual each year or have a source for current codes.

- The CPT codes available for massage therapists are all located in the Physical Medicine section of the CPT manual. The number of codes that a massage therapist may use is very limited.

In order to select a code there are 2 requirements that a therapist must meet:

- They must hold certification to perform the procedure which is described.
- They must have performed the procedure they select.

Reading the descriptions in the CPT manual requires a medical background and a familiarization with medical terminology and their uses. Units of work for massage therapy will be in 15-minute increments. The definitions and meanings of CPT codes is determined by the American Medical Association. Attempting to read this manual without some training in coding interpretation is not recommended.

When properly used, ICD and CPT codes accurately and concisely describe the condition treated as well as the methodology of treatment.

CPT codes are 5-digit numerical codes (eg,: 97124: Massage).

The implementation of HIPPA requires the use of CPT codes in all electronically transferred patient data in the United States.

For current CPT code information consult with AMTA or ABMP or the instructors of the modality of massage and/or bodywork for which you would like to submit bills.